Regional Anesthesia and Pain Management

Anesthesia Pocket Consult for iPod

Dell R. Burkey, MD
Department of Anesthesiology and Critical Care
University of Pennsylvania School of Medicine
Philadelphia, Pennsylvania

SERIES EDITOR

Lee A. Fleisher, MD
Robert D. Dripps Professor and Chair
Department of Anesthesiology and Critical Care
Professor of Medicine
University of Pennsylvania School of Medicine
Philadelphia, Pennsylvania

SAUNDERS

ELSEVIER

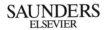

SAUNDERS
ELSEVIER

1600 John F. Kennedy Blvd.
Ste 1800
Philadelphia, PA 19103-2899

Regional Anesthesia and Pain Management   ISBN: 978-1-4160-3344-8

Notice

Knowledge and best practice in this field are constantly changing. As new research and experience broaden our knowledge, changes in practice, treatment and drug therapy may become necessary or appropriate. Readers are advised to check the most current information provided (i) on procedures featured or (ii) by the manu- facturer of each product to be administered, to verify the recommended dose or formula, the method and duration of administration, and contraindications. It is the responsibility of the practitioner, relying on their own experience and knowledge of the patient, to make diagnoses, to determine dosages and the best treatment for each individual patient, and to take all appropriate safety precautions. To the fullest extent of the law, neither the Publisher nor the Editors assume any liability for any injury and/or damage to persons or property arising out of or related to any use of the material contained in this book.

The Publisher

Library of Congress Cataloging-in-Publication Data
Burkey, Dell R.
    Regional anesthesia and pain management / Dell R. Burkey. – 1st ed.
        p. ; cm.
    Includes bibliographical references.
    ISBN 978-1-4160-3344-8
 1.   Conduction anesthesia.   I. Title.
    [DNLM: 1.   Anesthesia, Conduction–methods.   2.   Nerve Block–methods.
 3.   Pain–therapy.   WO 300 B959r 2009]
    RD84.B795 2009
    617.9'64–dc22
                                                                    2008050800

Acquisitions Editor: Natasha Andjelkovic
Developmental Editor: Isabel Trudeau
Project Manager: Bryan Hayward
Design Direction: Ellen Zanolle

Printed in the United States of America

Last digit is the print number: 9 8 7 6 5 4 3 2 1

Working together to grow
libraries in developing countries

www.elsevier.com | www.bookaid.org | www.sabre.org

ELSEVIER   BOOK AID International   Sabre Foundation

Dedication

*This book is dedicated to my wife, Marilyn, and my children,
Michele, Adam, and Jason.*

Contributors

Rahul Anand, MD
Private Practice
Fairfield, CT

Robert P. Brislin, DO
Department of Anesthesiology and Critical Care Management
Alfred I. DuPont Hospital for Children
Wilmington, DE

Dell R. Burkey, MD
Associate Professor of Anesthesiology and Critical Care
Associate Program Director, Pain Medicine Residency
Director, Acute Pain Services
Department of Anesthesiology and Critical Care
University of Pennsylvania School of Medicine
Philadelphia, PA

Vikash Dugar, MD
Private Practice
Elgin, IL

Andrew J. Engle, MD
Private Practice
Elgin, IL

Simon Galapo, MD
Private Practice
Meadowbrook, PA

Jonathan Gavrin, MD
Associate Professor
Department of Anesthesiology and Critical Care
University of Pennsylvania School of Medicine
Philadelphia, PA

Ankur Gosalia, MD
Assistant Professor, Department of Anesthesia and Critical Care
Western Pennsylvania Hospital
Pittsburgh, PA

Brett Gutsche, MD
Professor of Anesthesiology and Critical Care and Obstetrics
Department of Anesthesiology and Critical Care
University of Pennsylvania School of Medicine
Philadelphia, PA

Emily Joe, MD
Private Practice
Austin, TX

Benjamin Kohl, MD
Assistant Professor, Department of Medicine
Director of Critical Care Fellowship
University of Pennsylvania School of Medicine
Philadelphia, PA

Tony Ku, MD
Private Practice
Langhorne, PA

Robert Kuzel, MD
Private Practice
Phoenix, AZ

Tung Nguyen, MD
Private Practice
Thibodaux, LA

Natalia Ortiz, MD
Instructor, Department of Psychiatry
Temple University School of Medicine
Philadelphia, PA

Andrew Pierwola, MD
Private Practice
Philadelphia, PA

Rosemary Polomano, PhD, RN, FAAN
Associate Professor of Pain Practice, Clinician Educator
University of Pennsylvania School of Nursing
Philadelphia, PA

Abhijeet Rastogi, MD
Private Practice
Abingdon, MD

Joseph Richards, DO
Bryn Mawr Hospital
Bryn Mawr, PA
Paoli Hospital
Malvern, PA

Randy Robinson, MD
Private Practice
Meadowbrook, PA

John Rose, MD
Clinical Director, Pain Management Service
Children's Hospital of Philadelphia
Associate Professor, Department of Anesthesiology and Critical Care
University of Pennsylvania School of Medicine
Philadelphia, PA

Kieran Slevin, MD
Assistant Professor, Department of Anesthesiology and Critical Care
University of Pennsylvania School of Medicine
Philadelphia, PA

Kim Soo-Abboud, MD
Clinical Assistant Professor, Department of Otolaryngology
Head and Neck Surgery
University of Pennsylvania School of Medicine
Philadelphia, PA

Hari V. Sundram, MD
Vice President and Medical Director
Medical Capital Development
New York, NY

David Taylor, MD
Department of Psychiatry
University of Pennsylvania School of Medicine
Philadelphia, PA

Huy Tieu, MD
Private Practice
Hershey, PA

Gaurav Trehan, MD
Assistant Professor, Department of Anesthesiology
Temple University School of Medicine
Philadelphia, PA

Brian Weaver, MD
Department of Anesthesiology and Critical Care
University of Pennsylvania School of Medicine
Philadelphia, PA

Foreword

As anesthesiologists, we have a very diverse portfolio of procedures that we perform as part of our daily practice and care for patients with numerous diseases undergoing a wide variety of procedures. In an effort to provide the optimal care for these patients, access to information on best practices is essential. With the development of new technologies, this access has become even easier, and faculty of the Department of Anesthesiology and Critical Care at the University of Pennsylvania School of Medicine have chosen to develop programs to bring this information to the location of care.

In this portable resource, Dr. Burkey and his contributing authors provide practical coverage of regional anesthesia and pain management in a remarkably concise, at-a-glance manner. One can either carry and consult this compact book anytime, anywhere, or easily download and review the content on any standard click-wheel iPod and look up clinical questions rapidly, thanks to a consistent, bulleted, highly visual format. I am sure you will find the information contained herein helpful in your clinical practice.

Lee A. Fleisher, MD
Robert Dunning Dripps Professor and Chair
Department of Anesthesiology and Critical Care
University of Pennsylvania School of Medicine
Philadelphia, Pennsylvania

Preface

Regional anesthesia, including predominantly peripheral neural blockade techniques, is devoted its own section at the beginning of the book. A general approach to acute pain in the inpatient setting and perioperative period is then considered. The discussion of chronic pain opens with the neurophysiology and fundamentals of history-taking, physical examination, and questionnaire assessment. The medication-based treatment of chronic pain is then presented, followed by an overview of standard diagnostic and therapeutic interventions, with an emphasis on fluoroscopically guided spinal procedures. The psychiatric management of chronic pain, including the approach to patient education and emotional comorbidities, is devoted its own chapter. Finally, a taxonomy of common clinical pain syndromes is presented with a standard approach to initial diagnosis and management. Medico-legal considerations in chronic pain treatment are handled at the end.

Pain represents one of the greatest burdens to patients confronted by modern medicine. No longer is it considered merely a symptom; it impairs functional recovery and outcomes in the acute setting and multiple dimensions of quality of life in the chronic outpatient arena. An understanding of the fundamentals of pain therapy is a requirement for every healthcare practitioner today. This knowledge base includes the efficacy and side-effects of opioids and adjuvant pharmacotherapeutics; distinctions between nociceptive and neuropathic pain; and the special issues regarding the care of malignant pain and surgical patients. Newer agents, as they are developed, will still have to be applied with respect to these diagnostic entities and likely used in concert with already available agents.

The substance of this book developed out of years of clinical care and the teaching of residents and fellows at the Hospital of the University of Pennsylvania. It is designed to be a practical guide to assist decision-making for the nonspecialist who encounters these patients routinely. It could not have been accomplished without their input on innumerable rounds, in innumerable clinical situations, or without the mentorship of our Chairman, Lee Fleisher, MD.

Dell R. Burkey, MD

Contents

Section II. Pharmacotherapy

Section III. Diagnostic and Therapeutic Interventions for Chronic Pain

Section IV. Educational and Psychological Management

Part I

Regional Neural Blockade

1 Equipment and Patient Monitoring

1. GENERAL

a. Nerve block facility should have adequate space and equipment as well as a comfortable and relaxing environment to ensure proper care of the patient.

b. The physician and nurse should inform the patient as to the purpose of the procedure and how it is done, as well as risks, side effects, and expected outcomes.

2. FACILITIES

a. Peripheral nerve blocks can be performed in a separate block placement area, in the fluoroscopic suite, or in the operating room.

b. All drugs, supplies, and other equipment must be readily available regardless of where the procedure is done.

c. Supplies for the procedure include:
   i. Full monitoring equipment
   ii. Procedure tray(s)
   iii. Needles, catheters
   iv. Temperature probes, syringes, and medication

3. EMERGENCY DRUGS AND SUPPLIES

a. Although adverse events are relatively rare, the block placement location must have a source of oxygen, suction, airway equipment, and the ability to provide positive pressure ventilation.

b. In the event of an untoward outcome, the following emergency drugs and airway equipment must be available:
   i. Atropine: 0.2-0.4 mg incremental doses IV
   ii. Ephedrine: 5-10 mg IV; repeat as necessary
   iii. Epinephrine: 1-100 µg IV bolus(es)
   iv. Phenylephrine: 50-200 µg IV bolus(es)
   v. Propofol: 50-200 mg IV
   vi. Muscle relaxant: short-acting, mivacurium or Anectine

c. Airway equipment
   i. Oral airways: various sizes
   ii. Endotracheal tubes: various sizes
   iii. Laryngoscope handle and blades
   iv. Stylets
   v. Ambu bag, oxygen source, suction apparatus

4. NEEDLES FOR NERVE BLOCK PROCEDURES

a. Short-bevel needles are suggested rather than long (cutting) bevel needles to avoid needle-related nerve injury.

   b. Small-diameter needles cause a minimum of patient discomfort and tissue trauma.
   c. A needle appropriate for the procedure (not too long or too short) should be chosen to optimize precision needle control and avoid complications.

5. NERVE BLOCK TRAY

   a. Basic items should include:
      i. Items for sterile skin preparation and draping
      ii. Syringes: various sizes; skin infiltration of local, block performance
     iii. Needles: skin infiltration, block procedure
     iv. Marking pen, ruler
      v. Gauze sponges
     vi. Tubing

6. REGIONAL ANESTHESIA CART

   a. A well-organized and maintained cart is very useful.
   b. The cart should be stocked so that any regional block can be done efficiently in any location.
   c. The cart must be checked and restocked daily and locked when not in use.
   d. The cart should have six or seven drawers for storing the necessary supplies and equipment
      i. For example, a drawer for needles and syringes; a drawer with resuscitation equipment and cardiovascular drugs, etc.

7. PATIENT MONITORING

   a. For major conduction blocks
      i. Pulse oximetry
      ii. Electrocardiogram
     iii. Vital signs
     iv. Level of consciousness
   b. Post-procedure monitoring
      i. Routinely monitored in a designated recovery area for at least 30 minutes
      ii. Monitored after a major conduction block
     iii. Monitored principally for local anesthetic toxicity

SUGGESTED READINGS

Hadzic A, Vloka JD: Peripheral Nerve Blocks. New York, McGraw-Hill, 2004.
Raj PP: Textbook of Regional Anesthesia. London, England, Churchill Livingstone, 2002.

2 Peripheral Nerve Stimulators

1. GENERAL

a. The use of a nerve stimulator increases the specificity of peripheral neural blockade.

b. Stimulation of a particular nerve results in a specific motor response.

c. The technique of nerve stimulation was first described in 1912.

e. Insulated needles and localization of nerves with a specific motor response was described in 1955.

f. In 1973, the use of unsheathed (uninsulated) needles was commonplace. In a comparative study, the sheathed (insulated) needle was found to be superior in nerve localization.

2. CHARACTERISTICS OF A PERIPHERAL NERVE STIMULATOR

a. Constant current output. Current output does not change regardless of the different resistance applied to the output.

b. Linear output: percentage of output versus percentage of meter scale.

c. High and low output ranges allow the use of high output when the needle is a distance from the nerve and low output control as the needle is nearer the nerve.

d. Clearly marked polarity of the output. The cathode (−) must attach to the needle and the anode (+) to the surface of the patient.

e. A short stimulation pulse: more precise nerve localization.

f. Digital display, current output dial, digital current output meter, and a battery check.

g. Current range: 0 to 5 mA.

h. Frequency: 1 or 2 Hz.

3. TECHNIQUE OF PERIPHERAL NERVE STIMULATION

a. The anode (+) terminal of the stimulator is connected to an electrode on the patient's skin. The cathode (−) terminal is connected to the stimulator.

b. The stimulator output is set at 2 mA initially.

c. The needle is inserted and advanced toward the nerve to be blocked while observing or feeling for muscle contractions within the motor distribution of the nerve.

d. As the needle approaches the nerve, the lowest output that results in nerve stimulation (≤0.5 mA) and muscle contraction should place the needle proximate to the nerve.

   e. One to two milliliters of local anesthetic is injected, which should immediately abolish nerve stimulation and muscle contraction if the needle tip is at the site of the nerve.

   f. It is important to change only one variable at a time (voltage, angle of needle, depth, etc.) while attempting to localize the nerve.

   g. The use of nerve stimulators is rapidly increasing.

SUGGESTED READINGS

Cousins MJ, Bridenbaugh PO: Neural Blockade. Philadelphia, Lippincott-Raven, 1998.
Hadzic A, Vloka JD: Peripheral Nerve Blocks. New York, McGraw-Hill, 2004.

1. GENERAL

a. Local anesthetics interrupt nerve impulse generation and conduction by binding to a pore in the Na+ channel of the nerve, thus preventing or relieving pain.

2. STRUCTURE-ACTIVITY RELATIONSHIP

a. A typical local anesthetic contains hydrophilic and hydrophobic domains that are separated by an intermediate ester or amide linkage.
b. Hydrophobicity increases the potency and duration of action of the local anesthetic, but it also increases the toxicity of the local anesthetic.
c. Amino group: attached at the end of the molecule opposite the benzene ring lipophilic end. This unit determines the ionization and the hydrophilic activity of the drug.
d. pK_a: determines the ratio of ionized (cationic) and the uncharged (base) from of the drug. The pK_a is the pH at which 50% of the drug is ionized and 50% is base. It correlates with the speed of onset of the amide local anesthetics.
   i. Base form: penetrates nerve lipid membrane
   ii. Cationic form: This form is predominant and produces blockade of the sodium channel.
   iii. Local anesthetics act only from the inner surface of the cell membrane.
e. The ester or amide linkage determines the site of metabolic degradation of the drug.
   i. Ester-linked local anesthetics are inactivated in the plasma.
   ii. Amide-linked local anesthetics are inactivated in the liver.

3. NERVE FIBERS: SENSITIVITY TO LOCAL ANESTHETICS

a. C (pain sensation) and A delta (pain and temperature) fibers are blocked before A gamma, A beta, and A alpha fibers (postural, touch, pressure, and motor sensation).
   i. Small fibers are blocked first because the critical length over which an impulse can propagate passively is shorter.
   ii. The anesthetic action of local anesthetics is frequency dependent. Small sensory fibers propagate long action potentials at high frequency, which favors a faster onset of neural blockade.

4. PHYSICAL PROPERTIES AFFECTING LOCAL ANESTHETIC ACTION

   a. Potency: Correlates with an increase in lipid solubility.
   b. Onset of action: Correlates with the pK_a for amide-linked local anesthetics. The lower the pK_a, the shorter the onset.
   c. Protein binding: Local anesthetics bind to albumin and x-acid glycoprotein (AAG) in the plasma. The unbound form is the only active state.

5. FACTORS THAT DETERMINE PLASMA CONCENTRATION OF LOCAL ANESTHETICS

   a. Drug dosage
   b. Drug absorption from the site injected
   c. Biotransformation and drug elimination from the circulation

6. UNDESIRED EFFECTS OF LOCAL ANESTHETICS

   a. General: Local anesthetics interfere with the function of all organs in which nerve conduction impulse occurs.
   b. Central nervous system
      i. Depression: due to decreased neuronal activity
      ii. Stimulation: selective depression of inhibitory neurons
      iii. Drowsy: most frequent complaint
   c. Cardiovascular system
      i. Myocardium: primary site of action; decrease in conduction rate and contractility
      ii. Arteriolar dilatation
      iii. Cardiovascular adverse effects follow central nervous system effects
   d. Neuromuscular function and ganglionic synapse effect
      i. Effects are due to block of ion channel of the acetylcholine receptor
   e. Smooth muscle
      i. Depression of bowel contractions
      ii. Relaxation of bronchial and vascular smooth muscle
      iii. Increased tone of gastrointestinal musculature secondary to sympathetic nervous system paralysis

7. METABOLISM OF LOCAL ANESTHETICS

   a. Ester-type local anesthetics
      i. Hydrolysis in the plasma leads to the formation of para-aminobenzoic acid (PABA); potential for allergic reactions

   b. Amide-type local anesthetics
      i. Metabolized in the liver; clearance of the drug depends on hepatic blood flow and hepatic function.
   c. Renal clearance is a minor route of elimination of unchanged local anesthetics.

SUGGESTED READINGS

Barash PG, Cullen BF, Stoelting RK: Clinical Anesthesia. Philadelphia, Lippincott Williams & Wilkins, 2001.

Raj PP: Textbook of Regional Anesthesia. London, England, Churchill Livingstone, 2002.

1. GENERAL

a. Spinal, epidural, and caudal neuraxial blocks result in sympathetic block, sensory analgesia, and motor block, depending on dose, concentration, or volume of local anesthetic, after insertion of a needle in the plane of the neuraxis. Despite these similarities, there are significant physiologic and pharmacologic differences.

   i. Spinal anesthesia requires a small mass (i.e., volume) of drug, virtually devoid of systemic pharmacologic effect, to produce profound, reproducible sensory analgesia.

   ii. In contrast, epidural anesthesia necessitates use of a large mass of local anesthetic that produces pharmacologically active systemic blood levels, which may be associated with side effects and complications unknown with spinal anesthesia.

b. We are entering an exciting new era in the therapy of chronic pain conditions, with basic science providing a multitude of new intrathecal compounds to meet the needs of clinical practice. However, the only Food and Drug Administration (FDA)-approved compound for intrathecal use is morphine. All the other compounds described in this chapter are still experimental, and issues regarding long-term toxicity and drug interactions must be resolved. Nevertheless, the treatment landscape will soon be markedly altered with the introduction of many of these new compounds.

2. POSTOPERATIVE CENTRONEURAXIAL ANALGESIA

a. Contraindications and complications associated with postoperative epidural analgesia are similar to those associated with epidural anesthesia. These risks include:

   i. Epidural hematoma
   ii. Infection

b. These complications are rare and, in most cases, are offset by the superior analgesia associated with this technique. Catheter placement using strict aseptic technique and covering of the epidural catheter insertion site with a sterile occlusive dressing reduces the risk of epidural catheter–related infection.

   i. Epidural catheters at risk for bacterial "seeding" during a period of transient perioperative bacteremia should be removed and replaced.

   ii. Much controversy has developed surrounding the use of continuous epidural analgesia and perioperative thromboprophylaxis, especially with the low-molecular-weight heparins.

Current recommendations include attempting to ensure normal coagulation status at times of epidural catheter insertion and removal and avoiding the use of epidural analgesia and concomitantly administered low-molecular-weight heparins in all but individually selected cases.

iii. Guidelines for epidural catheterization and perioperative thromboprophylaxis have been recently developed and reviewed.

3. SPINAL ANALGESIA COMPLICATIONS

a. Nerve damage
b. Sympathetic block leading to hypotension
c. High-level spinal block (respiratory compromise)
d. Most complications are rare while paying attention to drug amount and adequately monitoring the patient.

SUGGESTED READINGS

Horlocker TT, Heit JA: Low molecular weight heparin: Biochemistry, pharmacology, perioperative prophylaxis regimens, and guidelines for regional anesthetic management. Anesth Analg 1997;85:874–885.

Horlocker TT, Wedel DJ: Spinal and epidural blockade and perioperative low molecular weight heparin: Smooth sailing on the Titanic. Anesth Analg 1998;86:1153–1156.

Miller R: Miller's Anesthesia, 6th ed. St. Louis, Mosby, 2005.

Raj PP: Practical Management of Pain, 3rd ed. St. Louis, Mosby, 2003.

5 | Cervical Plexus Block

1. GENERAL

a. Indications (deep cervical plexus block)
   i. Neck and supraclavicular fossa surgery
      (1) Neck dissection
      (2) Tracheal and laryngeal surgery
      (3) Carotid artery surgery: most common indication
      (4) Thyroid, parathyroid, and lymph glands
b. Unilateral deep cervical block is used for most of these procedures, unless the surgery extends to within 0.5 inch of the neck line (i.e., thyroid surgery and lymphatic gland excision).
c. Contraindications
   i. Patient refusal, coagulopathies, infection at the block site
   ii. Severe respiratory disease: potential blockade of phrenic nerve and diaphragmatic paralysis
d. Pertinent anatomy
   i. The anterior primary divisions of the first four cervical nerves make up the cervical plexus (C2-4).
   ii. The plexus emerges at the posterior border of the SCM (sternocleidomastoid muscle), deep to the internal jugular vein and anterior to the medial scalene muscle.
   iii. The cervical nerves exit from the cervical vertebrae through a gutter in the transverse process immediately posterior to the vertebral artery before regrouping to form the cervical plexus.
e. Position and technique
   i. Supine position, head and neck turned opposite the side to be blocked. The anesthesiologist stands approximately shoulder high on the side of the patient to be blocked.
   ii. A line is drawn between Chassaignac's tubercle, which is at the level of the cricoid cartilage (easily palpable on C6), and the mastoid process. A second line is drawn parallel to and 1 cm posterior to the first line.
   iii. The C2 transverse process is identified 1 to 2 cm caudad to the mastoid process; C3 (at the level of the body of the hyoid bone) is 1.5 cm caudad to C2; and C4 (located at the upper border of the thyroid cartilage) is identified 1.5 cm caudad to C3.
   iv. A 22-gauge, 5-cm needle is inserted medially and caudally immediately over the C4 transverse process and advanced until it contacts the process at a depth of 1.5 to 3.0 cm. At a depth greater than 3.0 cm, if there is bony contact, the needle is too far anteriorly or posteriorly and is most likely on the vertebral body.
   v. A nerve stimulator may be used. The needle is advanced until either a paresthesia is obtained or bony contact is encountered.

vi. After a negative aspiration for blood or cerebrospinal fluid (CSF), 15 to 20 mL of local anesthetic is injected by using this single-needle approach.

vii. Alternately, a single needle may be placed at the C2, C3, and C4 transverse processes and 5 mL of local anesthetic injected at each site. It has been suggested that the multiple-needle approach produces a more desirable block.

f. Concerns

   i. Inadequate block for the procedure
   ii. Accidental intravascular injection into the internal or external jugular vein or the vertebral artery
   iii. Injection into the epidural or subdural space by penetrating the dural sleeves or through the intervertebral foramina
   iv. Blockade of the vagus or phrenic nerve

SUGGESTED READINGS

Brown DL: Atlas of Regional Anesthesia, 2nd edition. Philadelphia, WB Saunders, 1999.

Raj P: Practical Management of Pain, 3rd ed. St. Louis, Mosby, 2000.

Waldman: Interventional Pain Management. Philadelphia, WB Saunders, 1996.

6 Genitofemoral Nerve Block

1. GENERAL

a. Consists of L1 and L2 ventral nerve roots, which pass through the psoas muscle and divide into two terminal branches: femoral and genital branches.

b. The femoral branch innervates a small area on the upper inner thigh, and the genital branch innervates the skin over the scrotum in males and the labia majora in females.

c. Clinical applications
   i. Can be combined with ilioinguinal and iliohypogastric nerve blocks for inguinal herniorrhaphy, orchiopexy, or hydrocelectomy.
   ii. Can be combined with femoral nerve block for long saphenous vein stripping.
   iii. Can be used to diagnose genitofemoral neuralgia.

d. Contraindications
   i. Patient refusal
   ii. Local anesthetic allergy
   iii. Severe coagulation disorders
   iv. Local infection

e. Technique: anterior approach
   i. The patient is placed in the supine position, and the groin is sterilely prepared. A 22-gauge, 5-cm b-bevel needle is placed through the skin just lateral to the pubic tubercle. The needle is advanced through the inguinal ligament, and 5 mL of local anesthetic solution is injected.
   ii. The genital branch of the genitofemoral nerve can be blocked independently by infiltration around the spermatic cord at its exit from the inguinal canal.

f. Alternative technique: trans-psoas approach
   i. With the patient in a prone position, a 21-gauge, 15-cm spinal needle is introduced paravertebrally, approximately 5 cm from the midline at the level of the L3-4 interspace. The needle is advanced toward the transverse processes of either L3 or L4.
   ii. After the depth of the processes is noted, the needle is redirected to pass between the transverse processes in perpendicular fashion. The loss of resistance is used to identify first the psoas muscle compartment and, after further advancement, the space located anteriorly to the psoas major muscle.
   iii. At this point, 2 to 3 mL of local anesthetic is injected to block the genitofemoral nerve.

g. Side effects and complications
   i. Intravascular injection and penetration of the peritoneum
   ii. Femoral nerve anesthesia by diffusion, which can compromise day case surgery

iii. Whole or partial failure is the main disadvantage of this block. Complement anesthesia is sometimes needed as a hernia orifice or spermatic cord infiltration.

SUGGESTED READINGS

DiFazio CA, Woods AM, Rowlingson JC: Drugs commonly used for nerve blocking: Pharmacology of local anesthetics. In Raj PP (ed): Practical Management of Pain, 3rd ed. St. Louis, Mosby, 2000, pp 557–575.

Genitofemoral block. Available at: http://www.nysora.com/techniques/genitofemoral_block/.

Hartrick C: Genitofemoral nerve block: A transpsoas technique. Reg Anesth 1994;19(6):432–433.

Vloka JD, Hadzic A, Mulcare R, et al: Femoral nerve block versus spinal anesthesia for outpatients undergoing long saphenous vein stripping surgery. Anesth Analg 1997;84:749–752.

1. GENERAL

a. Originate from L1 ventral nerve root, though it may include a contribution from the T12 nerve root. These nerves travel toward the iliac crest along the abdominal wall, where they perforate the transversus abdominis muscle.

b. The iliohypogastric nerve emerges from the lateral border of the psoas and runs obliquely adjacent to the posterior aspect of the internal oblique muscle. The nerve divides into two terminal cutaneous branches: the lateral branch supplies the buttocks, and the medial branch supplies the abdominal wall above the pubis after crossing the external oblique muscle.

c. The ilioinguinal nerve crosses the quadratus lumborum and the iliacus muscle obliquely, pierces the transversus abdominis (at the level of the iliac crest), crosses the internal then the external oblique muscles, and ends at the lower border of the spermatic cord or the round ligament of the uterus within the inguinal canal.

d. Sensory innervation to the upper medial part of the thigh and the upper part of the scrotum and penis or the labia major and the

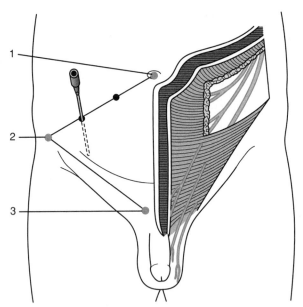

Figure 7–1 Iliohypogastric and ilioinguinal nerve blocks, with the sites indicated for the umbilicus (1), anterior iliac crest (2), and pubic spine (3). (From Miller's Anesthesia, 6th ed. Philadelphia, Elsevier, 2005.)

mons pubis are supplied by the ilioinguinal nerve. The ilioinguinal and iliohypogastric nerves, at the level of the medial part of the anterior wall of the abdomen, lie in the same fascial plane at the inner surface of the superficial aponeurosis of the external oblique muscle (**Fig. 7-1**).

2. CLINICAL APPLICATIONS

a. The ilioinguinal or iliohypogastric nerve block provides excellent pain relief for operations on the inguinal region, such as with herniorrhaphy, orchidopexy, hydrocele, and emergency procedures, such as for strangulated hernia with intestinal obstruction.
b. It should be preferred to caudal anesthesia for these procedures.

3. CONTRAINDICATIONS

a. Patient refusal
b. Local anesthetic allergy
c. Severe coagulation disorders
d. Local infection

4. TECHNIQUE: ANTERIOR APPROACH

a. The iliohypogastric and ilioinguinal nerves can be blocked as they pass the anterior–superior iliac spine. Place patient in supine position, and mark a point 3 cm medial to the anterior–superior iliac spine along a line between it and the umbilicus. This mark will illustrate the course that the iliohypogastric nerve takes. A second mark 3 cm caudal to the first will depict the ilioinguinal nerve's course.
b. The skin should be sterilely prepared. A 5-cm, 22-gauge b-bevel needle is then placed through the skin at the upper mark until it pierces the fascia of the internal oblique muscle, which is accompanied by a tactile "popping" sensation. Inject 5 to 10 mL of local anesthetic solution at this point. The solution should be injected in a fan because the course of the nerve can vary slightly. The needle is then inserted through the more caudal site, and the process is repeated.

5. ALTERNATIVE TECHNIQUES

a. The needle can be inserted through the more caudal site (3 cm medial and 3 cm caudal to the anterior–superior iliac spine) and then directed laterally until the inner edge of the iliac crest is contacted. Five to ten milliliters of local anesthetic is injected while pulling back the needle.
b. Another technique, the classic approach, used two sites of puncture, including one potentially dangerous site at the level of the

pubic tubercle, where three fascial planes had to be identified. It had a high failure rate. Intraoperative infiltration of the hernial sac (which is the same technique) effectively relieves postoperative pain, but does not protect against intraoperative pain.

6. SIDE EFFECTS AND COMPLICATIONS

   a. Intravascular injection and penetration of the peritoneum.
   b. Undesired nerve blocks (especially femoral nerve blocks) are occasionally observed, especially when too much local anesthetic is injected. The local anesthetic spreads caudad to the inguinal ligament. This can delay the discharge of the patient by 2 to 3 hours.

SUGGESTED READINGS

Bell E, Jones B, Olufolabi A, et al: Iliohypogastric-ilioinguinal peripheral nerve block. Can J Anesth 2002;49:694–700.

Brockwell RC, Andrews JJ: Inhaled anesthetic delivery systems. In Miller R (ed): Miller's Anesthesia, 6th ed. Philadelphia, Elsevier, 2005, pp 261–266.

DiFazio CA, Woods AM, Rowlingson JC: Drugs commonly used for nerve blocking: Pharmacology of local anesthetics. In Raj PP (ed): Practical Management of Pain, 3rd ed. St. Louis, Mosby, 2000, pp 561–564.

Genitofemoral block. Available at: http://www.nysora.com/techniques/genitofemoral_block/.

1. GENERAL

a. Thoracic nerves exit the spinal column through the intervertebral foramina, which are positioned midway between adjacent ribs. The posterior cutaneous nerve, which supplies the skin and muscles of the paraspinal area, immediately branches off. The intercostal nerve continues around the chest wall, where at the midaxillary line the lateral cutaneous nerve originates. These branches are the sensory supply to the anterior and posterior lateral chest wall.

b. The intercostal nerve runs with the vein and artery in the subcostal groove, located on the inferior edge of the ribs. Posteriorly, the pleura and a thin intercostal fascial layer separate the nerves from the lungs. When blocking the nerve posteriorly, be careful to avoid puncture of the thin fascia and underlying lung.

2. CLINICAL APPLICATIONS

a. Effective for post-thoracotomy pain with continuous analgesia via intercostals or paravertebral catheters. This technique is still inferior to epidural and other regional anesthetics.

b. Intercostal nerve blocks used on multiple rib fractures showed significant increases in arterial oxygen saturation (Sao_2) and peak expiratory flow rate (PEFR) as well as provided sustained analgesia, leading to improvement in respiratory mechanics.

c. Can be used alone or combined with celiac plexus blocks and light general anesthesia for intra-abdominal procedures if neuraxial blockade is contraindicated.

d. Intrathoracic surgery can be accomplished by using intercostal and stellate ganglion blocks if neuraxial blockade is contraindicated.

3. CONTRAINDICATIONS

a. Patient refusal
b. Local anesthetic allergy
c. Severe coagulation disorders
d. Local infection

4. TECHNIQUE: ANTERIOR APPROACH

a. Place patient in prone position with a pillow placed under the abdomen to reduce the lumbar curve. Provide patient with adequate anxiolytic and analgesia for tolerance of the procedure.

b. A line is drawn along the posterior vertebral spines. Along the posterior angles of the rib, which can be palpated 6 to 8 cm from the midline, nearly parallel lines are drawn. To prevent overlying of the scapula, the upper edges of these lines should angle medially. The inferior edge of each rib is palpated and is marked on the line intersecting the posterior angle of the rib.

c. After sterile preparation, inject skin wheals at each point. Attach a 10-mL syringe to a 22-gauge, short-bevel, 4-cm needle. Beginning at the lower rib, the index finger of the left hand displaces the skin up over the patient's rib. The needle is inserted at the tip of the finger until it rests on the rib.

d. The needle is walked 3 to 5 mm off the lower rib edge, where 3 to 5 mL of local anesthetic is injected.

e. Monitor blood pressure, electrocardiogram, respiratory rate, pulse oximetry, and level of consciousness. Differential diagnosis of dyspnea and chest pain, accentuated by deep breathing and coughing, should include pneumothorax; a chest x-ray should be obtained.

5. ALTERNATIVE TECHNIQUE

a. Can be performed by using a similar technique as above in a supine patient at the midaxillary line

6. SIDE EFFECTS AND COMPLICATIONS

a. Pneumothorax: Actual incidence was as low as 0.07% in a large series performed by anesthesiologists at all levels of training. Incidence of nonsymptomatic pneumothorax of 0.42% was seen on routine postoperative chest x-rays. Treatment usually involves observation, administration of oxygen, or needle aspiration. Chest tube drainage is rarely required.

b. Systemic local anesthetic uptake can occur secondary to the large volumes of local anesthetic used and to rapid absorption. Risk increases with multiple intercostal blocks. Use of epinephrine reduces intravascular absorption.

c. Patients with pleural fibrosis, pleural effusion, lung parenchymal disease associated with pleural disease, or bleeding diathesis should not receive interpleural block. Poor spread or rapid uptake of local anesthetic can occur in pleural disease or inflammation. Severe pulmonary disease can result in respiratory decompensation after bilateral intercostal blockade.

SUGGESTED READINGS

Osinowo OA, Zahrani M. Softah A: Effect of intercostal nerve block with 0.5% bupivacaine on peak expiratory flow rate and arterial oxygen saturation in rib fractures. J Trauma-Injury Infect Crit Care 2004;56(2):345–347.

Raj PP, Johnston M: Organization and function of the nerve block facility. In Raj PP (ed): Practical Management of Pain, 3rd ed. St. Louis, Mosby, 2000, pp 545–557.

Roberts J: Clinical Procedures in Emergency Medicine, 4th ed. Philadelphia, Elsevier, 2003, pp 571–575.

Savage C, McQuitty C, Wang D, et al: Postthoracotomy pain management. Chest Surg Clin North Am 2002;12(2):251–263.

Wedel DJ, Horlocker TT: Nerve blocks. In Miller R (ed): Miller's Anesthesia, 6th ed. Philadelphia, Elsevier, 2005, pp 1711–1713.

9 ■ Femoral Nerve Block

1. GENERAL

    a. The femoral nerve is the largest branch of the lumbar plexus.

    b. It emerges from the psoas major muscle in the groove separating the psoas and the iliacus muscles, passes behind the inguinal ligament, and enters the groin in the femoral triangle (i.e., Scarpa's triangle).

    c. It runs laterally to the femoral vessels from which it is separated by the lower part of the psoas major muscle and remains outside the sheath surrounding the femoral vessels.

    d. At this point, the nerve divides into multiple terminal branches, which have been classified as anterior and posterior. The anterior branches are primarily cutaneous, whereas the posterior branches are chiefly motor.

    e. The femoral nerve supplies the anterior compartment muscles of the thigh (i.e., quadriceps, sartorius) and the skin of the anterior thigh from the inguinal ligament to the knee. Its terminal branch is the saphenous nerve, which supplies an area of skin along the medial side of the leg from the knee to the big toe. *It is the sensory innervation component below the knee and does not arise from the sciatic nerve.*

2. CLINICAL APPLICATIONS

    a. Can be used as a solo block for quadriceps biopsies and in combination with general anesthesia for knee arthroscopy and mid-femur shaft fractures.

    b. In general, femoral block is combined with regional blocks of other nerves, including obturator, lateral femoral cutaneous, and sciatic, to provide regional anesthesia of varying distribution (i.e., combined with sciatic for below-the-knee procedure).

3. TECHNIQUE

    a. The patient is placed in the supine position. A line is drawn between the anterior–superior iliac spine and the pubic tubercle, identifying the inguinal ligament. The femoral artery is marked.

    b. A 22-gauge, 4-cm needle is advanced lateral to this line. When the needle reaches the depth of the artery, a pulsation of the hub is visible. Elicitation of a paresthesia or motor response verifies correct needle position.

    c. In general, the anterior branch of the femoral nerve is identified first. Stimulation of this branch leads to contraction of the sartorius muscle on the medial aspect of the thigh and should *not be accepted.*

d. The needle should be redirected slightly laterally, and with a deeper direction, to encounter the posterior branch of the femoral nerve. Stimulation of this branch is identified by patellar ascension as the quadriceps contract. Local anesthetic (20 mL) is injected at that site.

4. SIDE EFFECTS AND COMPLICATIONS

a. Intravascular injection and hematoma are possible because of the proximity of the femoral artery. Anatomically, the nerve and artery are located in separate sheaths approximately 1 cm apart. In most patients with normal anatomy, the femoral artery can be easily palpated, allowing correct, safe needle positioning lateral to the pulsation.
b. The presence of femoral vascular grafts is a relative contraindication to this block.
c. Nerve damage is rare with this technique.

SUGGESTED READINGS

Berry FR: Analgesia in patients with fractured shaft of femur. Anesthesia 1977;32:576–577.

Patel NJ, Flashburg MH, Paskin S, et al: A regional anesthetic technique compared to general anesthesia for outpatient knee arthroscopy. Anesth Analg 1986;65:185–187.

1. GENERAL

a. The sciatic nerve (L4 and L5, S1 through S3) is the largest of the four peripheral nerves of the lower extremity, with a width of 2 cm as it leaves the pelvis with the posterior cutaneous nerve of the thigh.

b. The sciatic nerve is composed of two nerves bound by a common sheath of connective tissue; the tibial component is medial and anterior, and the common peroneal component is lateral and slightly posterior.

c. After passing through the sacrosciatic foramen beneath the piriformis muscle, it lies between the greater trochanter of the femur and the ischial tuberosity.

d. The nerve becomes superficial at the lower border of the gluteus maximus muscle, where it begins its descent down the posterior aspect of the thigh to the popliteal fossa.

e. It supplies cutaneous innervation to the posterior thigh and all of the leg and foot below the knee, except a thin medial strip supplied by the saphenous nerve.

2. CLINICAL APPLICATIONS

a. Because of its wide sensory distribution, the sciatic nerve block can be used, together with a saphenous or femoral nerve block, for any surgical procedure below the knee that does not require a thigh tourniquet.

b. It can also be combined with other peripheral nerve blocks to provide anesthesia for surgical procedures involving the thigh and knee.

c. This form of anesthesia avoids the sympathectomy associated with neuraxial blocks and, therefore, may be advantageous when any shift in hemodynamics could be deleterious, such as in patients with significant aortic stenosis.

3. TECHNIQUE: CLASSIC (POSTERIOR) APPROACH OF LABAT

a. For the classic (posterior) approach of Labat, the patient is positioned laterally, with the leg to be *blocked* rolled forward onto the flexed knee as the heel rests on the knee of the dependent (nonoperative) leg.

b. A line is drawn to connect the posterior superior iliac spine to the greater trochanter of the femur. A perpendicular line is drawn bisecting this line and extending 5 cm caudad. A second line is drawn from the greater trochanter to the sacral hiatus. The intersection of this line with the perpendicular line indicates the point of needle entry and falls 3 to 5 cm along the line.

c. A 22-gauge, 10- to 12-cm needle is advanced until a paresthesia or nerve stimulator response is elicited or bone is contacted. If bone is encountered, the needle is redirected systematically in a lateral or medial direction.

d. After the needle is properly placed, a total of 20 to 30 mL of solution is injected.

4. TECHNIQUE: ANTERIOR APPROACH

a. A line is drawn along the inguinal ligament from the anterior–superior iliac crest to the pubic tubercle is trisected.

b. A second line is drawn parallel to the inguinal ligament, beginning at the tuberosity of the greater trochanter.

c. A 22-gauge, 10.5- to 12-cm needle is inserted perpendicularly with a slightly lateral angulation at the point where the line representing the juncture of the middle and medial thirds crosses the second line.

d. This needle is advanced until it contacts bone, the lesser trochanter of the femur. The needle is redirected medially past the femur, and a paresthesia or nerve stimulator response is sought at a depth of about 5 cm past the bone.

e. A total of 20 to 25 mL of solution is injected incrementally after careful aspiration.

f. The anterior approach is useful when the patient cannot be positioned for the classic posterior approach because of pain or lack of cooperation.

g. Initial blockade of the *femoral nerve* decreases the pain associated with this approach.

5. SIDE EFFECTS AND COMPLICATIONS

a. Attempts to place the needle in the middle of the sciatic nerve by identifying a specific motor end point (e.g., foot inversion) may increase success rates.

b. Another method is the concept of multiple injections. The two major components of the sciatic nerve are separately identified and blocked. The first block is done at the initial bifurcation (gluteal muscle) and the second is above the popliteal fossa.

c. Some experts recommend that sciatic nerve blocks be initiated well before the scheduled time of surgery to extend the dwell time and allow for long latencies.

d. The block is technically difficult to perform and can be quite painful.

e. Hematoma formation is possible. The risk of nerve damage is also reported, although persistent paresthesias are usually self-limited. A minimal degree of vasodilation may occur with sciatic nerve block.

SUGGESTED READINGS

Beck GP: Anterior approach to sciatic nerve. Anesthesiology 1963;24:222–224.

Labat G: Regional Anesthesia: Its Technic and Clinical Application. Philadelphia, WB Saunders, 1922.

Raj PP, Parks RI, Watson TD, et al: New single position supine approach to sciatic-femoral nerve block. Anesth Analg 1975;54:489–493.

Vloka JD, Hadzic A, April E, et al: The division of the sciatic nerve in the popliteal fossa: Anatomical implications for popliteal nerve blockade. Anesth Analg 2001;92: 215–217.

11 Obturator Nerve Block

1. GENERAL

a. The obturator nerve is derived primarily from the third and fourth lumbar nerves with an occasional minor contribution from L2. The nerve lies deep in the obturator canal, having descended from the medial border of the psoas muscle.

b. As the nerve leaves the obturator canal, it divides into anterior and posterior branches.

c. The anterior branch supplies an articular branch to the hip and the anterior adductor muscles and a variable cutaneous branch to the lower medial thigh. The posterior branch innervates the deep adductor muscles and may send an articular branch to the knee.

2. CLINICAL APPLICATIONS

a. The obturator nerve usually is blocked as part of regional anesthesia for knee surgery. Because it is primarily a motor nerve, it is rarely blocked on its own.

b. Obturator nerve block can be useful in treating or diagnosing the extent of adductor spasm in patients with cerebral palsy and other muscle or neurologic diseases affecting the lower extremities before surgical intervention (e.g., adductor tenotomy).

3. TECHNIQUE

a. The patient is placed in the supine position, and a mark is made 1 to 2 cm lateral and 1 to 2 cm caudad to the pubic tubercle. A skin wheal is raised, and a 22-gauge, 8- to 10-cm needle is advanced perpendicular to the skin entry site with a slight medial direction.

b. The inferior pubic ramus is encountered at a depth of 2 to 4 cm, and the needle is walked in a lateral and caudad direction, until it passes into the obturator canal. The obturator nerve is located 2 to 3 cm past the initial point of contact with the pubic ramus.

c. After negative aspiration, 10 to 15 mL of local anesthetic is injected. A nerve stimulator is helpful in locating the obturator nerve, and correct needle position is evidenced by contraction of the adductor muscles of the medial thigh.

d. This classic approach to obturator nerve block involves painful periosteal contact and multiple needle redirections.

4. ALTERNATIVE TECHNIQUE

a. The needle is inserted behind the adductor tendon, near its pubic insertion, and is directed laterally toward a mark on the skin 1 to

2 cm medial to the femoral artery and immediately below the inguinal ligament, representing the obturator canal.

b. The nerve is identified by a motor response to peripheral nerve stimulation in the adductor muscle

5. SIDE EFFECTS AND COMPLICATIONS

a. Of the lower extremity blocks, this block has the highest failure rate because of landmarks and technical difference.

b. The obturator canal contains vascular and neural structures, and there is a theoretical risk of intravascular injection, hematoma, and nerve damage.

c. Absence of anesthesia in the obturator nerve distribution can render an otherwise perfect lower extremity block inadequate for surgical procedures on the knee.

SUGGESTED READING

Wassef MR: Interadductor approach to obturator nerve blockade for spastic conditions of adductor thigh muscles. Reg Anesth 1993;18:13–17.

12 Popliteal Fossa Block

1. GENERAL

a. The posterior muscles of the thigh are the biceps femoris, the semi-membranosus, semitendinosus, and the posterior portion of the adductor magnus.

b. As these muscles are traced distally from their origin on the ischial tuberosity, they separate into medial (semimembranosus, semitendinosus) and lateral (biceps) musculature, and they form the upper border of the popliteal fossa.

c. The lower border of the popliteal fossa is defined by the two heads of the gastrocnemius.

d. In the upper part of the popliteal fossa, the sciatic nerve lies posterolateral to the popliteal vessels. The popliteal vein is medial to the nerve, and the popliteal artery is most anterior, lying on the popliteal surface of the femur.

e. Near the upper border of the popliteal fossa, the two components of the sciatic nerve separate. The peroneal nerve diverges laterally, and the larger tibial branch descends almost straight down through the fossa. The tibial nerve and popliteal vessels then disappear deep to the converging heads of the gastrocnemius muscle

2. CLINICAL APPLICATIONS

a. This block is chiefly used for foot and ankle surgery.

b. The block has also been successfully used in the pediatric population. Popliteal fossa block is preferable to ankle block for surgical procedures requiring the use of a calf tourniquet.

c. The components of the sciatic nerve may be blocked at the level of the popliteal fossa through posterior or lateral approaches.

d. Supplemental block of the saphenous nerve is required for surgical procedures to the medial aspect of the leg or when a calf tourniquet or Esmarch bandage is used.

3. TECHNIQUE: POSTERIOR APPROACH

a. The borders of the popliteal fossa are identified by flexing the knee joint. A triangle is constructed, with the base consisting of the skin crease behind the knee, and the two sides composed of the semimembranosus (medially) and the biceps (laterally).

b. A bisecting line is drawn from the apex to the base of the triangle, and a 5-cm needle is inserted at a site 5 to 10 cm above the skin fold and 0.5 to 1 cm lateral to the bisecting line. Classically, the 5-cm distance has been described. However, in an attempt to block the sciatic nerve before its division, a 7- to 10-cm distance has been recommended.

c. The needle is advanced at a 45-degree angle until a paresthesia or nerve stimulator response is elicited. With a nerve stimulator technique, inversion is the motor response that best predicts complete neural block of the foot. Injection of approximately 30 mL of local anesthetic solution is sufficient.

d. The success rate is typically 90% to 95%. No formal comparison between paresthesia and nerve stimulator techniques has been performed to assess efficacy and complications.

e. It is believed that incomplete block is the result of poor diffusion (because of the size of the sciatic nerve), the separate fascial coverings of the tibial and peroneal nerves, or blockade of only a single component of the sciatic nerve.

f. Identification of the tibial and peroneal components decreases onset time and improves the success rate.

4. ALTERNATIVE TECHNIQUE: LATERAL APPROACH

a. A lateral approach to blockade of the sciatic nerve in the popliteal fossa has been described. Although block time is somewhat longer, onset and quality of block are similar to the posterior approach.

b. The patient's leg is extended, with the long axis of the foot at a 90-degree angle to the table. The site of insertion is the intersection of the vertical line drawn from the upper edge of the patella and the groove between the lateral border of the biceps femoris and vastus lateralis.

c. A 10-cm needle is advanced at a 30-degree angle posterior to the horizontal plane. Because the common peroneal nerve is located lateral to the tibial nerve, the stimulating needle encounters the common peroneal nerve first with the lateral approach. As with the classic posterior approach, an elicited inversion response is sought.

d. If a response associated with common peroneal nerve stimulation (e.g., eversion) is elicited, the needle is redirected more posteriorly.

5. SIDE EFFECTS AND COMPLICATIONS

a. Neuropathy is the most common complication.

b. Intravascular injection may occur as a result of the presence of vascular structures within the popliteal fossa.

c. Performance of popliteal fossa block in patients with previous total-knee arthroplasty or vascular bypass (femoral-popliteal) should be done with care. However, there have been no cases of graft disruption or joint infections related to needle placement in these patients.

SUGGESTED READINGS

Hadzic A, Vloka JD: A comparison of the posterior versus lateral approaches to the block of the sciatic nerve in the popliteal fossa. Anesthesiology 1998;88: 1480–1486.

Paqueron X, Bouaziz H, Macalou D, et al: The lateral approach to the sciatic nerve at the popliteal fossa: One or two injections? Anesth Analg 1999;89:1221–1225.

Rorie DK, Byer DE, Nelson DO, et al: Assessment of block of the sciatic nerve in the popliteal fossa. Anesth Analg 1980;59:371–376.

Vloka JD, Hadzic A, April E, Thys DM: The division of the sciatic nerve in the popliteal fossa: Anatomical implications for popliteal nerve blockade. Anesth Analg 2001;92:215–217.

Zetlaoui PJ, Bouaziz H: Lateral approach to the sciatic nerve in the popliteal fossa. Anesth Analg 1998;87:79–82.

13 Sural Nerve Block at the Ankle

1. INDICATIONS

a. Anesthesia of the posterior aspect of the ankle and lateral foot
b. Part of an anesthetic for an ankle block; combined with a superficial and deep peroneal, tibial, and saphenous nerve blocks
c. Surgery of the foot or ankle in patients who will not tolerate the hemodynamic effects of neuraxial or general anesthetics
d. Postoperative pain in the foot
e. Foot trauma involving the heel or ankle
f. Palliation of distal peripheral neuropathies

2. ANATOMY

a. A branch of the posterior tibial nerve
b. Passes posteriorly, around the lateral malleolus
c. Sensory innervation to the lateral foot, plantar aspect of the heel, and into the lateral aspect of the fifth toe

3. CONTRAINDICATIONS

a. Patient refusal
b. Allergic reaction to the local anesthetic used
c. Inability to assess the patient's response during the procedure
d. Infection localized to the area, or a systemic infection
e. Pregnancy

4. TECHNIQUE

a. The patient's foot is placed in the decubitus position with the affected limb as the up limb, on a pillow.
b. The area between the Achilles tendon and the lateral malleolus is sterilely prepped and draped.
c. Using a 27-gauge, 1.5-inch needle, the needle is inserted at the midpoint between the Achilles tendon and the posterior aspect of the lateral malleolus, is aspirated to ensure no intravascular injection, and is injected in a deep "fan-wise" manner aiming toward the posterior malleolar grove.
d. A total of 4 mL of 0.25% bupivacaine is injected.
e. *Do not use epinephrine in the local anesthetic because this can compromise blood flow to the extremity.*

5. SIDE EFFECTS AND COMPLICATIONS

a. Hematoma
b. Ecchymosis
c. Neuritis
d. Infection

Superficial Peroneal Nerve Block at the Ankle

1. INDICATIONS

a. Anesthesia of the dorsal surface of the foot, excluding the web space between the first and second toes
b. Surgery of the foot or ankle in patients who will not tolerate the hemodynamic effects of neuraxial or general anesthetics
c. Part of an anesthetic for an ankle block; combined with deep peroneal, sural, tibial, and saphenous nerve blocks
d. Postoperative pain in the foot
e. Foot trauma involving the dorsum of the foot
f. Palliation of distal peripheral neuropathies

2. ANATOMY

a. A branch of the common peroneal nerve
b. Descends toward the ankle in the lateral compartment of the leg and enters the ankle just lateral to the extensor digitorum longus
c. Located lateral to the extensor digitorum longus at the adjacent level of the lateral malleolus, superficially

3. CONTRAINDICATIONS

a. Patient refusal
b. Allergic reaction to the local anesthetic used
c. Inability to assess the patient's response during the procedure
d. Infection localized to the area or a systemic infection
e. Pregnancy

4. TECHNIQUE

a. The patient's foot is placed in the supine position with the foot on a bump.
b. The extensor hallucis longus is identified by having the patient extend their big toe.
c. A point just medial to the tendon is marked and sterilely prepped and draped.
d. The 27-gauge, 1.5-inch needle is then advanced from this point subcutaneously toward the lateral malleolus.
e. A total of 6 mL of 0.25% bupivacaine is injected.
f. *Do not use epinephrine in the local anesthetic because this can compromise blood flow to the extremity.*

5. SIDE EFFECTS AND COMPLICATIONS

    a. Hematoma
    b. Ecchymosis
    c. Neuritis
    d. Infection

15 Saphenous Nerve Block

1. AT THE ANKLE

a. Indications
  i.   Anesthesia of the medial ankle and foot, excluding the big toe
  ii. Surgery of the foot or ankle in patients who will not tolerate the hemodynamic effects of neuraxial or general anesthetics
  iii. Part of an anesthetic for an ankle block; combined with a superficial and deep peroneal, sural, and tibial nerve blocks
  iv. Postoperative pain relief of the medial ankle and foot
  v.   Palliation of distal peripheral neuropathies
  vi. Foot trauma involving the medial aspect of the foot

b. Anatomy
  i.   The saphenous nerve is a branch of the femoral nerve.
  ii. It is the only nerve that enters the foot that does not derive from the sciatic nerve.
  iii. It gives superficial sensory innervation to the medial malleolus and the anteromedial foot, including the medial arch of the foot.
  iv. It traverses over the medial condyle of the foot.

c. Contraindications
  i.   Patient refusal
  ii. Allergic reaction to the local anesthetic used
  iii. Inability to assess the patient's response during the procedure
  iv. Infection localized to the area or a systemic infection
  v.   Pregnancy

d. Technique
  i.   The patient's foot is placed in the supine position on a pillow.
  ii. The patient is asked to extend their big toe elucidating the extensor hallucis longus tendon.
  iii. The point just medial to the tendon at the crease of the ankle, at the inferior border of the medial malleolus, is marked. A 27-gauge, 1.5-inch needle is advanced from this point toward the medial malleolus and 6 mL of 0.25% bupivacaine is injected subcutaneously, after careful aspiration, to rule out any intravascular injection.
  iv. Secondary to the proximity of the superficial peroneal nerve, it is most often blocked with the same injection technique.
  v.   *Do not use epinephrine in the local anesthetic because this can compromise blood flow to the extremity.*

e. Complications
  i.   Hematoma
  ii. Ecchymosis
  iii. Neuritis
  iv. Infection

2. AT THE KNEE

  a. Anatomy
     i. Provides sensory innervation to the medial calf, the medial malleolus, and the anteromedial foot
  b. Contraindications
     i. Patient refusal
     ii. Allergic reaction to the local anesthetic used
     iii. Inability to assess the patient's response during the procedure
     iv. Infection localized to the area or a systemic infection
     v. Pregnancy
  c. Technique
     i. The patient is put in a lateral decubitus position with the affected leg in the down position.
     ii. The down leg is slightly flexed and the medial condyle of the femur is palpated.
     iii. The point just anterior to the posterior edge of the medial condyle is marked. A 27-gauge, 1.5- to 3-inch needle is advanced toward the medial condyle and is touched down on os. Once on os, the needle is withdrawn slightly and a total of 5 mL of 0.25% bupivacaine is injected slowly.
     iv. *Do not use epinephrine in the local anesthetic because this can compromise blood flow to the extremity.*
  d. Complications
     i. Hematoma
     ii. Ecchymosis
     iii. Neuritis
     iv. Infection
     v. Intravascular injection. This occurs with a greater frequency than other blocks because of the close proximity of the saphenous artery and vein to the nerve. The syringe should be aspirated prior to injection to prevent injecting directly into the artery.

16   Lateral Femoral Cutaneous Nerve Block

1. GENERAL

a. The lateral femoral cutaneous nerve (L2 and L3) emerges at the lateral border of the psoas muscle immediately caudad to the ilio-inguinal nerve. It descends under the iliac fascia to enter the thigh deep to the inguinal ligament 1 to 2 cm medial to the anterior–superior iliac spine.

b. The nerve emerges from the fascia lata 7 to 10 cm below the spine and divides into anterior and posterior branches.

c. The skin of the lateral portion of the thigh from the hip to mid-thigh is supplied by the posterior branch; the anterior branch supplies the anterolateral thigh to the knee.

2. CLINICAL APPLICATIONS

a. This block is useful for skin graft harvesting.

b. It is also used in conjunction with other peripheral nerve blocks for complete anesthesia of the lower extremity.

c. Loss of sensation over anterolateral thigh is termed paresthesia paralytica. This phenomenon is observed after forceps delivery in parturients.

3. TECHNIQUE

a. A point is marked 2 cm medial and 2 cm caudad to the anterior–superior iliac spine.

b. A 22-gauge, 4-cm needle is advanced perpendicular to the skin entry site until a sudden release indicates passage through the fascia lata.

c. As the needle is moved in a fan-like pattern laterally and medially, 10 to 15 mL of solution is injected, depositing local anesthetic above and below the fascia.

4. ALTERNATIVE TECHNIQUE

a. The nerve can also be blocked just medial and posterior to the anterior–superior iliac spine with 10 mL of anesthetic solution.

b. Combining the two techniques (i.e., belt-and-suspenders method) increases the success rate, but the total volume of solution used may be limiting.

c. Because this is a pure sensory nerve, a nerve stimulator is not helpful in performing this block.

5. SIDE EFFECTS AND COMPLICATIONS

a. Neuritis of this nerve caused by needle trauma or drug toxicity is a potential but unlikely complication.

b. There are no large blood vessels in the vicinity of this nerve, and the likelihood of rapid uptake or intravascular injection is very small.

1. POSTERIOR TIBIAL NERVE BLOCK
AT THE ANKLE

a. Indications
   i. Part of an ankle block technique for surgery of the foot or ankle
b. Anatomy
   i. It is a branch of the sciatic nerve.
   ii. At the level of the ankle, the nerve is located posterior to the posterior tibial artery, midway between the medial malleolus and the Achilles tendon.
   iii. The posterior tibial nerve, via its calcaneal nerve branch, provides cutaneous coverage to the inner aspect of the heel, medial malleolus, sole of the foot, and Achilles tendon.
c. Contraindications
   i. Patient refusal
   ii. Infection at the block site
   iii. Allergy to the local anesthetic
d. Technique
   i. The patient is placed in the supine position with the leg externally rotated and the knee flexed.
   ii. The posterior tibial artery is palpated 1 to 2 cm anterior to the Achilles tendon at the inferior border of the medial malleolus.
   iii. The needle is directed posterior to the artery and advanced until contact with bone is felt in the groove behind the medial malleolus.
   iv. After a negative aspiration, 5 to 10 mL of local anesthetic is injected in a fan-wise manner.
e. Complications
   i. Hematoma
   ii. Ecchymosis
   iii. Nerve injury
   iv. Infection

2. DEEP PERONEAL NERVE BLOCK
OF THE ANKLE

a. Indications
   i. Part of an ankle block technique for surgery of the foot or ankle
b. Anatomy
   i. The deep peroneal nerve, a terminal branch of the common peroneal nerve, lies between the tendons of the extensor digitorum

longus and anterior tibial muscles at level of the ankle on the front of the leg. The dorsalis pedis artery is medial to the nerve.
  ii. As the medial branch of the deep peroneal nerve courses down the dorsum of the foot, it supplies sensory innervation of the first web space between the big toe and second toe.
c. Contraindications
  i. Local anesthetic allergy
  ii. Patient refusal
  iii. Uncooperative patient
  iv. Infection at the block site
d. Technique
  i. Patient is placed in the supine position.
  ii. The patient is asked to extend their foot and first toe against resistance. This allows for palpation of the extensor hallucis longus muscle.
  iii. At a point above the ankle and at the level of the malleoli, the palpating finger locates the dorsalis pedis artery.
  iv. A 25-gauge needle is directed perpendicular to the skin, medial to the artery, and between the tendons of the extensor digitorum and extensor hallucis longus until bony contact is made with the tibia.
  v. After a negative aspiration, 2 to 4 mL of local anesthetic is injected in a fan-wise manner. Epinephrine is not used because it may compromise the blood flow.
e. Complications
  i. Hematoma
  ii. Ecchymosis
  iii. Nerve injury
  iv. Infection

SUGGESTED READINGS

Chelly JE: Peripheral Nerve Blocks. A Color Atlas. Philadelphia, Lippincott Williams & Wilkins, 1999.

Hadzic A, Vloka J: Peripheral Nerve Blocks: Principles and Practice. New York, McGraw-Hill, 2004.

18 Popliteal Nerve Block

1. GENERAL

    a. Anesthesia of the foot and ankle when a calf tourniquet is adequate

    b. Surgery of the foot or ankle in patients who will not tolerate the hemodynamic effects of neuraxial or general anesthetics

    c. Postoperative pain relief of the foot and ankle

    d. Trauma involving the foot and ankle

    e. Palliation of distal peripheral neuropathies

    f. Useful for debridement or distal amputations

2. INDICATIONS

    a. It is indicated for procedures performed on the foot and ankle when a calf tourniquet is adequate.

    b. When combined with a saphenous nerve block, it provides total anesthesia to the foot and ankle.

3. ANATOMY

    a. Popliteal fossa

        i. The sciatic nerve divides into two major branches, mainly the tibial and common peroneal nerves at the most cephalad aspect of the popliteal fossa.

        ii. The upper area of the popliteal fossa is bounded by the biceps femoris tendon laterally and the semitendinosus and semimembranosus tendons medially.

        iii. At the most cephalad aspect of the popliteal fossa, the popliteal artery is located just lateral to the semitendinosus tendon and is followed by the popliteal vein and the tibial nerve and common peroneal nerves.

        iv. Both the tibial and common peroneal nerves lie within a sheath at this point.

        v. The tibial nerve continues deep to the gastrocnemius muscle, and the common peroneal nerve passes between the head and the neck of the fibula.

    b. Tibial nerve

        i. The tibial nerve provides sensory innervation to the posterior calf, the heel, and the medial plantar surface of the foot.

    c. Common peroneal nerve

        i. The common peroneal nerve provides sensory innervation to the lateral calf, lateral ankle, and the lateral dorsal surface of the foot.

4. CONTRAINDICATIONS

   a. Patient refusal
   b. Allergic reaction to the local anesthetic used
   c. Inability to assess the patient's response during the procedure
   d. Infection localized to the area or a systemic infection
   e. Pregnancy

5. TECHNIQUE

   a. The patient is put in a lateral decubitus position with the affected leg in the down position.
   b. The popliteal artery is palpated in the midline of the popliteal fossa at approximately 1 to 2 inches cephalad of the crease of the knee and is marked. If the popliteal artery cannot be palpated, a point at the midline of the posterior crease of the knee is made at approximately 2 inches cephalad to this point and is marked. This point is then sterilely prepped and draped.
   c. A 25-gauge, 1.5-inch spinal needle is inserted just lateral to the mark and is advanced 1 to 1.5 inches deep.
   d. The needle is then aspirated to rule out intravascular injection and is then injected with 20 to 30 mL of 0.25% bupivacaine.
   e. In the event that the common peroneal nerve is not anesthetized, it is necessary to block the nerve at the junction of the head and neck of the fibula just below the knee. Here, the common peroneal nerve can be blocked by just 5 mL of 0.25% bupivacaine.
   f. *Do not use epinephrine in the local anesthetic because this can compromise blood flow to the extremity.*

19 Bier Block

1. INDICATIONS

    a. Anesthesia for distal extremity surgery
    b. Drug administration for painful conditions (i.e., complex regional pain syndrome)

2. RELEVANT ANATOMY

    a. By sequestering drug in an extremity through the use of a tourniquet, the drug will diffuse into the soft tissue and nerves.
    b. Circulation time, occlusion of the extremity, and drug dosage are the limiting factors.

3. DEVICE-RELATED ASPECTS: UPPER EXTREMITY

    a. Most anesthesiologists (97%) exsanguinate the upper extremity by using an Esmarch bandage.
    b. The most commonly used tourniquet pressures are 250 mm Hg and 100 mm Hg greater than the systolic pressure.
    c. Most anesthesiologists (91%) use a dual bladder cuff.
       i. Decreased cuff pain
       ii. Improved safety
       iii. Decreased risk of accidental cuff deflation
       iv. Half of the anesthesiologists inflate the distal cuff first after exsanguination and the other half inflate the proximal cuff first.
    d. Most anesthesiologists (83%) do not perform intravenous regional anesthesia by using thigh or calf/ankle cuffs because of:
       i. Thigh cuff, calf/ankle blocks
       ii. No experience
       iii. Unsafe, large dose of local anesthetic (thigh cuff only)
       iv. Preference for epidural, spinal, or nerve block
       v. Unsuitable cases/no need
       vi. Cuffs not available
    e. Most anesthesiologists use either an electronic controller system (52%) or a mechanical or gas-powered system (29%).

4. TECHNIQUE: UPPER EXTREMITY

    a. The patient is placed in the supine position. Intravenous access is obtained in the other extremity.
    b. An intravenous catheter (22-gauge) is placed in the extremity to be treated.

c. The affected extremity is elevated to drain excess blood. Cotton cast padding is then wrapped around the arm prior to the placement of a double tourniquet.

d. After tightly placing the tourniquet, an Esmarch bandage is wrapped tightly around the extremity from the distal end (fingers) up to the tourniquet.

e. The upper portion of the double tourniquet is inflated to a pressure of 100 mm Hg above the patient's systolic pressure. The Esmarch is removed and the limb placed in a resting position. Preservative-free lidocaine 0.5% is slowly injected. A volume of 30 to 50 mL is adequate.

f. After 10 minutes, the area under the lower cuff is anesthetized. The lower cuff is then inflated.

g. After asserting that the lower cuff is adequately inflated (by absence of distal pulses), the upper cuff is deflated.

h. The lower cuff remains inflated for an additional 10 to 20 minutes.

i. To avoid possible local anesthetic toxicity, do not deflate the cuff for at least 25 to 30 minutes. When the lower cuff is deflated, do so for a few seconds before reinflating, while observing the patient for signs of local anesthetic toxicity. This step is done repeatedly to allow the local anesthetic to slowly wash out.

j. Initially, the cuff should be deflated to just below the systolic pressure.

5. SIDE EFFECTS AND COMPLICATIONS

a. Major side effect is phlebitis at the site of injection.

b. Local anesthetic toxicity is a major complication secondary to tourniquet failure or improper technique.

SUGGESTED READINGS

Raj P: Pain Medicine: A Comprehensive Review. St. Louis, Mosby, 2003.
Waldman S: Atlas of Intravenous Pain Management, 2nd ed. Philadelphia, WB Saunders, 2004.

Part II

Acute Pain

20 Rib Fractures

1. GENERAL

a. Rib fractures are a common component of traumatic injuries and motor vehicle accidents and are also a significant cause of pulmonary morbidity. In the acute pain setting, these injuries are most often seen after blunt trauma and have a reported incidence of 10% among patients admitted to one regional trauma center.

b. The greater the number of ribs fractured, the greater the degree of associated morbidity, with the presence of three or more fractures shown to be associated with increased mortality and duration of care in the in-patient and intensive care unit setting.

c. Patients older than 55 years have a 31% incidence of nosocomial pneumonia, whereas those as young as 45 years have been shown to suffer increased morbidity secondary to rib fractures.

2. PULMONARY MORBIDITY

a. Multiple pathophysiologic mechanisms are associated with the pulmonary morbidity following multiple rib fractures, including:
   i. Decreased phrenic nerve activity
   ii. Diaphragmatic dysfunction
   iii. Reflex increased spinal arc activity with increased intercostal tone
   iv. Decreased functional residual capacity and ventricular tachycardia, with these effects being compounded by concomitant administration of opioid analgesia
   v. Manifested ultimately as clinically significant V/Q mismatch, splinting, and hypoxemia

3. DIAGNOSIS

a. Rib fractures are commonly diagnosed by using chest x-ray (CXR).

b. Concomitant pulmonary contusions can be ruled in or out by using chest computed tomography (CT).

4. TREATMENT

a. Conservative management: Many patients with three or fewer rib fractures will be managed conservatively by using a combination of anti-inflammatory and intravenous opioid medications, the latter usually infused via patient-controlled analgesia (PCA). When these measures fail to manage the pain or do so suboptimally, then more invasive measures are used.

b. Multiple methods of pain control have been used to treat rib fractures, including:

    i. Anti-inflammatory medications
    ii. Intravenous narcotics
    iii. Epidural catheters
    iv. Intercostal blocks
    v. Intrapleural blocks.

c. The use of temporary mechanical ventilation has even been explored as a treatment for multiple rib fractures.

d. Physicians have traditionally based their choice for epidural analgesia on the presence of increasing age and number of rib fractures because these patients have been shown to be at increased risk of morbidity and mortality.

e. Treatment strategies depend on the number of rib fractures, the age of the patient, presence of any existing comorbidities and pulmonary disease, as well as analysis of blood gas parameters and coagulation status.

f. Epidural analgesia is associated with prolonged length of stay and increased complication in elderly patients (mean age, 77 years), particularly those with less significant injuries, regardless of cardiopulmonary comorbidities.

g. The method ultimately chosen depends significantly on the institution and varying degrees of success are seen.

5. NEURAXIAL ANESTHESIA

a. Neuraxial anesthesia options consist of epidural as well as intrapleural analgesia techniques. Epidural analgesia has been more extensively studied and is more widely used in clinical practice. Previous studies have shown that epidural analgesia provides superior pain relief and improves pulmonary function tests when compared with intravenous opioids for patients with rib fractures.

b. Recent studies have shown superior analgesia and pulmonary function as well as decreased levels of circulatory inflammatory mediators associated with acute lung injury in patients treated with an epidural versus those treated with PCA.

6. PRIOR TO EPIDURAL PLACEMENT

a. Coagulation studies: rule out the presence of coagulopathy

b. Blood gas analysis: assesses degree of respiratory compromise

c. CXR and chest CT: determine presence of rib fractures and pulmonary contusion

d. Complete blood count: rules out presence of systemic infection and bacteremia

e. Neurologic evaluation: For patient with altered mental status, any raised intracranial pressure must be ruled out prior to epidural placement to minimize the risk of dural puncture and, possibly, devastating brainstem herniation.

7. CONCLUSION

a. Epidural analgesia is an appropriate treatment modality for the pain of multiple rib fractures in patients who have failed a trial of conservative treatment and have been appropriately evaluated for suitability to and contraindications of epidural placement.

SUGGESTED READINGS

Bulger EM, Edwards T, Klotz P, et al: Epidural analgesia improves outcome after multiple rib fractures. Surgery 2004;136:426–430.

Holcomb JB, McMullins NR: Rib fracture pain and disability: Can we do better? J Trauma 2003;54:1058–1064.

Kieninger AN, Bair HA, Bendick PJ, et al: Epidural vs intravenous pain control in elderly patients with rib fractures. Am J Surg 2005;189:327–330.

Lee RB, Bass SM, Morris JA: Three or more rib fractures as an indicator for transfer to a level I trauma center: A population based study. J Trauma 1990;30:689–694.

Wu CL, Jani ND, Perkins FM: Thoracic epidural analgesia versus IV patient-controlled analgesia for the treatment of rib fracture pain after motor vehicle crash. J Trauma 1999;47:564–567.

Ziegler DW, Agarwal NN: The morbidity and mortality of rib fractures. J Trauma 1994;37:975–979.

21 Peripheral Nerve Injury

1. GENERAL

a. Peripheral nerves may be injured at a variety of peripheral locations.
   i. Ankle
   ii. Elbow
   iii. Brachial plexus
   iv. Wrist
b. Peripheral nerve injuries may be manifested in a variety of ways and the distribution of the injury, be it in the form of paresthesia, hypoesthesia, or neuralgia, may often be the key to the diagnosis of the nerve involved.

2. UPPER EXTREMITY INJURIES

a. Brachial plexus lesions
   i. Given the anatomic location of the brachial plexus and the close proximity of the axillary artery and subclavian artery, a host of causes may be responsible for brachial plexopathies, including:
      (1) Traumatic injury at birth
      (2) Traumatic injury following a motor vehicle accident (MVA) or gunshot injuries
      (3) Tumors
      (4) Iatrogenic injuries sustained while under general anesthesia or during cardiac catheterization
      (5) Vascular emboli or thoracic outlet syndrome
   ii. The exact anatomic location may usually be determined clinically, as can be seen in **Table 21-1.**
   iii. In general, all lesions of the brachial plexus can cause partial or total paralysis of the shoulder.

TABLE 21–1 Upper Extremity, Myotome, Dermatome, and Reflex Chart

Vertebral Level	Motor Deficit	Sensory Deficit	Reflex Affected
C5	Shoulder abduction, deltoids, biceps	Radial aspect of arm	Biceps
C6	Wrist extension	Lateral forearm	Brachioradialis
C7	Wrist flexion, finger extension	Middle finger	Triceps
C8	Finger flexion	Medial forearm	
T1	Finger abduction	Medial aspect of arm	

iv. Any lesion involving the T1 nerve root or sympathetic trunk will be accompanied by Horner syndrome.

v. Superior plexus lesions (Duchenne-Erb) result from damage to the fifth and sixth cervical roots.

   (1) The deltoid, biceps, and brachialis muscles are affected with a resulting inability to flex the elbow or pronate the forearm, and the arm hangs loose, internally rotated with the palm visible from behind.

vi. Lower plexus lesions are divided anatomically into three types: the posterior, lateral, and medial cord.

   (1) Posterior lesions cause sensory deficits along the distribution of the radial and axillary nerves, weakness of abduction of the arm, and inability to extend the wrist or fingers.

   (2) Medial cord lesions cause weakness of the muscles innervated by the ulnar nerve and medial head of the median nerve, thereby resulting in significant impairment of hand activity.

   (3) Lateral cord lesions involve the lateral head of the median nerve and the musculocutaneous nerve causing weakness of flexion and pronation of the forearm, wrist, and fingers.

vii. Because of its location, the brachial plexus is susceptible to traction and exogenous compression. Hematomas after anticoagulation or percutaneous axillary artery cannulation may also lead to plexus injuries.

viii. Peripheral nerve injuries may also occur following general anesthesia due to incorrect shoulder brace positioning, excessive arm abduction (>90 degrees).

ix. Additionally, radiation therapy can result in plexus injuries whereby paresthesias can be elicited by tapping the supraclavicular fossa.

3. LOWER EXTREMITY INJURIES

a. Lower extremity peripheral nerves can also be adversely affected following traumatic events such as lacerations or MVAs.

b. Peripheral nerves can be injured, resulting in neuropathic pain, paresthesias, and hypoesthesias. For example, such nerves as those supplying the ankle joint, including:

   i. Saphenous

   ii. Superficial peroneal

   iii. Sural nerves

c. Such injuries can also result from open reduction and internal fixation of ankle joint fractures.

d. The common peroneal nerve, which, along with the tibial nerve, comprises the sciatic nerve, arises from the posterior divisions of L4, L5, S1, and S2. Along its course it travels superficially around

the fibular neck, and it is at this location that it is most susceptible to injury, as can occur during general anesthesia in the lithotomy position or during coma.
e. Less common etiologies include squatting and crossing of the legs.
f. Affected patients may have footdrop as well as sensory deficits over the anterolateral aspect of the lower leg and dorsum of the foot.
g. Specific sural neuropathy can cause paresthesias and pain over the lateral aspect of the foot and ankle.

4. MANAGEMENT: KEYS TO SUCCESSFUL RECOVERY FROM PLEXOPATHIES

a. Initial rest
b. Early mobilization
c. Therapeutic rehabilitation
d. Thorough history and physical examination can eliminate the need for additional invasive tests.
e. However, electromyography can be useful in identifying the paths of the involved nerves.
f. Regular occupational and physical therapy are often necessary to help patients regain full use of the limb following a significant brachial plexus lesion and can often reduce or offset significant impairment and disuse atrophy.
g. Orthotic devices can also be used to assist in rehabilitation as in the treatment of footdrop.
h. Tendon transfer surgery is a viable and often successful treatment for severe nerve injuries that have resulted in disuse atrophy and contracture of a limb or part thereof.

SUGGESTED READING

Salam AA: Brachial plexus paralysis: An unusual complication of anticoagulant therapy. Am Surg 1972;38(8):454–455.

22 Amputation Pain

1. GENERAL

a. Amputation pain can result from the amputation of any appendage, and phantom sensation of the tongue, penis, breast, and nose have all been reported, but is most often described in the extremities.
  i. Phantom sensation is the perception of the continued presence of the amputated part.
  ii. Phantom pain is a term used to describe painful sensations that are not perceived to originate in the amputated portion of the extremity.
b. Amputation sensation is almost a universal occurrence at some time during the first month after surgery or traumatic severing of a limb or appendage.
  i. However, amputation and phantom limb pain have been shown in large studies to carry an incidence of 72% to 85%.
  ii. Amputation pain has been reported to occur as early as 1 week after amputation.
  iii. Although the incidence certainly does decrease with time, data reveal that 60% of amputees experience pain 6 months following amputation. Of these, about 27% have phantom limb pain more than 15 hours per day, more than 20 days of the month.
  iv. The incidence of amputation pain increases with more proximal lesions.
  v. Phantom limb pain may begin months to years after an amputation, but pain beginning more than 1 year after the initial insult occurs in fewer than 10% of patients.

2. SIGNS AND SYMPTOMS

a. Amputation pain is usually described as burning, aching, or cramping.
b. One-third of patients may report sharp, shock-like pains that are excruciating but brief.
c. Pain exacerbations may be produced by trivial physical or emotional stimuli.
d. Fifty percent of patients have pain that is induced by urination, coughing, or sexual activity, suggesting that autonomic input increases internuncial neuron activity and, thereby, precipitates amputation pain.
e. Many patients report that exposure to a cold environment or changes in weather also worsen pain.
f. Amputation pain may also be triggered by recurrence of cancer or reactivation of herpes zoster.

g. The usual course of amputation pain is to remain unchanged or to improve.
h. Physical examination is unrevealing although the stump should be examined for trigger areas reproducing pain.
i. Neuromas are found in only 20% of patients.

3. ETIOLOGY

a. The cause of amputation pain is not clearly defined.
b. Proposed models suggest an interaction of central and peripheral mechanisms.
c. Peripheral theories suggest that spontaneous firing occurs from neuromas, with an increase in the rate of spontaneous discharge originating in the neuroma, occurring on sympathetic stimulation of injection of epinephrine.
d. The gate-control theory of pain is commonly used to explain amputation pain: following destruction of sensory neurons by amputation, wide dynamic neurons are freed by inhibitory control, with self-sustaining neuronal activity then free to occur in neurons. Should this spontaneous activity exceed a critical level, pain may occur in the phantom limb.
e. No consistent personality disorder has been shown in patients with amputation pain, and there does not appear to be an increased incidence of neurosis or other psychological disorder in amputees with phantom pain.
f. It is possible that phantom or amputation pain exists only as the psychopathic interpretation of phantom or amputation sensation because the same adjectives are used for both the pain and the normal amputation sensation.

4. TREATMENT

a. Physical therapy
   i. Because amputation pain occurs more frequently in patients who are unable to use a prosthesis within 6 months, attention to healing, early prosthesis fitting, and intensive physical therapy are key pain treatment and prevention areas.
b. Transcutaneous electrical nerve stimulation (TENS)
   i. TENS has been used extensively with varied reported response rates.
   ii. Long-term success reported in five of six patients treated, while Shealy found good to excellent results in only 25% of patients treated with TENS.
   iii. Stimulation of the contralateral extremity with TENS has also shown a favorable response in some patients.
c. Acupuncture
   i. Relief of amputation pain of the arm with electroacupuncture has been reported in the Western literature by Monga.

    ii. Levine and colleagues reported short-term relief with the first few acupuncture treatments, but found no long-term improvement in patients with a history amputation pain.

d. Psychological therapies

    i. Individual psychotherapy and relaxation techniques have been reported to benefit patients with amputation pain.

    ii. Sherman reported relief in 2 patients with acute pain and significant improvement in 12 of 14 patients with chronic amputation pain. Patients required an average of six treatments to produce a lessening of pain, with an increase in pain relief associated with a decrease in anxiety level.

e. Medications

    i. The most commonly used classes of medications are *antidepressants* and *anticonvulsants*.

       (1) Historically, carbamazepine is the most commonly used anticonvulsant, but gabapentin currently appears to be the most commonly used anticonvulsant for amputation and other neuropathic pain syndromes.

       (2) Gabapentin is obviously an attractive choice given its low toxicity, ability to titrate to high doses to achieve analgesia, and the absence of requiring blood tests to monitor while treating.

    ii. *β-adrenergic blockers* have also been suggested as a treatment option based on several cases reported by Marsland et al., where patients' pain was greatly improved after treatment with propranolol and metoprolol. However, in a double-blind crossover trial of propranolol (up to 240 mg daily), Scadding et al. were unable to show significant improvement in neuralgias.

f. Nerve blocks

    i. Trigger point or direct stump injections and sympathetic, peripheral nerve, and major conduction blocks have all been used with success in the treatment of pain.

    ii. Given the theories discussed above regarding sympathetic discharge, a series of sympathetic blocks seems an appropriate interventional tool.

    iii. Random case reports also revealed the resolution of symptoms after epidural blockade and epidural meperidine.

g. Neurostimulation

    i. Stimulation of the posterior columns of the spinal cord is the most common neurosurgical technique for the treatment of phantom limb pain.

    ii. To improve success rates, patients with evidence of drug dependence or psychological disturbances should be omitted.

    iii. The success rate of dorsal column stimulation declines over time, and greater than 50% long-term pain reduction is present in only one-third of patients originally showing improvement.

5. CONCLUSION

Early intervention, counseling about phantom stimulation and pain before amputation where possible, and a multidisciplinary treatment regimen are the keys to diagnosing and treating this devastating condition, where patients not only have to cope with trauma surrounding the amputation but also with pain in a limb that is physically absent.

SUGGESTED READINGS

Carabelli RA, Kellerman WC: Phantom limb pain: Relief by application of TENS to contralateral extremity. Arch Phys Med Rehabil 1985;66:466–467.

Jensen TS, Krebs B, Nielsen J, et al: Immediate and long-term phantom limb pain in amputees: Incidence, clinical characteristics and relationship to pre-amputation limb pain. Pain 1985;21:267–278.

Matzer O, Devor M: Contrasting thermal sensitivity of spontaneously active A- and C-fibers in experimental nerve-end neuromas. Pain 1987;30:373–384.

Saris SC, Iacono RP: Dorsal root entry zone lesions for post-amputation pain. J Neurosurg 1985;62:72–76.

Sherman RA, Sherman CJ: Chronic phantom and stump pain among American veterans: Results of a survey. Pain 1984;18:83–95.

23 Extremity Injury

1. GENERAL

a. Trauma-related pain of the extremities can present along the same paths and mechanisms as those described in the section on Soft Tissue Pain.

b. In addition, an important subset exists of extremity-related painful conditions that are related to trauma and are discussed below.

2. VASCULAR PAIN

a. Vascular insufficiency

  i. The pain associated with the acute onset of arterial insufficiency is characterized by its sudden onset.

  ii. Classically, such arterial insufficiency is associated with the 5 P's: pain, pallor, paresthesias, paralysis, and pulselessness.

b. Traumatic injury

  i. After a traumatic vascular injury, the pulses are usually absent distal to the site of the injury, the extremity will appear pale, and the veins may appear to be empty. The muscles begin to feel firm and inelastic as the ischemia progresses.

c. Traumatic aneurysms

  i. These are false aneurysms that are produced from arterial penetration.

  ii. Perivascular hematomas that result may be classified as follows:

    (1) Acute traumatic hematomas: Total vessel wall disruption occurs leading to a gradually enlarging hematoma contained by surrounding tissues.

    (2) Chronic traumatic aneurysms: Absorption of the perivascular hematoma occurs and surrounding fibrosis provides boundaries.

  iii. Traumatic aneurysms may be the result of radiologic procedures, penetrating injuries, and vascular procedures, such as the placement of infra-aortic balloon pumps as well as internal fixation of bone fractures.

    (1) The interval period from injury to detection of the lesion is longer than 1 month in greater than 50% of cases.

    (2) A systolic bruit is heard on examination and compression of the expanding aneurysm may result in secondary neuropathy or venous occlusion.

3. NEUROGENIC PAIN

a. Myriad causes of traumatic brachial plexopathies exist.

  i. The anatomic location of the plexus is important when considering and understanding these disorders.

      ii. The plexus itself is superficial in the supraclavicular fossa where it lies in close proximity to the subclavian artery, with both structures lying close to the apex of the lung.

      iii. More distally, the plexus lies close to the first and second parts of the axillary artery with a fat pad surrounding both.

  b. Common causes of traumatic injury to the plexus occur after:

      i. Birth injuries

      ii. Stab and gunshot wounds

      iii. Motor vehicle accidents

      iv. Sports injuries in football or rugby players

      v. Repetitive strain injuries in laborers carrying heavy loads

      vi. Injuries seen in travelers carrying heavy backpacks

  c. Specific lesions following such injuries are often characterized as being superior or inferior, clinically comprising.

  d. Superior plexus lesions

      i. Erb-Duchenne palsy

      ii. Results from damage to the 5th and 6th cervical roots

      iii. Affects the deltoid, brachioradialis, biceps, and brachialis muscles

      iv. Inability to abduct and externally rotate the shoulder

      v. Inability to flex the elbow or pronate the forearm

      vi. Associated with sensory loss over the deltoid and radial forearm

  e. Isolated middle plexus lesions (C7) are unusual.

  f. Inferior plexus lesions

      i. May occur following sudden upward pulling on the shoulder

      ii. Occur following damage to C8 and T1 nerve roots

      iii. Paralysis of small hand muscles and finger flexors

      iv. Associated with preservation of wrist and finger extensors

      v. Result in hyperextension at the metacarpophalangeal (MCP) joints and flexion at the interphalangeal (IP) joints

      vi. May be associated with Horner syndrome

  g. Cervical disc disease

      i. Common cause of shoulder and arm pain

      ii. The radiculopathy usually follow a descending order, C5, C6, C7, and C8, with the symptoms being commonly seen after trauma or sudden hyperextension.

      iii. One common syndrome involves lateral disc protrusions between C5 and C6 and, clinically, is represented by pain at the trapezium ridge, tip of the shoulder, radial forearm, and thumb. Motor and sensory loss occurs in the same distribution.

      iv. Another common syndrome occurs with lateral disc protrusion between the sixth and seventh cervical vertebrae, affecting the seventh cervical root. In this instance, there is pain in the shoulder that radiates down the elbow and dorsal forearm to the index and middle fingers. Associated tenderness occurs over the third and fourth thoracic spinous processes and triceps.

v. Common patient complaints, regardless of the nerve root involved, include a history of chronic sharp pain.
vi. On examination, turning the head to one side and hyperextending the neck produce neck pain and characteristic radicular paresthesias.
vii. Treatment options
(1) Conservative management
(2) Selective nerve root blocks
(3) Facet joint injections
(4) Dorsal rhizotomies
(5) Spinal cord stimulator trials

4. SCIATIC NERVE SYNDROMES

a. The sciatic nerve comprises two distinct nerves, the tibial and common peroneal, arising from L4-5, S1-3, and L4-5, S1-2, respectively. Aside from penetrating trauma, most injuries to these structures occur as a result of fracture dislocations of the hip joint.
b. Piriformis syndrome is caused by spasm of the piriformis muscle. Affected patients have symptoms that are radicular in nature due to muscle irritation of the underlying nerve roots; presents clinically as buttock pain and burning dysesthesias down the back of the leg.
c. Anterior tibial syndrome involves compression of the deep peroneal nerve caused by muscle swelling in the anterior compartment of the leg. These patients have exquisite anterior lower leg pain and motor dysfunction. Often seen following trauma, reperfusion injury, and excessive exercise.
d. Tarsal tunnel syndrome is characterized by diffuse foot pain and paresthesias on the sole of the foot. Physical examination will exhibit both weakness of foot muscles and plantar sensory nerve abnormalities. Compression over the Achilles tendon may elicit pain. Causes include ill-fitting footwear or tendon sheath compression.

SUGGESTED READINGS

Adams JA: The piriformis syndrome-report of four cases and review of the literature. S Afr J Surg 1980;18:13.

Bullard DE: Cervical disc lesions. In Sabiston DC Jr (ed) Textbook of Surgery: The Biological Basis of Modern Surgical Practice, 14th ed. Philadelphia, WB Saunders, 1994, p 1392.

Lloyd K, Agarwal A: Tarsal tunnel syndrome, a presenting feature of rheumatoid arthritis. Br J Med 1990;3:32.

Perry MO: Acute arterial insufficiency. In Rutherford RB (ed) Vascular Surgery, 3rd ed. Philadelphia, WB Saunders, 2004.

24 Soft Tissue Injuries

1. OVERVIEW

a. Soft tissue injuries include those sustained to muscles, tendons, ligaments, bone and joints, as well as the skin and nail beds on all extremities.

b. Many of these injuries are sustained through sporting activities, but others are secondary to traumas.

2. TENDONS

a. Tendonitis and muscle strains account for 30% to 50% of all sports injuries.

b. The forces applied to the tendon itself can be either extrinsic to the tendon itself, causing an impingement syndrome on the tendon, or intrinsic, related to excessive stretch forces on the tendon during activity.

   i. An example of an *extrinsic* tendonitis is shoulder impingement syndrome, where there is inadequate space between the humeral head and the acromion for free passage of the rotator cuff tendons during overhead activity (throwing and swimming), leading to direct tendon trauma.

   ii. *Intrinsic* tendonitis is seen following repetitive type activity or sudden excessive loading as is seen with weight lifting.

3. LIGAMENTS

a. Ligament injuries or sprains commonly occur in the knees and ankles of athletes.

b. The etiology of such injuries is almost always the result of excessive sudden force on the ligament.

c. For example, a sudden valgus stress to the knee following a football tackle, causing disruption of the medial collateral ligament, or the sudden change on a tennis court when the foot is firmly planted, can lead to anterior cruciate ligament injury.

d. Serious ligamentous injury can, if improperly treated, lead to chronic stress to the supporting muscles and tendons.

4. MUSCLES

a. Muscle injuries are probably the most common of all soft tissue injuries and can occur from either acute excessive load or excessive chronic use.

b. When adequately severe, muscle and tendon tears can occur and be associated with hematomas.

c. Those muscles crossing two joints have a higher percentage of type II fibers and are more prone to strain-type injuries.

i. Examples of such muscle groups include the hamstrings, rectus femoris, and gastrocnemius.

d. Delayed onset muscle soreness is more common after eccentric loading; this condition usually appears 24 to 48 hours after an exercise bout and is associated with high serum levels of intramuscular enzymes such as creatine kinase.

e. Other significant causes of muscle injuries include muscular contusions by blunt trauma and exertional rhabdomyolysis, seen with or without trauma, which is potentially fatal. This can occur following compartment syndrome in the affected limb due to excessive muscle swelling and renal failure.

5. BONE AND JOINT

a. Bone injury is most frequently seen in athletes in the form of stress fracture-type injuries.

b. In runners, stress fractures account for nearly 25% of all injuries.

c. The most common joints injured in sports are the shoulder and the knee.

d. The shoulder is the most unstable joint in the body and depends almost exclusively on ligaments and the tendons of the intrinsic muscles to maintain a balance between the extremes of range of motion and stability. As a result, these structures are commonly injured in sports, with both acute and chronic repetitive injuries being seen.

e. The knee is typically injured acutely because of sudden forces that overwhelm the supporting ligaments.

f. Common causes of knee pain include meniscal tears, patellofemoral pain syndrome, ligamentous injuries, and patellar tendonitis.

g. Among juveniles, Osgood-Schlatter syndrome is often seen, i.e., apophysitis of the tibia.

6. ASSESSMENT

The vast majority of soft tissue injuries can be managed conservatively assuming that a thorough and thoughtful history and physical examination is performed.

a. History

i. A thorough history is often the key to diagnosis and treatment options and must address:

(1) Acute vs. chronic type of injury

(2) Exact mechanism of injury, for instance, motor vehicle accident vs. inversion sprains or decelerating injuries

(3) Presence of associated disease states including osteoarthritis, rheumatoid arthritis, peripheral vascular disease (PVD), and a prior history of injuries

(4) Appropriately grading any overuse injuries

b. Examination
   i. Key points not to be missed include:
      (1) Full examination, making sure not to focus too narrowly on the affected area alone.
      (2) For joint problems, joints involved at least one level above and below the area of pain must be assessed.
      (3) Bilateral exam of any injured muscle, tendon, or joint aids toward detecting any imbalances, while remembering that in some sports injuries involving asymmetrical extremity use, such as tennis or baseball, significant differences may exist but can also be problematic.
      (4) For ligamentous sprain injuries, grading is important to help with the clinical decision-making regarding immobilization, rehabilitation, and surgical intervention.
      (5) Peripheral vascular and neurologic examination assesses their integrity and may indicate presence of other undiagnosed comorbidities.
c. Imaging studies
   i. Can usually be delayed until treatment response is assessed
   ii. Plain radiographs for the detection of stress fractures will be negative two-thirds of the time when done initially, with triple-phase bone scanning being the modality of choice, with 100% sensitivity. Infection and arthritic disease will also be deemed positive, and clinical correlation is recommended.
   iii. Magnetic resonance imaging (MRI) has significant advantages over computed tomography scanning because of its excellent sensitivity and superior specificity for bone abnormalities.
   iv. MRI can differentiate between stress fractures and bone tumors or infectious processes.
   v. Diagnostic ultrasound has well-documented sensitivity and specificity in soft tissue injury.

7. TREATMENT OPTIONS

a. Acute injuries
   i. Basic treatment protocols follow the RICE acronym: rest, ice, elevation, and compression.
   ii. Immobilization is required for more severe sprains, grade II and above, i.e., anything involving greater than minimal swelling, discomfort, and functional loss.
   iii. Ice is applied for periods of 15 to 20 minutes at a time while range of motion within the limits of pain is preferred.
   iv. Relative rather than complete rest is preferred to avoid deconditioning.
   v. Heat is applied to the affected area following the initial icing period of 24 to 48 hours because this allows improved circulation and ease of stretching of the affected area.

b. Medications
  i. Nonsteroidal anti-inflammatory drugs (NSAIDs) provide the cornerstone of conservative medical management for acute soft tissue injuries.
  ii. Most NSAIDs inhibit cyclooxygenase (COX-1 and COX-2), nonspecifically limiting the production of PGE1 and PGE2.
  iii. Both NSAIDs and corticosteroids are known to have suppressive effects on the inflammatory response to injury.
  iv. Short-term use of NSAIDs (3 to 5 days) appears to be most successful in control of pain, reduction of swelling, and early mobilization post injury.
  v. Most evidence suggests that corticosteroids inhibit tendon and ligament healing following injury.
c. Injections
  i. Appropriate injection into tendon sheaths, bursa, muscle trigger points, and other soft tissue structures has both diagnostic and therapeutic benefit.
  ii. Conservative approaches allow for only two tendon sheath injections and three joint injections annually.
  iii. Bursa can be injected safely up to 3 times in a 6-month period.
  iv. Local anesthetic solution may be injected alone first to determine a therapeutic benefit prior to injection of steroid.
  v. Known risk factors of corticosteroid injection include transient hyperglycemia in diabetics, allergic reactions, systemic infection, and suppression of the pituitary-adrenal axis, as well as avascular necrosis of the hip.
  vi. Conservative injection frequency as well as proper sterile and hemostatic technique can prevent complications.

SUGGESTED READINGS

Arrington ED, Miller MD: Skeletal muscle injuries. Sports Med 1995;26:411.

El-Khoury GY, Brandser EA, Kathol MH, et al: Imaging of muscle injuries. Skeletal Radiol 1996;25(1):3.

Fredericson M: Common injuries in runners: Diagnosis, rehabilitation and prevention. Sports Med 1995;26(3):547.

Garrett WE: Muscle strain injuries. Am J Sports Med 1996;24:S2.

25 Whiplash

1. GENERAL

a. The clinical spectrum of whiplash-associated syndromes includes neck pain and stiffness, arm pain and paresthesias, temporomandibular joint (TMJ) dysfunction, headache, dizziness, visual disturbances, and memory and concentration problems, as well as multiple psychological stressors.

b. The scope of the syndrome extends beyond the actual physical manifestations, seen clinically to include significant public health problems, morbidity, and a significant cause of chronic disability.

c. Pathophysiology

  i. Forces acting on the head and neck during a motor vehicle accident (MVA)

    (1) Rear-end collisions result in forward acceleration of the trunk and shoulders caused by the impact. This leads to forced extensions of the lower cervical spine as the head is moved posterior in relation to T1. These types of injury have received the most attention.

    (2) The spine assumes an S-curve with the upper spinal levels in flexion and the lower spinal levels in extension.

    (3) The sternocleidomastoid lengthens and becomes active electrophysiologically prior to activation of the paraspinal musculature.

    (4) Following extension, the head is also accelerated forward, forcing the entire neck into an abnormal flexed position.

  ii. Zygapophyseal joints

    (1) The facet joints are richly innervated and are a source of much referred pain and, given the mechanism of whiplash, these joints are at risk for overload and injury.

    (2) In a recent randomized, controlled, double-blinded study using blocks of the medial branch of the cervical dorsal rami, 60% of patients had complete relief of neck pain after the injections with local anesthetic compared with no relief after the injection of normal saline, thus identifying these injections as a significant therapeutic intervention.

    (3) Among patients with neck pain and headache in which headache was the dominant symptom, the prevalence of C2-C3 facet joint pain was 50%.

    (4) Referred pain from the facet joints is also considered a source of headache, with the symptoms being exacerbated by referred pain from the third occipital nerve, which supplies the C2-C3 facet joint and the back of the head.

  iii. Ligaments

    (1) Magnetic resonance imaging (MRI) scans show significant ligamentous injury, but this is not as well appreciated in groups with mild whiplash-associated disorders.

(2) Whiplash-related ligamentous injuries are focused at the ligaments between the skull and C1, thus explaining the symptom of decreased extension of the head seen in many patients with whiplash injuries who lack visible injury to the structure.

iv. Disk injury and nerve roots

(1) No evidence exists regarding the role of de novo disc injury or radicular symptoms in whiplash disorders, given the prevalence of disc disease in the asymptomatic population.

v. Muscle injuries

(1) Patients who have received MRI scans between 2 days and 3 weeks after injury have generally not shown signs of muscle damage. Numerous studies suggest that the amount of muscular injury to the neck muscles is proportional to the forces sustained in the accident. It has been hypothesized that the increased muscle pain represents central hyperexcitability.

d. Diagnosis

i. The diagnosis of whiplash is made based on a review of the patient's symptoms and after consideration of the mechanism of the injury. The clinical symptoms associated with whiplash disorder are noted above. Imaging studies are generally helpful only in excluding fractures as well as severe ligamentous and disc injury, but the results are normal, in general, and not helpful unless severe injury has been sustained.

ii. There are no specific blood tests, neuropsychological, or electrophysiologic studies that can diagnose whiplash.

e. Treatment

i. Treatment options can be considered on an acute (less than 2 weeks), subacute (2 weeks to 6 months), and chronic (greater than 6 months) stage of injury.

ii. Acute treatment

(1) Oral analgesics, soft collars, prescribed rest, and anti-inflammatory medications form the mainstay of most acute injuries, most of which present to the primary care practitioner.

(2) Studies have shown that wearing a soft collar neither shortens nor prolongs the duration of neck pain when used acutely after whiplash injury. High-dose methylprednisolone compared with placebo has been shown not to be advantageous clinically for patients with grade 2 or 3 whiplash-associated syndrome within 8 hours of an MVA.

iii. Subacute treatment

(1) Active, as opposed to passive, treatment may result in improved outcome in the subacute period. Patients who were enrolled in a multimodal program consisting of passive ultrasound, transcutaneous electrical nerve stimulation

(TENS), counseling to reduce anxiety, active exercises, and manual massage returned to work earlier and had both less severe pain and improved perception of function compared with passive ultrasound and TENS alone.

    (2) Acupuncture has been studied only as a tool for treatment of balance disorders after whiplash, in a study involving small numbers of patients, but has long been used clinically with success for treatment of acute and chronic pain.

f. Chronic pain states

    i. Percutaneous radiofrequency neurotomy: There is now good evidence that neurotomy of the facet innervation can relieve pain in the patient with chronic pain associated with whiplash injuries.

    ii. Intra-articular steroids/local anesthetics: Betamethasone has not been shown to be more successful than 0.5% bupivacaine in terms of time to return to preinjection level of pain following injection.

    iii. Exercise: Many studies support active rather than passive treatments following chronic whiplash injuries.

    iv. Botulinum toxin: Randomized controlled studies have shown improvement in Visual Analog Scale (VAS) pain scores for headaches following the injection of 100 units of Botulinum Toxin A into trigger points compared with a saline control. Increased range of motion was also noted in the Botox group.

g. Prognosis

    i. Marked variability in prognosis for recovery in patients with whiplash injuries has been noted, with some studies showing that the majority of patients have long-term disability, whereas others report an undetectable rate of chronic symptoms.

    ii. Societal expectations reflect the different outcomes seen when comparing studies from different countries.

    iii. Individual prognostic factors have been identified in a number of areas, such as collision-related factors, early signs and symptoms, as well as sociodemographic and psychological factors, whereas the findings on diagnostic imaging appear to have no prognostic values in whiplash injuries of grades 1 to 3.

h. Conclusions

    i. Active approaches to management by using exercise seem to result in better outcomes.

    ii. The facet joint appears to be the source of neck pain in many patients with chronic whiplash disorder.

    iii. Percutaneous radiofrequency neurotomy of selected facet joints can reduce pain for many months in properly selected patients.

    iv. Multimodal rehabilitation programs result in improved outcomes in patients with chronic whiplash injuries.

SUGGESTED READINGS

Holcomb JB, McMullins NR, Kozar RA, et al: Morbidity from rib fractures increases after age 45. J Am Coll Surg 2003;196:549–555.

Lee RB, Bass SM, Morris JA: Three or more rib fractures as an indicator for transfer to a Level I trauma center: A population-based study. J Trauma 1999;30:689–694.

Wu CL, Jani ND, Perkins FM, et al: Thoracic epidural analgesia versus intravenous PCA for the treatment of rib fracture pain after motor vehicle crash. J Trauma 1999;47:564–567.

Ziegler DW, Agarwal NN: The morbidity and mortality of rib fractures. J Trauma 1999;37:975–979.

Principles for Pharmacologic Management of Perioperative Pain

1. GENERAL

a. Anesthesiologists who manage perioperative pain should consider all therapeutic options, such as epidural or intrathecal opioids, systemic therapy (e.g., IV opioid patient-controlled analgesia [PCA], intermittent IV opioids, nonsteroidal anti-inflammatory drugs [NSAIDs]), and regional analgesia techniques, after thorough evaluation of the patient's health, type of surgical procedure, anticipated length of hospitalization and recovery, and risks and benefits of pain treatment options.

b. Principles for postoperative pain control include:
   i. Whenever possible, anesthesiologists should employ multimodal pain management therapy.
   ii. Multimodal therapy involves at least two analgesic agents that act by different mechanisms via a single route for providing superior analgesic efficacy with equivalent or reduced adverse effects.
   iii. Unless contraindicated, all patients should receive an around-the-clock regimen of NSAIDs, cyclooxygenase 2 (COX2) inhibitors or acetaminophen.
   iv. In addition, regional blockade with local anesthetics should be considered.
   v. Dosing regimens should be administered to optimize effectiveness.

c. Patients who are at special risk for inadequate pain control and who require additional analgesic considerations include:
   i. Pediatric patients
   ii. Elderly or geriatric patients
   iii. Critically ill or hemodynamically unstable patients
   iv. Patients with cognitive impairments or patients having difficulty communicating
   v. Health care disparities that may exist based on gender, race, ethnicity, culture, and socioeconomic status influence access to treatment as well as pain assessment by health care providers.

d. IV PCA
   i. Acceptable opioids include morphine, hydromorphone, or fentanyl.
   ii. Indicated for patients who can understand the underlying principles of therapy and can self-administer demand doses.
   iii. For opioid-naïve patients:
      (1) PCA demand dosing only: No basal or background infusion should be prescribed until after 24 hours of therapy and opioid requirements can be determined.

(2) Lockout interval 8 to 15 minutes. Ten minutes is the accepted standard; shorter lockout intervals are recommended for fentanyl.

(3) Initiate therapy with the demand dose at the usual starting dose:

    (a) Morphine: 1 mg

    (b) Hydromorphone: 0.15 to 0.2 mg

    (c) Fentanyl: 10 to 15 µg

(4) A basal rate along with the demand dose

    (a) For severe pain unrelieved by demand dosing

    (b) Once the 24-hour requirement has been established and pain is likely to last longer than 3 days

    (c) Use caution with basal rates in the elderly.

(5) Supplemental intermittent IV nurse-administered doses can be prescribed for times of increased pain (e.g., activity, procedures) or to prevent gaps in analgesia (after awakening from sleep).

(6) IV nurse-administered dose is ½ to 1 hour of the PCA dose given as needed (PRN) every 2 hours

iv. For opioid-dependent patients:

(1) Basal infusions may be necessary.

(2) Important to prevent life-threatening physiologic withdrawal if physical dependence has developed.

(3) Always adjust for the preoperative chronic opioid use (i.e., longer than 1 to 2 weeks).

(4) Average daily opioid requirements should be calculated and converted to a 24-hour dose of an IV opioid, then divided by 24, and this can be the minimum hourly basal rate infusion.

(5) Along with basal infusion, PCA demand dose should be initiated.

    (a) Half of the basal rate can be available in demand dosing with a lockout interval of every 10 to 15 minutes, or;

    (b) Two percent to 5% of the total 24-hour dose (converted to IV) with a lockout interval of every 15 to 20 minutes

e. Intermittent IV nurse- or staff-administered analgesia

  i. For opioid-naïve patients, initiate therapy with usual starting doses for IV opioids every 1 to 3 hours.

  ii. For opioid-dependent patients with chronic pain:

(1) Start intermittent doses at 20% to 25% of the total 24-hour requirement given every 2 or 3 hours.

(2) Order medication "Around the clock (ATC) – patient may refuse" rather than "PRN."

(3) Additional doses should be available for unrelieved pain and to determine the optimal dose and dosing interval.

f. Acute unrelieved pain: always an emergency
  i. Evaluate the patient for new problems or sources of pain, but at the same time treat the pain.
  ii. Titrate IV opioids quickly considering the pharmacology, onset of action, peak effect, and duration.
  iii. ALWAYS adjust dose if previous doses provide inadequate relief.
  iv. Monitor patient frequently at least every 4 hours, and more frequently, if necessary, including respiratory rate, heart rate, blood pressure, and O_2 saturation.
  v. Remember about differences in potency of opioids.
    (1) Avoid administering naloxone (Narcan), unless absolutely necessary.
      (a) If needed, dilute 1 mL with 9 mL of normal saline and administer very slowly.
g. General principles for pharmacologic management of chronic pain
  i. Prevent the worsening or recurrence of pain
  ii. Administration should be "by the clock" and "ATC."
  iii. Assess patients for "breakthrough pain" and prescribe a PRN regimen for control of episodic pain.
  iv. Consider both nonopioids, opioids, and adjuvant agents.
  v. Manage any adverse effects of analgesic therapy.

27 **Preemptive Analgesia**

1. GENERAL

a. An antinociceptive treatment that prevents the establishment of altered central processing of afferent input, thereby leading to a reduced postoperative pain state.

b. At present, the clinical relevance of such treatment is controversial. Only in animal studies is the evidence convincing.

c. Through a large number of investigations, it has become more evident that multiple variables influence postoperative pain as well as the limitations in outcomes studies.

d. A series of animal studies has shown that nociception produces an altered central processing of afferent input, resulting in neural plasticity and sensitization. This leads to an abnormal amplification of future incoming impulses.

e. Pain intensity measured by the patient may be the most reliable estimate of treatment efficacy.

f. Total analgesic consumption is perhaps the most adequate outcome measure for showing a true preemptive effect.

2. PREVENTION OF CENTRAL SENSITIZATION

a. Analgesic interventions

   i. N-Methyl-D-aspartate (NMDA) antagonists (ketamine) have not consistently been shown to reduce postoperative pain scores or analgesic requirements.

   ii. Opioids

     (1) Spinally and systemically administered opioids have given inconsistent results in preemptive trials. Tolerance to opioids can develop rapidly.

   iii. Nonsteroidal anti-inflammatory drugs (NSAIDs)

     (1) Improved analgesic consumption and time to first rescue analgesia but not postoperative pain scores.

   iv. Local anesthetics

     (1) Preoperative epidural analgesic treatment may be more effective in managing acute postoperative pain, attenuating pain scores, decreasing total supplemental analgesic consumption, and prolonging the time to first-rescue analgesia.

     (2) Preoperative local wound infiltration: The timing of a single analgesic intervention (pre- vs. postincisional), defined as preemptive analgesia, does not have a clinically significant effect on postoperative pain intensity.

3. PREEMPTIVE ANALGESIA DILEMMA

a. The differences in the efficacy of various analgesic interventions for a preemptive effect may be due to the degree of afferent blockade, the nature of the pain, and its inflammatory component.

b. Preemptive analgesia cannot be effective if the analgesic intervention is not dense enough and of sufficient duration to block afferent noxious stimuli from the peripheries to the spinal cord and brain.

c. Opioid consumption as a measure of outcome has multiple confounding factors.
   i. Anxiety, depression, perception of the surgical outcome, and overall care may contribute to opioid use.

d. Inhaled anesthetics are known to suppress spinal cord sensitization; the degree of suppression varies depending on the agent used. Thus, they may have a preemptive effect.

e. Once adequate afferent blockade to the spinal cord is lost, postsurgical inflammatory response may establish central sensitization.

f. The immediate postoperative period, as yet an undefined length of time, must be covered.

SUGGESTED READINGS

Australian and New Zealand College of Anaesthetists, Faculty of Pain Medicine: Acute Pain Management: Scientific Evidence, 2nd ed. Melbourne, Australian and New Zealand College of Anaesthetists, 2005:50–51.

Benson HT, Raja SN, Molly RE, et al: Essentials of Pain Medicine and Regional Anesthesia, 2nd ed. Philadelphia, Elsevier, 2005.

Ong Cliff K-S, Lirk P, Seymour PA, et al: The efficacy of preemptive analgesia for acute postoperative pain management: A meta-analysis. Anesth Analg 2005;100:757–773.

1. GENERAL

a. Allows the patient to titrate their analgesic medications against sedation and other side effects of the administered drug.
b. Types of patient-controlled analgesia (PCA)
   i. Intravenous, intramuscular, subcutaneous, epidural, oral, sublingual, inhaled, intranasal, transcutaneous, transmucosal
c. This section focuses on intravenous PCA, the most frequently used postoperative modality.

2. INTRAVENOUS PATIENT-CONTROLLED ANALGESIA

a. Eliminates the variable absorption of the opioid from the injection site and bypasses unavoidable delays when an opioid is requested.
b. Adjustable PCA parameters
   i. Programmable infusion device
      (1) Bolus dose: amount of analgesic drug the patient receives after a successful demand
      (2) Lockout interval: the time during which the machine will not administer another dose despite further demands by the patient
      (3) Background infusion: continuous drug delivery that requires no action by the patient
      (4) Dose limit: total amount of drug the machine will deliver within a given time (commonly, 4 hours)
c. Indications
   i. Adults and some children where there is the likelihood of the need for parental opioid analgesia for 24 hours or more
      (1) Following surgery, trauma, acute pain from some medical conditions
d. Contraindications
   i. Patient rejection
   ii. Patient unable to safely comprehend the technique
   iii. Extremes of age (children older than 7 years do well)
   iv. Lack of appropriately trained nursing staff
e. Standard orders
   i. A statement eliminating the concurrent use of other opioids or sedatives
   ii. Oxygen orders
   iii. Whom to contact for problems
   iv. The variables (bolus-demand-background infusion) to be programmed into the machine
   v. Monitoring and documentation
   vi. Orders for adverse events

f. Monitoring requirements
   i. Pain scores at rest and movement: ideally ≤3
   ii. Sedation scores: most important, precedes respiratory depression
   iii. Respiratory rate: rate ≤8 demands intervention
   iv. Total amount of opioid used in 24 hours: essential when converting to oral opioids
   v. Side effects:
      (1) Respiratory depression, prurities urinary retention, sedation, nausea or vomiting
      (2) If treatment needed and was it successful
   vi. Changes made in the PCA program
g. Intravenous PCA: helpful hints
   i. Managed by a dedicated service: acute pain service (APS)
   ii. Staff education: nurses, interns, residents, attendings
   iii. Institutional policies, a standardized preprinted PCA order form that provides guidelines to ensure consistency in the use of PCA
   iv. Patient and family education
h. Stopping PCA and subsequent analgesia
   i. Depending on the type of surgery or severity of trauma, the opioid requirement, continuous severe pain, and the ability of the patient to ingest liquids.
   ii. Usually when normal gastrointestinal function is restored and opioid need is about 50 mg parental morphine equivalents for previous 24 hours.
   iii. The first oral dose is given while the patient still has access to the PCA pump. If, at the peak of the oral medication effect, the patient is comfortable, the pump may be removed.
   iv. Those patients with severe pain or higher documented opioid requirement are started on a long-acting or sustained-release oral opioid.
   v. If they cannot take enteral medications, they are started on a Duragesic patch.
   vi. Once the long-acting agent is begun, the patient will still have access to the demand feature of the PCA pump only for another 24 hours.
   vii. Finally, the 24-hour requirement: long-acting opioid + PCA demand dosages, successfully given. This total is then converted to an equianalgesic oral dose; the ¾ of 24 requirement is met by long-acting opioid, the remainder by a short-acting or immediate-release opioid.

SUGGESTED READING

Benson HT, Raja SN, Molly RE, et al: Essentials of Pain Medicine and Regional Anesthesia, 2nd ed. Philadelphia, Elsevier, 2005.
Rowbotham DJ, MacIntyre PE: Acute Pain. London, Arnold Publishers, 2003.
Wallace MS, Staats PS: Pain Medicine and Management. New York, McGraw-Hill, 2005.

29 Patient-Controlled Analgesia: Epidural

1. EPIDURAL ANALGESIA

a. Pharmacologic agents are given into the epidural space via an indwelling catheter for the management of acute pain in adults or children, in particular; after surgery and trauma; and in obstetrics.

2. PHARMACOLOGY OF EPIDURAL OPIOIDS

a. Produce effect by either a supraspinal, systemic, or spinal mechanism
   i. Supraspinal: absorbed into the plasma and are redistributed to the brainstem via the bloodstream
   ii. Spinal: diffuse into the cerebrospinal fluid (CSF), penetrate the meninges, and interact with opioid receptors located in lamina II of the spinal cord dorsal horn
   iii. Lipophilic agents (fentanyl, sufentanil): may produce effect primarily by systemic uptake and redistribution to the brainstem opioid receptors
   iv. Hydrophilic opioids (morphine): selective spinal site for analgesic effect

3. EFFICACY

a. Epidural analgesia, opioid plus local anesthetic, provides better pain relief than parenteral opioid administration in all clinical settings.

4. DRUGS USED FOR EPIDURAL ANALGESIA

a. Opioids: alone have no advantage over parenteral opioids.
b. Local anesthetics (opioid combinations): provide pain relief consistently superior to either of the drugs alone.
c. Adjuvant drugs: Addition of epinephrine has resulted in improved analgesia and decreased systemic opioid levels.

5. LEVEL OF ADMINISTRATION

a. Thoracic: pain after thoracic and abdominal surgery
   i. Improved bowel recovery with thoracic but not lumbar administration.
   ii. Reduction in the incidence of postoperative myocardial infarction when used for more than 24 hours.
   iii. Rib fractures: reduced risk of nosocomial pneumonia and number of ventilation days

    iv. High thoracic epidural analgesia: reduced postoperative pain and risk of dysrhythmias, pulmonary complications, and time to extubation when used for coronary artery bypass graft surgery

  b. Lumbar

    i. Provides analgesia after orthopedic and vascular operations to the lower limbs and the pelvis

    ii. Hip and knee replacement: provides better analgesia than parental opioids

    iii. Vascular surgery: reduces the incidence of graft occlusion

6. SIDE EFFECTS OF EPIDURAL OPIOIDS

  a. Respiratory depression: same as parental opioids, 0.1% to 0.9%. Increased risk is seen in thoracic surgery, increasing age, opioid-naïve patients, and concomitant use of systemic opioids and sedatives.

  b. Nausea and vomiting: dose-dependent, continuous infusion 45% to 80%; single dose, 20% to 50%.

  c. Pruritus

    i. Not associated with peripheral histamine release; may or may not be dose-dependent

    ii. Occurrence: as many as 60% of patients compared with 15% to 18% with systemic opioid

  d. Urinary retention

    i. Appears to be as high as 70% to 80% compared with 18% for systemic opioids

    ii. Does not appear to be dose-dependent

7. ADVERSE EFFECTS

  a. Neurologic injury

    i. Transient neuropathy: 0.013% to 0.023%

    ii. Severe neurologic injury, possibly 0.0003%

  b. Epidural hematoma: in the order of 0.00001% (1 in 100,000)

  c. Epidural abscess

    i. In one large series, where the majority of the patients were immunocompromised: 0.015% to 0.05%

    ii. Long duration of epidural catheterization (mean, 11 days)

      (1) Classic triad—fever, back pain, neurologic deficit: 13%

      (2) Back pain: 71%

      (3) Febrile: 66%

  d. Hypotension

    i. Depends on the dose of local anesthetic: 5.6% (3.0% to 10.2%)

    ii. It is often the result of hypovolemia.

e. Postdural puncture headache
   i. Incidence of 0.4% to 24%
   ii. Postural in mature; more common in patients younger than 50 years
f. Treatment failure
   i. Patients had premature termination of postoperative epidural infusions (22%), dislodgement (10%), inadequate analgesia (3.5%), sensory or motor deficit (2.2%).
   ii. Most failures occurred on or after postoperative day 2.

SUGGESTED READINGS

Australian and New Zealand College of Anaesthetists, Faculty of Pain Medicine: Acute Pain Management: Scientific Evidence, 2nd ed. Melbourne, Australian and New Zealand College of Anaesthetists, 2005.

Benson HT, Raja SN, Molly RE, et al: Essentials of Pain Medicine and Regional Anesthesia, 2nd ed. Philadelphia, Elsevier, 2005.

Continuous Peripheral Nerve Blocks for Postoperative Analgesia

1. GENERAL

a. Also called "perineural local anesthetic infusions"

b. Percutaneous insertion of a catheter directly adjacent to the peripheral nerve innervating a surgical site

c. The infusion of local anesthetic provides site-specific pain relief.

d. Advantages
   i. Improved postoperative analgesia
   ii. Increased patient satisfaction
   iii. Decreases the need for supplemental opioid requirements
   iv. Eliminates concerns over interactions of anticoagulants and central neuraxial techniques
   v. Useful for outpatient pain control

e. Interscalene brachial plexus block
   i. One of the most commonly performed regional techniques
   ii. The gold standard in shoulder analgesia
   iii. Fifty percent reduction in verbal analog scales
   iv. Delayed time to first opioid use and reduced total amount of opioid needed
   v. Other beneficial effects
      (1) Reduced incidence of postoperative nausea and vomiting
      (2) Improved postprocedure mood
      (3) Faster discharge of ambulatory patient; reduced in-patient length of stay

f. Lumbar plexus
   i. Femoral nerve sheath approach
      (1) Used for continuous femoral analgesia after total knee replacement
         (a) Comparable or better analgesia with fewer side effects than either in patient-controlled analgesia (PCA) or epidural analgesia for 48 hours or longer after surgery.
         (b) Faster short-term recovery of knee flexion than IV PCA
         (c) Twenty percent reduction in physical rehabilitation and hospital stay
      (2) Use after total hip replacement
         (a) Significant morphine-sparing effects
         (b) Less nausea, vomiting, pruritus, and sedation than IV PCA
         (c) Decreased urinary retention and hypotension versus epidural analgesia

        (3) Complications
           (a) Catheter colonization (57%)
              (i) 208 patients monitored
              (ii) Three presented with fever and bacteremia, no antibiotic given
              (iii) One case of persistent femoral nerve dysesthesia that lasted 1 year
           (b) No vascular complications
      ii Fascia iliaca approach
        (1) No obvious superiority for fascia iliaca approach compared with the femoral nerve approach
      iii. Psoas compartment approach
        (1) More consistent block of obturator nerve than either the femoral or fascia iliaca approach
        (2) Paucity of clinical trials comparing its efficacy compared with the femoral approach
        (3) Approach has variable success, depending on catheter placement
        (4) Concept of a true psoas compartment has been questioned
        (5) Lumbar nerves often lie within the psoas muscle at the L 4-5 vertebrae level
      iv. Sciatic nerve
        (1) Continuous popliteal sciatic nerve block
           (a) Sixty patients (foot surgery) compared with IV PCA
              (i) Superior analgesia
              (ii) Less frequent side effects
              (iii) No immediate or long-term side effects
              (iv) Twenty-five percent incidence of either broken or kinked catheters: mobile joint
        (2) Lateral approach to the popliteal block
           (a) Advantages: supine patient, more secure catheter placement
           (b) No clinical trials to show that this approach is optimal for continuous sciatic analgesia
        (3) Parasacral approach, posterior approach of Labat, posterior subgluteal approach
           (a) Surgery on the lower leg and foot
           (b) Clinical trials needed to compare the efficacy and superiority of these approaches to continuous sciatic perineural analgesia
  g. Drugs for continuous perineural analgesia
    i. Local anesthetics
      (1) No optimal analgesic solution
      (2) Bupivacaine (0.1% to 0.25%): safe for postoperative analgesia for 24 to 72 hours in current regimens

            (3) Ropivacaine (0.2%) less motor block and equivalent anal-
                gesia compared with bupivacaine decreased cardiotoxicity
                potential from a large initial loading dose.
        ii. Adjuvants
            (1) Reduce the total dose of the local anesthetic, thus decreas-
                ing the degree of motor and sensory blockade. Adjuvant
                agents may also improve the quality of analgesia.
            (2) Examples of adjuvant agents are epinephrine, clonidine,
                and the opioids.
    h. Delivery of continuous peripheral nerve blocks
        i. Background infusion and PCA boluses
            (1) Decreased consumption (~30%) compared with other in-
                fusion techniques
        ii. Boluses, continuous infusion, or PCA
            (1) Probably less advantageous than background infusion and
                PCA boluses
    i. Contraindications
        i. Infection at the block site
        ii. Allergy to medications
        iii. Safe in anticoagulated patient

SUGGESTED READINGS

Evans H: Peripheral nerve blocks and continuous catheter techniques. Anesthesiol
    Clin North Am 2005;23:141–162.
Liu SS, Salinas FV: Continuous plexus and peripheral nerve blocks for postopera-
    tive analgesia. Anesth Anal 2003;96:263–272.

1. PREVALENCE OF PAIN IN THE INTENSIVE CARE UNIT

a. Very high prevalence
   i. Within 5 days of discharge from intensive care unit (ICU), as many as 63% of surgical patients rated their ICU pain as moderate to severe; 42% of cardiothoracic patients rated pain from chest tubes or incision as "worst memory" of hospital stay.
   ii. Study to Understand Prognoses and Preferences for Outcomes and Risks of Treatment (SUPPORT) reported "pain" in 50% of seriously ill patients.

2. HOW PATIENTS IN THE ICU DIFFER FROM OTHER PATIENT POPULATIONS

a. Plethora of painful stimuli
b. Frequently intubated
   i. Inability to communicate
      (1) Assumption of "pain-free"
   ii. Frequent suction
   iii. Anxiety (in addition to pain)
c. Sleep deprivation
d. Changes in physiologic variables (e.g., heart rate, blood pressure, respiratory rate) notoriously inaccurate
e. Frequent drug interactions

3. ASSESSMENT/QUANTIFICATION OF PAIN AND ANXIETY

a. Must differentiate pain vs. anxiety
   i. Pain frequently causes and/or augments anxiety.
   ii. Is patient "bucking the vent" agitated or in pain?
      (1) Must assess at bedside!
   iii. Differentiating pain and anxiety can only occur in a conscious patient.
b. Assessment of consciousness in patient in ICU
   i. Multiple algorithms/scales published
   ii. Most popular are Ramsay criteria and Richmond Agitation-Sedation Scale (RASS)
      (1) Most literature uses Ramsay criteria
      (2) RASS is newer

        (a) Takes into account "consciousness"
           (i) Arousal
           (ii) Content of thought
     (3) Studies of reliability show excellent inter-rater correlation with RASS.
  iii. Quantification of pain
     (1) Poor subjective measurements
        (a) 35% to 55% of nurses underrate patient's pain.
        (b) Family members assess presence (or absence) of pain in nonintubated patients only 53% of the time.
     (2) Several linear scales
        (a) Adjective Rating Scale (ARS)
        (b) Numerical Rating Scale (NRS)
        (c) Visual Analog Scale (VAS)
     (3) Sedation-agitation scales (such as Ramsay and RASS) used in mechanically ventilated patients have been shown not to be useful in guiding analgesia.
     (4) Behavioral Pain Scale (BPS)
        (a) Based on behavioral indicators
           (i) Movements
           (ii) Facial expressions
           (iii) Posturing
        (b) Influenced by sedation/analgesia regimens

4. RATIONAL APPROACH TO MANAGING PAIN AND SEDATION IN THE ICU

a. Intercostal nerve blocks
  i. Good for patients with unilateral or abdominal wall somatic pain
  ii. Superior analgesia when compared with systemic opioids
  iii. Requires local anesthetic plus epinephrine
     (1) Brief duration of action necessitates repeated injections
        (a) Increased risk of pneumothorax and intravascular injections
b. PRN opioids
  i. Numerous studies showing ineffectiveness and dissatisfaction
  ii. Inadequate dosing at infrequent intervals
     (1) Drug levels must decrease in order for patient to become uncomfortable.
     (2) Nurses frequently are delayed with other patients.
  iii. Central nervous system depression
  iv. Respiratory depression
c. Patient-controlled analgesia (PCA)
  i. Demand dose + basal dose
     (1) Gives patient satisfactory level of pain relief in addition to autonomy with self-regulation

(2) "Demand" permits titration to a minimum effective analgesic concentration

(3) "Basal" prevents decreased plasma concentrations during sleep

    (a) Has also been shown to increase opioid use without improving Visual Analog Pain Scales (VAPS)

    (b) Increases risk of respiratory depression (usually not a problem if patient on positive pressure ventilation)

ii. Earlier ambulation (when compared with PRN opioids), shorter ICU stay and hospital length of stay

d. Patient-controlled epidural analgesia (PCEA)

  i. Extreme satisfaction for patient

  ii. Selective suppression of activity in substantia gelatinosa

  iii. Controversial whether or not affects perioperative morbidity and mortality

  iv. Less respiratory depression than PCA

  v. Faster weaning of mechanical ventilation

  vi. Patient better able to participate in his/her recovery (moving around, larger tidal volumes, increased bowel function, etc.)

  vii. May cause hypotension (but can easily be reversed by α agonists)

    (1) Pain control more important than hypotension (which can be treated)

5. FUTURE AREAS OF ICU PAIN MANAGEMENT

a. Need better appreciation regarding mechanism of action of analgesics and anxiolytics

b. Specific ICU rotations for pain fellows

c. Continued research into mechanisms of pain

  i. New medications: Dexmedetomidine

    (1) Highly selective α_2-adrenoceptor agonist

    (2) Potent analgesic

    (3) Causes sedation akin to "natural" sleep

    (4) Little to no ventilatory depression

d. Research into potentiation of existing drugs

  i. Ketamine + morphine

SUGGESTED READINGS

Desbiens NA, Mueller-Rizner N: How well do surrogates assess the pain of seriously ill patients? Crit Care Med 2000;28:1347–1352.

Desbiens NA, Wu AW, Broste SK: Pain and satisfaction with pain control in seriously ill hospitalized adults: Findings from the SUPPORT research investigations. For the SUPPORT investigators. Study to Understand Prognoses and Preferences for Outcomes and Risks of Treatment. Crit Care Med 1996;24:1953–1961.

Ely EW, Truman B, Shintani A, et al: Monitoring sedation status over time in ICU patients: Reliability and validity of the Richmond Agitation-Sedation Scale (RASS). JAMA 2003;289:2983–2991.

Guillou N, Tanguy M, Seguin P, et al: The effects of small-dose ketamine on morphine consumption in surgical intensive care unit patients after major abdominal surgery. Anesth Analg 2003;97:843–847.

Hamill-Ruth RJ, Marohn ML: Evaluation of pain in the critically ill patient. Crit Care Clin 1999;15:35–54.

Hogarth DK, Hall J: Management of sedation in mechanically ventilated patients. Curr Opin Crit Care 2004;10:40–46.

Hsu YW, Cortinez LI, Robertson KM, et al: Dexmedetomidine pharmacodynamics: part I: Crossover comparison of the respiratory effects of dexmedetomidine and remifentanil in healthy volunteers. Anesthesiology 2004;101:1066–1076.

Loper KA, Butler S, Nessly M, et al: Paralyzed with pain: The need for education. Pain 1989;37:315–316.

Paiement B, Boulanger M, Jones CW, et al: Intubation and other experiences in cardiac surgery: The consumer's views. Can Anaesth Soc J 1979;26:173–180.

Payen JF, Bru O, Bosson JL, et al: Assessing pain in critically ill sedated patients by using a behavioral pain scale. Crit Care Med 2001;29:2258–2263.

Peyton PJ, Myles PS, Silbert BS, et al: Perioperative epidural analgesia and outcome after major abdominal surgery in high-risk patients. Anesth Analg 2003;96:548–554.

Puntillo KA: Pain experiences of intensive care unit patients. Heart Lung 1990;19:526–533.

Rodgers A, Walker N, Schug S, et al: Reduction of postoperative mortality and morbidity with epidural or spinal anaesthesia: Results from overview of randomised trials. BMJ 2000;321:1493.

Venn RM, Hell J, Grounds RM: Respiratory effects of dexmedetomidine in the surgical patient requiring intensive care. Crit Care 2000;4:302–309.

Part III

Chronic Pain

Section I

OVERVIEW AND CLINICAL ASSESSMENT

32 Neurophysiology of Pain

1. THE KEY PLAYERS

a. Main pain pathways
   i. Three neuron pathways via spinothalamic tract
   ii. Dorsal root ganglion → contralateral thalamus → post-central gyrus of parietal cortex (somatosensory areas I and II)
   iii. Second-order neurons are either nociceptive specific or wide dynamic range (WDR)
   iv. Spinal cord gray matter is 10 lamina
   v. Substantia gelatinosa (lamina II) believed to have a major role in processing and modulating nociceptive input and to be a major site of opioid action
b. Alternate pathways
   i. May mediate arousal and autonomic responses (spinoreticular tract)
   ii. Pathways integrated with skeletal motor and sympathetic systems
   iii. Dorsal column pathways carry light touch/proprioception response to pain
   iv. Spinomesencephalic, spinohypothalamic, spinotelencephalic tracts may be responsible for emotional behavior

2. PHYSIOLOGY OF NOCICEPTION

a. Nociceptors
   i. A delta fibers (first pain): fast, sharp, well-localized, myelinated, small, short latency (0.1 sec)
   ii. C fibers (second pain): duller, slower, poorly localized, unmyelinated
   iii. Most peripheral nociceptors are free nerve endings that sense heat, mechanical, and chemical tissue damage.
   iv. Cutaneous and deep nociceptors
   v. Deep nociceptors are less sensitive and characterized by dull and poor localization.
   vi. Visceral nociceptors are insensitive tissues that respond to smooth muscle spasm, ischemia, and inflammation.

b. Chemical mediators
  i. Neurotransmitters → neuropeptides + amino acids
  ii. Most important are substance P and calcitonin gene-related peptide (CGRP)
  iii. Glutamate: most important excitatory amino acid
c. Modulation of pain
  i. Occurs peripherally at the nociceptor, spinal cord, and supraspinal structure
  ii. Peripheral
    (1) Primary hyperalgesia results in decrease in threshold, increase in frequency, and spontaneous firing even after cessation around site of injury.
    (2) Mediated by histamine, cox pathway, bradykinin
    (3) Secondary hyperalgesia—neurogenic inflammation, long-term response
  iii. Central
    (1) Excitatory
      (a) Three mechanisms
      (b) Windup and sensitization by WDR neurons by increasing their firing rate exponentially and prolonged discharge
      (c) Receptor field expansion
      (d) Hyperexcitability of flexion reflexes
      (e) Neurochemicals include substance P, CGRP, and vasoactive intestinal peptide (VIP).
      (f) Glutamate and aspartate play important role in windup via N-methyl-D-aspartate (NMDA) receptors
      (g) NMDA receptor activation leads to prostaglandin and nitric oxide formation
    (2) Inhibition
      (a) Occurs via segmental activity in the spinal cord and descending neural activity from supraspinal centers
      (b) Segmental
        (i) "Gate" theory: Pain in one part of the body inhibits pain in other parts.
        (ii) Glycine and γ-aminobutyric acid (GABA) as inhibitory neurotransmitters.
        (iii) Antagonism results in activation of WDR neurons producing allodynia and hyperesthesia.
      (c) Supraspinal
        (i) Results from fibers down the spinal cord from periaqueductal gray matter, reticular formation, and nucleus raphe magnus
        (ii) Mediated by α_2-adrenergic, serotonin, opiate receptor mechanisms (μ, δ, and κ)

SUGGESTED READINGS

Baker K: Recent advances in the neurophysiology of chronic pain. *Emerg Med Australasia* 2005;17:65–72.

Bennett GJ: Update on the neurophysiology of pain transmission and modulation: Focus on the NMDA-receptor. *J Pain Sympt Manage* 2000;19(1):S2–S6.

Morgan GE, Mikhail MS, Murray MJ: Clinical Anesthesiology, 3rd ed. New York, McGraw-Hill, 2002, pp 309–318.

Wilkinson PR: Neurophysiology of pain. Part I: Mechanisms of pain in the peripheral nervous system. *CPD Anaesth* 2001;3(3):103–108.

33 Taxonomy of Pain

1. THE NEED FOR TAXONOMY

a. Most common reason for patients to seek help is pain
b. Many pain syndromes
c. Standardized treatments and composed outcomes
d. Communication

2. CLASSIFICATION IN PAIN MEDICINE

a. Neurophysiologic
   i. Nociceptive
      (1) Unpleasant sensation mediated by nociceptors, stimulated by a noxious stimuli, and transmitted via pain fibers
      (2) Somatic (intense and discrete) and visceral (diffuse and poorly localized) pain
      (3) Easy to diagnose and manage
   ii. Neuropathic
      (1) Non-nociceptive produced by alteration of neurologic structure or function
      (2) Absence of a continuous nociceptive input
      (3) Mechanisms include possible "gate" malfunction, ectopic impulse, cross-talk between large or small fibers, or damage in central processing function
      (4) Central → lesions in central nervous system (CNS) that are difficult to manage
      (5) Peripheral → lesions in peripheral nervous system (PNS), which leads to persistent pain state (i.e., complex regional pain syndrome II [causalgia], postherpetic neuralgia)
   iii. Psychogenic
      (1) Must exclude all somatic pathology
      (2) Diagnostic and Statistical Manual of Mental Disorders, 4th edition (DSM IV-TR) guideline
b. Temporal pain (acute and chronic)
   i. Acute
      (1) Caused by internal disease that prompts an individual to seek help
      (2) Associated with psychological, autonomous, and behavioral responses
      (3) May be abolished in days or weeks by effective treatment
      (4) Improper treatment results in chronic pain
   ii. Chronic
      (1) Associated with cognitive-behavioral aspects, not duration
      (2) Physical, emotional, and socioeconomic stresses on the patient, family, and society

(3) Difficult to treat
(4) International Association for the Study of Pain (IASP) uses a five-axial system to classify chronic pain:
    (a) Five-axial system
        (i) Anatomic region
        (ii) Organ system
        (iii) Temporal characteristics
        (iv) Patient's statement of intensity and time of onset
        (v) Etiology
(5) Other classification systems for chronic pain have been proposed, such as the Multiaxial Assessment of Pain.
  c. Etiologic
    i. Most important cause is pain associated with cancer, either directly or as a result of its treatment.
    ii. Other causes include postherpetic neuralgia, sickle cell disease, and arthritis.
  d. Regional pain
    i. Classification includes headache, orofacial pain, low-back pain, pelvic pain.

SUGGESTED READING

Derasari M: Taxonomy of pain syndromes: Classification of chronic pain syndromes. In Raj PP (ed): Practical Management of Pain. St. Louis, Mosby, 2000, pp 10–17.

1. HISTORY

  a. Conduct a face-to-face interview at an unhurried pace.
  b. Use open-ended questions but guide the patient through the interview.
  c. Need to cover certain topics
      i. Chief complaint
     ii. History of presenting complaint
    iii. Past medical history
    iv. Systems review
     v. Family history
    vi. Occupational/social history

2. PHYSICAL EXAMINATION

  a. Vital signs at each visit
  b. General description
      i. Appropriateness of dress
     ii. Anxiety and comfort level
    iii. Posture
  c. Gait
      i. Pelvic rotation/tilt
     ii. Knee flexion/motion
    iii. Center-of-gravity motion
  d Reflexes (2/4 physiologic reflexes)
  e. Sensory examination
      i. Dysesthesia
     ii. Hyperesthesia
    iii. Paresthesia
  f. Trophic examination
      i. Visual examination for edema, atrophy, and discoloration
     ii. Physical examination for temperature changes
  g. Cervical spine examination
      i. Visual inspection and palpation
     ii. Lateral bending to 45 degrees
    iii. Rotation to 80 degrees
    iv. Flexion to 60 degrees
     v. Extension to 75 degrees
  h. Thoracolumbar spine examination
      i. Visual inspection and palpation
     ii. Flexion-extension to 90 degrees
    iii. Lateral flexion to 25 degrees
    iv. Spinal extension to 30 degrees
  i. Shoulder examination
      i. Visual inspection and palpation
     ii. Range of motion in flexion and extension to 180 degrees

   iii. Range of motion in abduction and adduction to 180 degrees
   iv. Range of motion in external rotation to 90 degrees
   v. Range of motion in internal rotation to 40 degrees
   vi. Yergason test for biceps tendon stability
   vii. Drop arm test for rotator cuff competence
 j. Elbow examination
   i. Visual inspection and palpation
   ii. Range of motion in extension to 180 degrees
   iii. Range of motion in flexion to 30 degrees
   iv. Lateral epicondylitis test
 k. Wrist examination
   i. Visual inspection and palpation
   ii. Range of motion in dorsiflexion to 60 degrees
   iii. Range of motion in plantiflexion to 70 degrees
   iv. Phalen and reverse Phalen maneuver
 l. Finger examination
   i. Visual inspection and palpation
   ii. Proximal interphalangeal (PIP) joints range of motion to 120 degrees
   iii. Distal interphalangeal (DIP) joints range of motion to 35 degrees
 m. Hip examination
   i. Visual inspection and palpation
   ii. Hip flexion (T12 to L3, iliopsoas)
   iii. Hip extension (S1, inferior gluteal nerve, gluteus maximus)
   iv. Hip adduction (L2 to L4, obturator nerve, adductor magnus, longus, brevis)
   v. Fabere test
   vi. Leg length discrepancy
   vii. Straight-leg-raising test: Lasègue sign and Gowers sign
   viii. Ober test
   ix. Thomas test
 n. Knee evaluation
   i. Visual inspection and palpation
   ii. Knee extension (L2 to L4, femoral nerve, quadriceps)
   iii. Knee flexion (L5 to S1, sciatic nerve, hamstrings)
 o. Ankle evaluation
   i. Visual inspection and palpation
   ii. Ankle inversion (L4, deep peroneal nerve, tibialis anterior muscle)
   iii. Ankle eversion (S1, superficial peroneal nerve, peroneus longus, brevis muscles)
   iv. Ankle dorsiflexion (L4 and L5, deep peroneal nerve, tibialis anterior and extensor hallucis longus muscles)
   v. Ankle plantiflexion (L5 to S2, tibial nerve, gastrocnemius-soleus, and flexor digitorum longus and hallucis longus muscle)

SUGGESTED READING

Abrams BM: History taking in the patient in pain. In Raj PP (ed): Practical Management of Pain, 3rd ed. St. Louis, Mosby, 2000, pp 333–359.

35 Pain Questionnaires and Assessment Tools

1. DESCRIPTION

    a. There are many sensations attributed to pain.
        i. Quality
        ii. Intensity
        iii. Location
        iv. Frequency
    b. Intensity is considered the most relevant to the clinical experience.

2. UNIDIMENSIONAL PAIN MEASUREMENT TOOLS

    a. Three tools are well validated in the cancer pain population.
        i. Visual analog scales (VAS)
        ii. Categorical verbal rating scales
        iii. Categorical numerical rating scales
    b. Numeric rating scales are considered to have better compliance than VAS.
    c. The aforementioned scales can be used for chronic nonmalignant pain or cancer pain.

3. MULTIDIMENSIONAL PAIN MEASUREMENT TOOLS

    a. McGill Pain Questionnaire (MPQ)
        i. Validated in cancer pain
        ii. Provides scores that reflect sensory, affective, and evaluative components of pain
        iii. Includes the verbal rating scale and a VAS
    b. Brief Pain Inventory
        i. Validated in many different languages
        ii. Numeric scale for pain intensity
        iii. Figure to represent area of the body in pain
    c. Memorial Pain Assessment Card (MPAC)
        i. Only validated in English

4. HEALTH-RELATED, QUALITY-OF-LIFE MEASURES

    a. European Organization for Research and Treatment of Cancer (EORTC)
        i. Designed for clinical trials
        ii. Assess physical, psychological, and social function

5. PEDIATRIC PAIN

    a. Children with no cognitive impairment and who can understand directions
        i. VAS, Faces scale, and MPQ
    b. Children with cognitive impairment
        i. Behavioral pain assessment tools, such as the Douleur Enfant Gustave-Roussy (DEGR) and San Salvador Scales
    c. Children unable to communicate
        i. DEGR scale

6. CRITERIA FOR FUTURE SCALES

    a. Future scales need to meet the following criteria:
        i. Ease of administration
        ii. Sensitivity to treatment effect
        iii. Multilingual validity
        iv. Internal validity
        v. Reliability

SUGGESTED READING

Caraceni A, Chemy N, Fainsinger R, et al: Pain measurement tools and methods in clinical research in palliative care: Recommendations of an expert working group of the European Association of Palliative Care. J Pain Sympt Manage 2002;23:239–255.

36 Psychological Assessment of Pain

1. GENERAL MEDICAL EXAMINATION

a. General medical and family history
b. Review of current medications
   i. Special emphasis on opiates
   ii. History of drug and alcohol abuse
c. Mental status
   i. Assessment of memory and concentration
   ii. Evaluation of psychological state, including depression, anxiety, anger, and irritability
d. Psychological history
   i. Socioeconomic background
   ii. Educational history
   iii. Family dynamics

2. PSYCHOLOGICAL TESTING

a. Minnesota Multiphasic Personality Inventory (MMPI)
   i. Most useful to gain a general psychological assessment for a patient with pain
   ii. Contains 3 validity and 10 clinical scales
   iii. A modernized MMPI-2 also exists
b. Pain Assessment Index
   i. Attempts to predict surgical outcome in patients with low-back pain
   ii. Combines MMPI scales
c. Personality Assessment Inventory
   i. Self-reporting scale of personality traits
   ii. Useful for people older than 18 years
   iii. Takes up to 1 hour to complete
   iv. Contains 4 validity and 11 clinical scales
d. Symptom Checklist-90
   i. A screen for psychological symptoms
   ii. Useful for patients older than 13 years
   iii. Takes 15 minutes of interview time
   iv. Contains no validity scales
e. Sickness Impact Profile
   i. Patient's report of his/her perception of illness
   ii. Very limited usefulness in patients with chronic pain
f. Millon Behavioral Health Inventory
   i. Addresses psychological symptoms in medical patients
   ii. Useful for patients older than 18 years
   iii. Takes 30 minutes to complete

iv. Scores of patients with chronic pain match those of patients with general medical issues, except for their higher depression and anxiety ratings

3. MOOD STATES

a. Beck Depression Inventory
   i. Takes 10 minutes to complete
   ii. Correlates with the depression scales on the MMPI
   iii. No validity measures
b. Spielberger State-Trait Anxiety Inventory
   i. Measures trait (stable personality characteristic) and state (situation dependent) anxiety
   ii. Correlates with affective index on McGill Pain Questionnaire
   iii. No validity scales

4. MALINGERING

a. Need to approach this conclusion with caution
b. MMPI-2 has validity scales
   i. Could help determine the test-taking motives
   ii. Currently considered experimental
c. Structured Interview of Reported Symptoms
   i. Assesses malingering psychological symptoms
   ii. Need to combine with MMPI validity scales

SUGGESTED READING

Doleys DM, Doherty DC: Psychological and behavioral assessment. In Raj PP (ed): Practical Management of Pain, 3rd ed. St. Louis, Mosby, 2000, pp 408–426.

1. GENERAL

a. Electrodiagnostic testing
b. Functional information of the nervous system, both central and peripheral
c. Localization of the problems: its chronicity, severity, and prognostic information
d. Electrodiagnostic testing includes nerve conduction studies (NCS) and electromyography (EMG)
e. NCS and EMG together provide information about the peripheral nerves and muscles.

2. NERVE CONDUCTION STUDIES

a. Done before EMG, provides quantitative information
b. Nerves routinely studied: medical, radial, ulnar posterior tibial, deep peroneal, sural, and, occasionally, the facial and trigeminal nerves

3. MOTOR NERVE CONDUCTION STUDIES

a. After electrode placement near the insertion of the muscles, the nerve is stimulated at gradually increasing intensity until the motor response no longer increases in amplitude (compound motor action potential [CMAP])
b. A conduction velocity is calculated for each nerve segment tested.
c. F responses (named for the foot where first identified)
   i. After discharges that occur normally in motor nerves as a result of proximal stimulation that reaches the spinal cord, the F response results in a new descending nerve depolarization.
   ii. The F response measures the integrity of the entire motor nerve.
   iii. F-response study: The most accepted use is in early suspected Guillain-Barré syndrome.
   iv. Its use in evaluating radiculopathy is highly controversial.

4. REFLEX STUDIES: HOFFMAN REFLEX (H REFLEX)

a. Electrostimulation of the posterior tibial nerve in the popliteal space: Recording surface electrodes are placed over the gastrocnemius muscle. Impulses are mostly carried in the SI nerve root distribution, the electrical equivalent of the ankle jerk.
b. The main value of the test is when a SI radiculopathy is suspected and the results of the EMG are normal.

5. ELECTROMYOGRAPHY

   a. Indications
      i. Painful peripheral neuropathies
      ii. Traumatic nerve injuries
      iii. Lumbar spinal stenosis
      iv. Arachnoiditis
      v. Nerve entrapment
   b. Painful myopathies
   c. Evaluates the physiologic state and anatomic integrity of the lower motor neuron

6. NORMAL MUSCLE

   a. Insertional response
   b. Needle insertion evokes a brief burst of electrical activity: 2 to 3 msec, 50 to 250 mV in amplitude
   c. Activity at rest
   d. Normal muscle should remain stable and silent after needle movement.
   e. Voluntary activity
   f. Number of motor units recruited determined by the force of contraction
   g. One motor unit—a nerve plus the number of muscle fibers it innervates

7. WAVEFORM

   a. Most are biphasic or triphasic
   b. Fifteen percent are polyphasic: cross the baseline or have more than 5 phases

8. AMPLITUDE

   a. Dependent on the number of fibers in the motor unit and EMG needles used
   b. Normal amplitude: 1 to 5 mV

9. INTERFERENCE PATTERNS

   a. A result of a large number of motor units that tend to interfere with each other such that they are not recognized as undivided units. This is a normal pattern.

10. CLINICAL CORRELATES

   a. EMG, NCD: best for separating neuropathy from myopathy
   b. Neuropathy: distinguishes between generalized axonal, demyelinating mixed, or focal

11. NERVE TRAUMA

a. Neurapraxia: no structural change, mildest form of axonal injury
b. Axonotmesis: axon disruption, total recovery
c. Neurotmesis: very severe injury, severe disruption or transection of the nerve.
d. Nontraumatic neuropathies and polyneuropathy
e. Entrapment neuropathies: medial, ulnar, radial, common peroneal, and tibial
f. Radiculopathies: nerve root diseases, plexopathies

12. LIMITATIONS OF EMG

a. Cannot give the evaluated sympathetic and small nerves better function
b. Early nerve injury (0 to 14 days): electrical silence
c. Fibrillation potentials appear only after 2 to 3 weeks
d. Cost-containment insurers have developed guidelines as to when it is appropriate to test for various conditions.

SUGGESTED READINGS

Abrams BM: Electromyography in the diagnosis and management of pain. In Raj PP (ed): Practical Management of Pain, 3rd ed. St. Louis, Mosby, 2000, pp 361–376.
Warfield C, Bajwa Z: Principles and Practice of Pain Medicine, 2nd ed. New York, McGraw-Hill, 2004, 113–114.

38 Imaging of the Spine

1. PLAIN RADIOGRAPHY (X-RAYS)

a. Quick, inexpensive, readily available, excellent spatial resolution
b. Screening of the spine
c. Bony pathology
d. Fractures
e. Vertebral misalignment
f. Spondylolisthesis
g. Spondylolysis
h. Dynamic, weight-bearing upright flexion and extension views
i. Degenerative disc changes
j. Hardware failure (fractures)

2. MAGNETIC RESONANCE IMAGING (MRI)

a. Most useful and versatile tool in the evaluation of the spine
b. Provides the best definition of tissue type
c. MRI protocols: sagittal and axial images
   i. T1-weighted sequences: High signal intensity represents fat, whereas low signal intensity represents fluid.
      (1) End-plate reactive changes
      (2) Osteophytic narrowing
      (3) Lateral disc herniation
      (4) Postoperative scarring, infiltrative disease
   ii. T2-weighted sequences: Fat-containing structures are less bright, whereas fluid-containing structures appear hyperintense (bright).
      (1) Intramedullary disease
      (2) Inflammation
      (3) Infection
   iii. Contraindications
      (1) Cardiac pacemaker
      (2) Ferromagnetic aneurysm clips
      (3) Ferromagnetic cochlear implants
      (4) Intraocular metallic foreign bodies
   iv. Gadolinium contrast
      (1) Postoperative patient-differentiated scarring from intervertebral discs
      (2) Patients with cancer, inflammation, or infection
      (3) Used with computer tomography (CT)
      (4) Provides the best possible definition of bone detail
      (5) Equivalent to MRI in facilitating the diagnosis of spinal stenosis or disc herniation
      (6) Actively depicts nerve root impingement
      (7) Useful in patients with ferromagnetic devices

v. Myelography
   (1) Radiographic technique used to identify the contents of the spinal canal by the introduction of an iodinated contrast material into the spinal subarachnoid space. This is usually followed by CT scanning.
   (2) Indications
      (a) CT or MRI contraindicated, equivocal, or limited because of surgical hardware artifacts
      (b) Definitive preoperative study
      (c) Postmyelography CT: high sensitivity in detecting arachnoiditis, subarachnoid tumor spread, disc herniation, osteophytic impingement
   (3) Complications
      (a) Postdural puncture headache (most common)
      (b) Contrast-related seizure
      (c) Infection
vi. Arteriography (spinal arteries)
   (1) Indications
      (a) Improves preoperative or preembolization visualization
      (b) Identifies possible cause of a vascular tumor or malformation revealed by MRI
   (2) Risks
      (a) Complications associated with invasive vascular procedure
      (b) Spinal infarction
vii. Discography
   (1) Identifies a disc as a potential source of a patient's pain by the fluoroscopically guided injection of contrast into the center of the nucleus pulposus
   (2) Concordance-duplication of the patient's pain by the force of injection of the contrast material
viii. Radionuclide scanning
   (1) Injection of technetium 99m-labeled phosphate followed by a whole-body bone scan
   (2) Indications
      (a) Detection of early osteomyelitis, skeletal metastasis, malignancy, compression, small stress fractures
   (3) Disadvantages
      (a) Poor detail and specificity
      (b) Usually requires further studies to confirm diagnosis if a positive result is obtained

SUGGESTED READINGS

Raj P: Pain Medicine: A Comprehensive Review. St. Louis, Mosby, 2003, 192–194.
Wallace M, Staats P: Pain Medicine and Management. New York, McGraw-Hill, 2005, 28–30.

Section II
_____

PHARMACOTHERAPY

39 Opioids

1. CATEGORIES OF OPIOID ANALGESICS

a. Pure (full) agonists: preferred for chronic pain
  i. Bind to opioid receptor(s)
  ii. No antagonist activity
  iii. No ceiling effect
b. Agonist-antagonists
  i. Ceiling effect for analgesia
  ii. Can reverse effects of pure agonists
    (1) Mixed agonist-antagonists (butorphanol, nalbuphine, pentazocine, dezocine)
    (2) Partial agonists (buprenorphine)
c. Antagonists
  i. Reverse or block agonist effects of pure opioids
  ii. Naloxone (Narcan) has been used to treat opioid overdose, addiction.
d. Short-acting opioid agonists
  i. Hydrocodone/N-acetyl-p-aminophenol acetaminophen (APAP)
  ii. Hydromorphone
  iii. Morphine
  iv. Oxycodone with or without APAP
  v. Oral transmucosal fentanyl (Actiq)
  vi. Tramadol (Ultram, Ultracet)
e. Long-acting opioids
  i. Transdermal fentanyl (Duragesic)
  ii. Methadone
  iii. Controlled and extended-release morphine
  iv. Controlled-release oxycodone (OxyContin)
  v. Levorphanol

2. IF A TRIAL OF OPIOIDS IS CONSIDERED

a. Ensure that the patient and/or family/primary guardian or caregiver is informed of the risks and benefits of chronic opioid use.
b. Inform about possible side effects.
c. Set realistic expectations.
d. Explain the conditions under which opioids will be prescribed.
e. Provide instructions for follow-up.
f. For elders, "Start low" and "Go slow."
g. Offer alternative therapeutic options.

3. PRINCIPLES OF EQUIANALGESIC CONVERSIONS

a. Ensure that an adequate trial of titration has been attempted prior to switching to another opioid due to unrelieved pain or suspected ineffectiveness.
b. Response to opioids is variable among individuals.
c. Side-effect profile vs. benefit of opioid should be considered when switching from one opioid to another.
d. Equianalgesic conversion guidelines differ according to available references.
e. When converting from one opioid to another, decrease the dose of the new opioid by 25% to 50% to account for incomplete cross-tolerance.
f. Provide adequate short-acting breakthrough medications when converting from one drug to another and titrate as indicated.
g. Avoid transdermal fentanyl patches (Duragesic) in opioid-naive patients.
h. Conversion to methadone should be undertaken by personnel experienced with high-dose conversions of opioids.

4. ADVERSE EFFECTS AND PATIENT MONITORING

a. Respiratory depression
   i. Tends to be short-lived
   ii. Typically occurs in the opioid-naive patients
   iii. Pain is a potent respiratory stimulant.
   iv. Withholding the appropriate use of opioids from a patient who is experiencing pain on the basis of respiratory concerns is unwarranted.
b. Constipation managed by:
   i. Attention to diet
   ii. Regular use of stool softeners and laxatives; however, stool softeners alone do little to prevent opioid induced constipation.
c. Sedation
   i. Typically subsides after a few days because patients generally become tolerant with continued use.
   ii. Escalate doses slowly.
   iii. Avoid using more sedating opioids (morphine, methadone) in the elderly population.
d. Nausea
   i. Possible early side effect, but usually dissipates with continued use
   ii. Concomitant therapy with antiemetics should be considered.

5. CONSIDERATIONS WITH OPIOID THERAPY

a. Intra- and interpatient variability
b. Sensitivity to adverse effects

c. Organ function or dysfunction
d. Hepatic
e. Renal
f. Ability to manage adverse effects or multiple analgesics
g. Patient adherence
h. Ability to titrate medication or self-manage pain
i. Chronic pain unresponsive to nonopioid therapy
j. Response to previous trials of opioids
k. History of substance abuse
l. Potential for functional gains
m. Ability to respond to limit setting and comply with a patient agreement
n. Ability to maintain the necessary level of care
o. Whether or not opioid therapy is appropriate for patients with chronic nonmalignant pain

6. BASIC PRINCIPLES OF "ACCEPTABLE" OPIOID MANAGEMENT

a. The American Academy of Pain Medicine and American Pain Society recommend the following guidelines for prescribing opioids.
b. Initial evaluation
   i. Pain history
   ii. Assessment of the impact of pain
   iii. Physical examination
   iv. Review of previous diagnostic studies and previous interventions
   v. Drug history
   vi. Assessment of coexisting diseases or conditions
c. Treatment plan
   i. Should be tailored to both the individual and the presenting problem.
   ii. Consider different treatment modalities (e.g., formal pain rehabilitation program, behavioral strategies, noninvasive techniques, or other classes of medications).
   iii. Ensure that patients and their guardians are informed of the risks and benefits of opioid.
   iv. Explain conditions under which opioids will be prescribed, which may include a written agreement specifying these conditions.
   v. Opioid trial should not be done in the absence of a complete assessment of the pain complaint.
d. Arrange consultation with a specialist in pain medicine or with a psychologist as needed.
e. Periodically review of treatment for efficacy.
f. Provide documentation of the evaluation, the reason for opioid therapy, overall pain management treatment plan, any consultations received, and periodic review of the status of the patient.

7. SPECIFIC ASPECTS OF CLINICAL CARE

a. Provide trials of alternative therapies and results.
b. Document indication for treatment.
c. Document regular history and physical examination.
d. Assess and document pain outcomes (intensity, perceptions of relief, functional gains).
e. Require regular visits (at least once a month).
f. Document patient teaching/instructions, e.g., risks and benefits.
g. Document need for modifications in prescription.
h. Establish plans to monitor patient.
i. If a trial of opioids is considered, physicians must ensure that patients, families/primary guardians, or caregivers are informed of:
   i. Risks and benefits of chronic opioid use
   ii. Conditions under which the opioids will be prescribed, including monitoring and follow-up care, and other alternative treatments
   iii. Criteria for chronic opioid therapy
     (1) Chronic pain unresponsive to nonopioid therapy
     (2) Response to previous trials of opioids
     (3) Consideration of history of substance abuse
     (4) Potential for functional gains
     (5) Ability to respond to limit setting and comply with a patient agreement
     (6) Ability to maintain the necessary level of care
j. The American Academy of Pain Medicine, the American Pain Society, and the American Society of Addiction Medicine have agreed on the following definitions:
   i. Addiction is a primary, chronic, neurobiologic disease, with genetic, psychosocial, and environmental factors influencing its development and manifestations. It is characterized by behaviors that include one or more of the following: impaired control over drug use, compulsive use, continued use despite harm, and craving.
   ii. Physical dependence is a state of adaptation that is manifested by a drug class–specific withdrawal syndrome that can be produced by abrupt cessation, rapid dose reduction, decreasing blood level of the drug, and/or administration of an antagonist.
   iii. Tolerance is a state of adaptation in which exposure to a drug induces changes that result in a diminution of one or more of the drug's effects over time.

SUGGESTED READINGS

Raj P: Pain Medicine: A Comprehensive Review. St. Louis, Mosby, 2003, pp 88, 113–115, 208.

Wallace M, Staats P: Pain Medicine and Management. New York, McGraw-Hill, 2005, pp 28–30.

40 Nonopioid Analgesics

1. ASPIRIN

a. Useful in the treatment of acute and chronic pain
b. Dosing range: 500 to 1000 mg every 4 to 6 hours
c. Exerts a minimal anti-inflammatory effect
d. Indicated for mild to moderate pain
e. Possesses fewer adverse effects than other nonopioid analgesics
f. Adverse effects: tinnitus, stomach or gastrointestinal bleeding, under 16 (children): Reye's syndrome.

2. ACETAMINOPHEN

a. Exerts a minimal anti-inflammatory effect
b. Exerts a dose-sparing effect with systemically administered opioids
c. Indicated for mild to moderate pain
d. Possesses fewer adverse effects than other nonopioid analgesics
e. Adverse effects include:
   i. Risk for hepatotoxicity at high doses exceeding 4000 mg/day and at lower doses with chronic use; increased risk with preexisting liver disease/impairment or chronic alcoholism
   ii. Renal toxicity
f. No effect on platelet function

3. SALICYLATES

a. Exerts a minimal anti-inflammatory effect
b. Indicated for mild to moderate pain
c. Possesses fewer adverse effects than other nonopioid analgesics
d. Adverse effects include:
   i. Risk for hepatotoxicity at high doses exceeding 4000 mg/day and at lower doses with chronic use; increased risk with preexisting liver disease/impairment or chronic alcoholism
   ii. Renal toxicity
e. No effect on platelet function

4. NONSTEROIDAL ANTI-INFLAMMATORY DRUGS (NSAIDs)

a. Mechanism of action
   i. Inhibit both peripheral and central cyclooxygenase, reducing prostaglandin formation
   ii. NSAIDs and cyclooxygenase 2 (COX-2) inhibitors exert a dose-sparing effect for systemically administered opioids
   iii. Preparations

    iv. Two isoforms of COX:
      (1) COX-1: constitutive, physiologic
      (2) COX-2: inducible, inflammatory
    v. Newer agents: COX-2-selective NSAIDs
    vi. COX-2-selective inhibitors have better gastrointestinal (GI) safety profile; no change in platelet function

b. Selection of therapy
    i. Start at a low but therapeutic dose.
    ii. Consider side-effect profile.
      (1) COX-1: GI effects
      (2) COX-2: platelet effect
      (3) Both: renal
    iii. Increase dose with expected therapeutic response attained or side effects occur.
    iv. Effect is additive to opioid therapy.
    v. Monitor for renal dysfunction and GI bleeding in long-term use.
    vi. Drug selection should be influenced by drug-selective toxicities, prior experience, convenience, and cost.
    vii. Great individual variation in response to different drugs.

c. Adverse effects
    i. Use with caution in patients with renal insufficiency, congestive heart failure, or volume overload.
    ii. GI side effects
      (1) Use with caution when patient has a history of NSAID-induced peptic ulcer disease and prior peptic ulcer disease.
      (2) Avoid concomitant therapy with corticosteroids.
      (3) Avoid use with anticoagulant therapy.
      (4) Use the lowest effective dose.
      (5) Switch to another NSAID with lower GI toxicity profile.
      (6) Use in conjunction with a H_2 blocker (ranitidine), gastroprotectant (misoprostol), or sucralfate.
      (7) Instruct patients to take with food and to avoid taking antacids with NSAIDs that may interfere with absorption.
    iii. Hematologic effects
      (1) Instruct patients to avoid taking over-the-counter medications with aspirin-containing compounds.
      (2) For patients at risk for bleeding, prescribe COX-2 NSAIDs or agents with minimal to no platelet effect (choline magnesium trisalicylate, salsalate, or nabumetone).
    iv. Renal effects
      (1) Assess renal function prior to therapy.
      (2) Monitor renal function with chronic NSAID use.
      (3) NSAID-induced renal insufficiency and renal failure are rare but can occur with chronic use of high doses.
    v. Central nervous system effects
      (1) Assess patients for dizziness and drowsiness.
      (2) Assess patients for cognitive impairment, decreased attention span, and short-term memory loss.
      (3) Discontinue use or reduce dose if these occur.

41 Antidepressants

1. TRICYCLIC ANTIDEPRESSANTS (TCAs)

a. Best evidence is for the use of TCAs in the treatment of neuropathic pain syndromes
  i. Diabetic neuropathy
  ii. Postherpetic neuralgia (PHN)
  iii. Central pain
  iv. HIV-related neuropathy
  v. Atypical facial pain
  vi. Postsurgical pain syndromes (postmastectomy, post-thoracotomy)
  vii. Other peripheral neuropathies
b. A TCA is the preferred initial therapy if the patient has coexisting insomnia, anxiety, or depression, or if cost is a consideration.
c. Titrate the selected medication to achieve clinical effect or to the maximum tolerated dosage.
d. A Cochrane Collaboration review of 50 randomized controlled trials documents the effectiveness of TCAs.
  i. Doses up to 150 mg/day demonstrated that the number needed to treat (NNT) was 2 (95%, CI 1.7 to 2.5), meaning 1 of 2 patients treated will obtain at least moderate pain relief.
  ii. Twenty percent of participants withdrew from studies because of intolerable side effects.
  iii. Often effective for continuous dysesthesias
  iv. Analgesic doses for TCAs are typically less than the antidepressant dose.
  v. Dose-response data have not been established.
  vi. Selection of agents is based on their side-effect profiles.
  vii. May need lower doses than those used to treat depression.
  viii. Careful titration is necessary for elderly patients.

2. SELECTION OF THERAPY

a. Dose-response data have not been established.
b. Selection of agents is based on their side-effect profiles.
c. May need lower doses than those used to treat depression.

3. ADVERSE EFFECTS OF TCAs

a. Sedation
b. Orthostatic hypotension
c. Confusion
d. Arrhythmias
e. Anticholinergic effects (dry mouth, constipation, urinary retention, blurred vision)

4. COMMONLY PRESCRIBED ANTIDEPRESSANT FOR NEUROPATHIC PAIN

a. *Amitriptyline* (Elavil) (tertiary amine)
  i. Initial starting dose: 10 to 25 mg at bedtime
  ii. Effective dosing ranges: 50 to 150 mg at bedtime
  iii. Clinical considerations
    (1) Produces more sedation, confusion, orthostatic hypotension, and anticholinergic effects
    (2) Must be used with extreme caution in the elderly
    (3) Slow titration often required
b. *Doxepin* (Sinequan) (tertiary amine)
  i. Initial starting dose: 10 to 25 mg at bedtime
  ii. Effective dosing ranges: 50 to 150 mg at bedtime
  iii. Clinical considerations
    (1) Less anticholinergic effects and slightly less sedation compared with amitriptyline
c. *Nortriptyline* (Pamelor, Aventyl) (secondary amine)
  i. Initial starting dose: 10 to 25 mg at bedtime
  ii. Effective dosing ranges: 50 to 150 mg at bedtime
  iii. Clinical considerations
    (1) Better tolerated than amitriptyline with fewer sedation and anticholinergic effects
d. *Desipramine* (Norpramine) (secondary amine)
  i. Initial starting dose: 10 to 25 mg at bedtime
  ii. Effective dosing ranges: 50 to 150 mg at bedtime
  iii. Clinical considerations
    (1) Significantly fewer sedation and anticholinergic effects compared with amitriptyline
    (2) Better tolerated in the elderly
e. *Trazodone* (Desyrel, Trialodine, Trazon)
  i. Initial starting dose: 50 to 100 mg/day
  ii. Effective dosing ranges: 50 to 100 mg/day in 3 divided doses
  iii. Clinical considerations
    (1) Not to exceed 400 mg/day in outpatients
    (2) Must be used with caution in patients with cardiovascular disease
    (3) Lower doses may be used to treat insomnia: 25 to 100 mg at bedtime

5. SELECTIVE SEROTONIN REUPTAKE INHIBITORS (SSRIs)

a. Although better tolerated, limited evidence suggests similar efficacy for SSRIs and SNRIs (serotonin-norepinephrine reuptake inhibitors)

b. In a single study, paroxetine (Paxil) was effective for diabetic neuropathy.
c. In a randomized controlled trial, fluoxetine (Prozac) failed to demonstrate efficacy with painful diabetic neuropathy.
d. Bupropion (Wellbutrin): 75 to 150 mg, twice daily
e. Citalopram (Celexa): 20 to 40 mg/day
f. Fluoxetine (Prozac): 20 to 60 mg/day
g. Paroxetine (Paxil): 20 to 40 mg/day
h. Sertraline (Zoloft): 50 to 200 mg/day

6. SEROTONIN-NOREPINEPHRINE REUPTAKE INHIBITORS (SNRI)

a. SNRIs seem to be helpful in relieving chronic pain associated with and independent of depression.
b. Duloxetine (Cymbalta) and milnacipran appear to be better tolerated and essentially devoid of cardiovascular toxicity.
c. Duloxetine (Cymbalta): 20 to 60 mg/day, twice daily
d. Milnacipran: 50 mg/day first week, then up to 100 mg/day
e. Venlafaxine (Effexor): 37.5 to 112.5 mg/day, twice daily

42 Anticonvulsants

1. GENERAL

a. Anticonvulsants are commonly used in neuropathic pain.
b. They raise the threshold for nerve depolarization and, thus, suppress abnormal neuronal discharges.
c. In general, pain relief obtained from these agents requires a trial period of at least 4 to 8 weeks.
d. Starting at the lower end, the doses are slowly titrated up to therapeutic levels.

2. SODIUM CHANNEL BLOCKERS

a. *Carbamazepine* (Tegretol)
   i. Dosing: initial dose 100 mg, twice daily, titrated to effect; typically 300 to 1000 mg/day
   ii. Mechanism of action (MoA): may inhibit pain via peripheral and central mechanisms
   iii. Indications: primary therapy for trigeminal neuralgia (*tic douloureux*), diabetic neuropathy, postherpetic neuralgia, thalamic mediated poststroke pain
   iv. Side effects (SE): Blood tests are advisable every 2 to 4 months because side effects include aplastic anemia (in 1:200,000) and agranulocytosis. Reversible leukopenia and thrombocytopenia are more common. Other adverse effects include sedation and gait alterations.
b. *Oxcarbazepine* (keto-analog of carbamazepine)
   i. Dosing: initial dose of 300 mg at bedtime; titrate up by 300 to 600 mg/day weekly, to a maximum of 1200 to 2400 mg/day
   ii. MoA: does not affect γ-aminobutyric acid (GABA) receptors, may modulate voltage-activated calcium currents
   iii. Plasma levels and hematologic monitoring not necessary
   iv. Less likely than carbamazepine to cause dizziness and other central nervous system (CNS) side effects or leukopenia
   v. SE: Severe hyponatremia (<125 mmol/L) can occur within the first 3 months, with normalization within a few days of discontinuation.
c. *Lamotrigine* (Lamictal)
   i. Dosing: initial dose 20 to 50 mg at bedtime, slowly titrated to 300 to 500 mg/day divided twice daily; drug should be slowly tapered off over 2 weeks
   ii. MoA: prevents release of excitatory neurotransmitter, glutamate
   iii. Indications: second-line agent for trigeminal neuralgia, cold-induced pain, diabetic neuropathy, HIV-associated polyneuropathy

      iv. SE: rash, more common in pediatric population and with rapid titration

d. *Levetiracetam* (Keppra)
   i. Dosing: initially 500 mg by mouth twice daily, titrated up to goal of 1500 mg, twice daily
   ii. MoA: not yet elucidated
   iii. SE: rash, hives, itching, dizziness

e. *Phenytoin* (Dilantin)
   i. Dosing: initial dose 100 mg, two to three times daily
   ii. MoA: prevents release of excitatory glutamate, activates the P450 system
   iii. SE: sedation, confusion, nystagmus, diplopia, ataxia, giddiness, slowing of mentation, facial alterations including gum hyperplasia, Stevens-Johnson syndrome

f. *Topiramate* (Topamax)
   i. Dosing: initial dose 50 mg at bedtime, titrated to maximum of 200 mg, twice daily
   ii. MoA: enhances action of GABA (inhibitory) neurotransmitter and inhibits the α-amino-3-hydroxy-5-methylisoxazole-4-propionic acid (AMPA)-type glutamate (excitatory) neurotransmitter
   iii. Indications: adjunct in treating diabetic neuropathy, postherpetic neuralgia, intercostal neuralgia, complex regional pain syndrome (CRPS)
   iv. SE: primarily sedation; also, carbonic anhydrase enzyme inhibitor, which may predispose to ocular glaucoma and renal calculi

g. *Valproic acid*
   i. Dosing: 800 mg/day in migraine therapy
   ii. MoA: acts on GABA-A receptor
   iii. Efficacy in neuropathic pain is controversial
   iv. SE: sedation, dizziness, gastrointestinal upset

3. CALCIUM CHANNEL BLOCKERS

a. *Gabapentin* (Neurontin)
   i. Dosing: initially 100 to 300 mg by mouth at bedtime, slowly titrated up to usual dose of 1800 to 3600 mg/day, with a maximum of 4800 mg/day, divided three times daily; dose adjustment necessary for renal impairment
   ii. MoA: membrane stabilizer by binding at alpha-2-delta subunit of L-type calcium channel
   iii. Indications: neuropathic pain disorders including CRPS, postherpetic neuralgia, postlaminectomy syndrome, radiculopathy, poststroke syndrome, and phantom limb pain
   iv. Effective in reducing multiple sclerosis-associated paroxysmal pain, specifically throbbing, pricking, and cramping quality.
   v. SE: dizziness, somnolence, fatigue which may decrease with slow drug titration, peripheral edema

b. *Pregabalin* (Lyrica)
   i. Dosing: usually initiated at 50 mg three times daily, which can be increased to 300 mg/day in a week if tolerated; minimally metabolized, almost entirely renally excreted; dose adjustment necessary for renal impairment
   ii. MoA: Unclear; however, Pregabalin binds with high affinity to the alpha-2-delta site (an auxiliary subunit of voltage-gated calcium channels) in CNS. This may be involved in Pregabalin's antinociceptive and antiseizure effects in animal models.
   iii. Indications: partial-onset seizures, neuropathic pain associated with diabetic neuropathy, postherpetic neuralgia
   iv. SE: dizziness (23%), somnolence, euphoria, vertigo, ataxia, constipation, dry mouth, peripheral edema, asthenia
c. *Zonisamide* (Zonegran)
   i. Dosing: initial dose 100 mg/day, slowly titrated up by 200 mg/week to a goal of 600 mg/day
   ii. MoA: increases GABA release
   iii. Indication: Used for neuropathic pain
   iv. SE: ataxia, rash, reduced appetite, renal calculi (carbonic anhydrase inhibitor), and oligohidrosis and susceptibility to hyperthermia (in children).

SUGGESTED READINGS

Rana M, Benzon HT, Molloy RE: Membrane stabilizers. In Benzon HT, et al (eds): Essentials of Pain Medicine and Regional Anesthesia, 2nd ed. Philadelphia, Elsevier, 2005, pp 134–140.

Strasser F, Driver LC, Burton AW: Update on adjuvant medications for chronic non-malignant pain. Pain Pract 2003;3:282–297.

43 Anxiolytics

1. GENERAL

a. Generalized anxiety disorder is characterized by a maladaptive response to various stressful stimuli.

b. Neurotransmitters primarily indicated include serotonin, norepinephrine, and γ-aminobutyric acid (GABA).

c. Pathologic anxiety is prevalent in about 30% to 60% of the pain clinic population.

d. Benzodiazepines and tricyclic antidepressants (TCAs) are traditionally the most commonly used agents.

2. BENZODIAZEPINES

a. Mechanism of action (MoA): Bind to GABA (inhibitory) receptor; suppress central nervous system (CNS) at the levels of the limbic system, brainstem reticular formation, and cortex.

b. Acute anxiety can be treated with short-acting benzodiazepines, but many patients may suffer significant rebound anxiety.

c. All benzodiazepines can cause confusion, sedation, and respiratory depression. Overdose can be fatal. These side effects can be synergistically compounded by the concomitant use of opioids.

d. Abrupt discontinuation can cause insomnia, anxiety, delirium, and, in severe cases, seizures.

e. All benzodiazepines cause physical and psychological dependence. Addiction potential is very real.

   i. *Alprazolam* (Xanax)

     (1) Intermediate onset. Half-life: 6 to 20 hours

     (2) Dosage: 0.5 to 4 mg/day by mouth in divided doses, titrated slowly

   ii. *Clonazepam* (Klonopin)

     (1) Intermediate onset. Half-life: 18 to 50 hours

     (2) Dosage: 0.25 to 2 mg by mouth twice daily, titrated slowly to 0.125- to 0.25-mg increments. Maximum: 4 mg/day.

   iii. *Diazepam* (Valium)

     (1) Rapid onset. Half-life: 30 to 100 hours

     (2) Dosage: 2 to 10 mg by mouth, two to four times daily (maximum, 20 mg/day)

   iv. *Lorazepam* (Ativan)

     (1) Intermediate onset. Half-life: 10 to 20 hours.

     (2) Dosage: 0.5 to 1 mg by mouth, two to three times daily; usual dose: 2 to 6 mg/day in divided doses

   v. *Midazolam* (Versed)

     (1) Rapid onset. Half-life: 2 to 3 hours

     (2) Causes anterograde amnesia

    vi. *Oxazepam* (Serax)
       (1) Intermediate-slow onset. Half-life: 8 to 12 hours
       (2) Dosage: 10 to 30 mg by mouth, three to four times daily and titrated slowly
    vii. *Temazepam* (Restoril)
       (1) Intermediate onset. Half-life: 8 to 20 hours
    viii. *Triazolam* (Halcion)
       (1) Intermediate onset. Half-life: 1.5 to 5 hours

3. BUSPIRONE

a. MoA: Serotonin agonist
b. Especially useful in treating patients with a history of substance abuse who may abuse benzodiazepines
c. Does not impair psychomotor or cognitive functions; no addictive potential
d. Dosage: started at 5 mg, three times daily; can be increased to 10 mg, three times daily
e. May take 1 to 4 weeks for the anxiolytic benefits.
f. SE: Headache, fatigue, dizziness, gastrointestinal upset, paresthesias.

4. ANTIDEPRESSANTS

a. Serotonin-norepinephrine reuptake inhibitors (SNRIs)
    i. *Venlafaxine* (Effexor) may have some benefit in generalized anxiety. Start at 37.5 mg/day for 4 to 7days, can increase by 75 mg every 4 days to a maximum of 225 mg/day.
b. Selective serotonin reuptake inhibitors (SSRIs)
    i. Of all antidepressants, SSRIs are the most effective anxiolytics, with typical doses higher than used for depression.
    ii. Paroxetine started at 5 to 10 mg/day, in particular, tends to have greater anxiolytic effects.
    iii. Other SSRIs, including sertraline 12.5 to 25 mg/day , fluoxetine 5 mg/day, or citalopram 10 mg/day, can also be started and slowly titrated up.
c. TCAs
    i. *Clomipramine* (Anafranil) is most useful in obsessive-compulsive disorder.
    ii. *Mirtazapine* (Remeron) has anxiolytic properties at lower, sedating doses; doses higher than 45 to 60 mg may worsen the anxiety.

SUGGESTED READINGS

Gelenberg AJ, Lydiard RB, Rudolph RL, et al: Efficacy of venlafaxine extended-release capsules in non-depressed outpatients with generalized anxiety disorder: A 6-month randomized controlled trial. JAMA 2000;283(23):3082–3088.

Rickels K, Zaninelli R, McCafferty J, et al: Paroxetine treatment of generalized anxiety disorder: A double-blind, placebo-controlled study. Am J Psychiatry 2003;160(4):749–756.

Wasan AD, Gallagher RM: Psychopharmacology for pain medicine. Chapter 14 of Essentials of Pain Medicine and Regional Anesthesia, 2nd ed, Philadelphia, Elsevier, 2005.

44 Muscle Relaxants

1. CENTRALLY ACTING MUSCLE RELAXANTS

a. Benzodiazepines: diazepam, clonazepam
   i. Mechanism of action (MoA): Act presynaptically on the interneurons to facilitate release of γ-aminobutyric acid (GABA) (inhibitory neurotransmitter) and its binding to GABA-A receptor. This leads to opening of chloride channels and hyperpolarization of I-a afferent terminals at their synapses with GABAergic interneurons in the spinal cord.
   ii. *Diazepam* (Valium)
      (1) Dosage: initial dose 2 mg twice daily, may be titrated up by 2 to 4 mg/week to a maximum of 20 to 30 mg
      (2) Long-term use predisposes to dependence. Abrupt termination may lead to serious withdrawal symptoms, such as seizures and delirium.
      (3) Side effects (SE): somnolence, dizziness, confusion, memory loss, increased reaction time, ataxia, gastrointestinal disturbance. Occasional paradoxical responses include euphoria, anxiety, irritability, hypomania, depression, paranoia, and suicidal ideation.
      (4) Concomitant use of other centrally acting drugs may potentiate side effects.
   iii. *Clonazepam* (Klonopin)
      (1) Dosage available as 0.125-, 0.25-, 0.5-, 1-, or 2-mg tablets.
      (2) Indications: primarily for myoclonus and petit mal seizures. Has a role in alleviating nocturnal spasms, reducing spasticity in children with cerebral palsy. Cautious use in pregnant women.
      (3) SE: sedation, seizures due to abrupt withdrawal, hypersalivation, dizziness, nervousness, ataxia
b. *Baclofen*
   i. Dosage: initial dose of 5 mg three times daily, can be doubled every 3 to 4 days to maximum of 80 to 100 mg/day; available in 10-mg tablets
   ii. MoA: structurally similar to GABA
      (1) Binds to presynaptic GABA-B receptors in spinal cord, brain, and other CNS sites.
      (2) It suppresses the release of excitatory neurotransmitters and inhibits excitatory afferent terminals involved in monosynaptic and polysynaptic reflex activity at the spinal cord level.
      (3) Additionally, there may be an inhibitory effect on the release of excitatory neurotransmitters from nociceptive afferent neural endings that originate in the skin.
      (4) High baclofen concentration may block postsynaptic action of excitatory neurotransmitters.

   iii. Indications
     (1) Primarily for spasticity of spinal cord origin: spinal cord injury (SCI) and multiple sclerosis (MS)
     (2) May be useful in cervical dystonia, upper motor neuron disease, and stiff-person syndrome
     (3) Provides long-term reduction in spasticity and decreases the pain associated with and frequency of flexor spasms
   iv. Intrathecal baclofen is an effective alternative, primarily for SCI and MS. Offers the advantage of achieving rapid and sustainable cerebrospinal fluid levels, also reaching the receptor sites in the spinal cord and CNS without systemic side effects.
   v. SE: modest muscle weakness without overall interference with locomotion
     (1) CNS: somnolence, dizziness common
     (2) Confusion, hallucinations, ataxia in higher doses
   vi. Abrupt withdrawal may predispose to seizures, hallucinations, and increased flexor spasms.

  c. *Tizanidine* (Zanaflex)
   i. Dosage: initial dose 4 mg/day, may be titrated up by 4 to 6 mg/week to a maximum of 36 mg/day; available in 4-mg tablets
   ii. MoA: α_2-adrenergic agonist; may inhibit locus ceruleus firing and subsequent inhibition of cerulospinal pathway
   iii. Indications: MS, SCI, motor neuron disease, and stroke. More effective in reducing muscle spasm and clonus, but less consistent in decreasing muscle tone.
   iv. SE: sedation and muscle weakness, but much better SE profile than baclofen and diazepam
     (1) Asthenia, headaches, hallucinations, and dry mouth
     (2) Careful administration when used with other antihypertensives

2. PERIPHERALLY ACTING ANTISPASTIC AGENTS

  a. *Carisoprodol* (Soma)
   i. Dosage: available as 350-mg tablets. Usual recommended dose is 350 mg, three or four times daily. Also available as a combination of 200 mg of carisoprodol and 325 mg of aspirin
   ii. MoA: likely acts by inhibiting interneuronal activity in descending reticular activating system and the spinal cord.
   iii. Indications: in acute musculoskeletal conditions, for relief of discomfort and pain; not indicated in spasticity
   iv. SE: sedation, confusion, disorientation, ataxia, tremor, irritability, insomnia, and, rarely, tachycardia and postural hypotension

b. *Cyclobenzaprine* (Flexeril)
   i. Dosage: standard dose 30 to 40 mg/day for 2 to 3 weeks; available in 10-mg tablets
   ii. MoA: relieves muscle strain of local origin without interfering with muscle strength
   iii. Indications
       (1) Recommended for short-term treatment
       (2) Improves signs and symptoms of skeletal muscle spasm, reduces local pain and tenderness
       (3) May help improve range of motion
   iv. SE: drowsiness, dizziness, and dry mouth; interaction with monoamine oxidase inhibitors (MAOIs) possible
c. *Dantrolene*
   i. Dosage: Initial dose for chronic spasticity is 25 mg by mouth twice daily. May be slowly titrated up to maximum 400 mg/day over 3 to 4 weeks. Drug should be discontinued if no response in 1 month.
   ii. MoA: blocks the release of calcium from sarcoplasmic reticulum and dissociates excitation-contraction coupling leading to hypotonia and muscle weakness
   iii. Indications
       (1) Primarily used to treat spasticity in SCI, MS, cerebral palsy, and stroke
       (2) Not indicated for skeletal muscle spasms or pain of rheumatologic origin
       (3) May be less helpful in ambulatory patients because of muscle weakness
   iv. Dantrolene IV is indicated in treatment of malignant hyperthermia. IV or PO form used as an adjunct to dopamine agonists for treatment of neuroleptic malignant syndrome.
   v. SE: confusion, dizziness, mental depression, muscle weakness; may cause fatal or nonfatal hepatotoxicity

SUGGESTED READINGS

Melen O: Muscle relaxants. In Benzon HT, et al (eds): Essentials of Pain Medicine and Regional Anesthesia, 2nd ed. Philadelphia, Elsevier, 2005, pp 159–165.
Strasser F, Driver LC, Burton AW: Update on adjuvant medications for chronic nonmalignant pain. Pain Pract 2003;3:282–297.

45 Oral and Topical Anesthetics/Analgesics

1. ORAL LOCAL ANESTHETICS

a. *Mexiletine* (Mexitil)
   i. Initial starting dose: 150 mg daily
   ii. Effective dosing ranges: 100 to 300 mg, three times daily
   iii. Clinical considerations
      (1) It is used as a second-line agent if there is no response to other antineuropathic pain agents.
      (2) The predictive value of a local anesthetic infusion to determine response to oral local anesthetics has not been established.
      (3) High rate of adverse effects (nausea, vomiting, tremor, unsteadiness) necessitates its use in almost half of patients.

2. TOPICAL ANESTHETICS

a. Actions and properties
   i. Target free nerve endings by inhibiting transport of ions across neural membranes, preventing initiation and conduction of nerve impulses.
   ii. Factors that influence cutaneous analgesia include anesthetic's lipid solubility, protein binding, pK_a (active base form responsible for diffusion), and vasodilatory action.
   iii. Higher lipid solubility is generally associated with potent effects.
   iv. Duration of anesthesia is a function of degree of protein binding.
   v. Action is more rapid on mucous membranes than skin.
   vi. Consult drug information for recommended areas of application.
      (1) Apply to intact skin.
      (2) Avoid contact with nontreated skin surfaces.
      (3) Use cautiously with:
         (a) Repeated use or coverage of large areas
         (b) Elderly or acutely ill
         (c) Severe liver disease
         (d) Any conditions related to methoglobinemia (e.g., glucose-6-phosphate dehydrogenase deficiency)
      (4) Discontinue use if erythema, blanching, swelling, edema, or other signs of local skin reaction appear.

b. Brand preparations
  i. *EMLA cream or anesthetic disc* (2.5% lidocaine/2.5% prilocaine)
    (1) Must be applied under an occlusive dressing
    (2) Onset of action: 15 to 120 minutes
    (3) Peak effect 3 hours with occlusive dressing
    (4) Duration 1 to 2 hours after removal of occlusive dressing
  ii. *ELA-Max cream* (4% lidocaine)
    (1) Onset of action is rapid
    (2) Peak effect unknown
    (3) Duration up to 4 hours
    (4) Systemic absorption directly related to the duration of use, surface area of application, and time of exposure
    (5) Safe dosing recommendations not available for application on mucous membranes
  iii. *Lidoderm patch* (5% lidocaine)
    (1) Indicated for treatment of postherpetic neuralgia (PHN) and effective for other neuropathic and myofascial pain syndromes
    (2) Onset of action is rapid
    (3) Peak effect unknown
    (4) Duration up to 4 hours
    (5) Duration 1 to 2 hours after removal of occlusive dressing
  iv. *Amethocaine* (4% tetracaine)
    (1) Must be applied under an occlusive dressing
    (2) More lipophilic than lidocaine
    (3) Faster onset of action (40 minutes)
    (4) Good tolerability with repeated exposures
    (5) Limited data for use on mucous membranes
    (6) Duration up to 4 hours

3. TOPICAL ANALGESICS

a. *Capsaicin*
  i. Vanilloid receptor agonist
  ii. Derived from cayenne pepper
  iii. Depletes substance P in nerve terminals
  iv. Useful in diabetic neuropathy, PHN, phantom limb, postmastectomy pain, and osteoarthritis (OA)
  v. 0.025% to 0.075% cream 2 to 4 times per day
  vi. Repeated consistent applications are required.
  vii. Long-term use can result in irreversible damage to nerve terminals.

46 Botulinum Toxin

1. GENERAL

a. There is evidence to support its use with headache syndromes, cervical dystonia, pain associated with spasticity, and myofascial pain syndromes.

b. Suggested mechanism of action of direct analgesic botulinum toxin is possibly mediated by blockade of substance P, glutamate, and calcitonin gene-related peptide.

c. It is used only for chronic myofascial pain syndromes that are resistant to physical therapy and oral pharmacotherapy.

d. The toxin should be applied only by physicians who are experienced in its use.

e. Discontinue use if erythema, blanching, swelling, edema, or other signs of local skin reaction appear.

SUGGESTED READINGS

American Academy of Pain Medicine and the American Pain Society: Consensus statement. The Use of Opioids for the Treatment of Chronic Pain. http://www.painmed.org/productpub/statements/pdfs/opioids.pdf. Accessed 1 December 2005.

American Pain Society: Principles of Analgesic Use in the Treatment of Acute and Cancer Pain, 5th ed. Glenview, II, American Pain Society, 2005.

American Pain Society and American Academy of Pain Medicine: Definitions Related to the Use of Opioids for the Treatment of Pain. http://www.painmed.org/productpub/statements/pdfs/definition.pdf. Accessed 1 December 2005.

American Society of Anesthesiology: Practice Guidelines for Acute Pain Management in the Perioperative Setting. http://www.asahq.org/publicationsServices.htm#practice. Accessed 30 October 2005.

Cordivari C, Misra P, Catania S, Lees AJ: New therapeutic indications for botulinum toxins. Movement Disorders 2004;19(Suppl 8):S157–S161.

Dalpiaz AS, Lordon SP, Lipman AG: Topical patch therapy for myofascial pain. J Pain Palliat Care Pharmacother 2004;18:15–34.

Dworkin RH, Backonja M, Rowbotham MC, et al: Advances in neuropathic pain: Diagnosis, mechanisms, and treatment recommendations. Arch Neurol 2003;60(11):1524–1534.

Gammaitoni AR, Alvarez ND, Galer BS: Safety and tolerability of the lidocaine patch 5%, a targeted peripheral analgesic: A review of the literature. J Clin Pharmacol 2003;43:111–117.

Huang W, Vidimos A: Topical anesthetics in dermatology. J Am Acad Dermatol 2000;43:286–298.

Maizels M, McCarberg B: Antidepressants and antiepileptic drugs for chronic noncancer pain. Am Fam Physician 2005;71:483–490.

Raj PP: Botulinum toxin therapy in pain management. Anesthesiol Clin N Am 2003;21:715–731.

Reilich P, Fheodoroff K, Kern U, et al: Consensus statement: Botulinum toxin in myofascial pain. J Neurol 2004;251(Suppl 1):I36–I38.

Wiffen ST: Antidepressants for neuropathic pain. The Cochrane Collaboration. The Cochrane Library Issue 2005;3:1–49.

1. OPIOID-INDUCED SEDATION FOR MALIGNANT PAIN

a. Opioids are mainstay of therapy.
b. Require increased dosing secondary to tolerance.
c. With initiation or increased dose, side effects develop.
d. Sedation may diminish quality of life and lead to noncompliance.
e. Dose reduction may decrease sedation, but also decreases analgesia.
f. Treatment
   i. Central nervous system (CNS) stimulants
      (1) Caffeine
         (a) Advantages
            (i) Inexpensive
            (ii) Easily attainable
            (iii) Well-tolerated
         (b) Disadvantages
            (i) No data to support efficacy
            (ii) Dosing range unknown
      (2) Methylphenidate (Ritalin)
         (a) Advantages
            (i) Rapid onset of action
            (ii) Inexpensive
            (iii) Known dosing: 10 to 15 mg/day
         (b) Disadvantages
            (i) Abuse potential
            (ii) Anxiety
            (iii) Agitation
            (iv) Psychosis
            (v) Tachycardia
            (vi) Hypertension
      (3) Dextroamphetamine (Dexedrine)
         (a) Advantages
            (i) None when compared with other CNS stimulants
            (ii) Known dosing: 5 to 30 mg/day
         (b) Disadvantages
            (i) Abuse potential
            (ii) Anxiety
            (iii) Agitation
            (iv) Psychosis
            (v) Tachycardia
            (vi) Hypertension

(4) Modafinil (Provigil)
  (a) Advantages
    (i) Well-tolerated
    (ii) Low abuse potential
    (iii) Known dosing: 100 to 600 mg/day
  (b) Disadvantages
    (i) Cost
    (ii) Limited clinical trials
    (iii) Affects CYP450 enzyme
    (iv) Anxiety
    (v) Agitation
    (vi) Psychosis
    (vii) Tachycardia
    (viii) Hypertension
ii. Acetylcholinesterase inhibitor
  (1) Donepezil (Aricept)
    (a) Advantages
      (i) Well-tolerated
      (ii) Once daily dosing
      (iii) Nonscheduled medication
      (iv) May improve constipation
      (v) Known dosing: 2.5 to 15 mg/day
    (b) Disadvantages
      (i) Cost
      (ii) Limited clinical trials
      (iii) Nausea
      (iv) Vomiting
      (v) Diarrhea

2. OPIOID-INDUCED SEDATION FOR NONMALIGNANT PAIN

a. Controversial topic
  i. If patients are sedated with nonmalignant pathology, are we overprescribing?
  ii. Clinical trials have been done mainly on patients with malignant pathology.
  iii. Medications
    (1) Same as for malignant pain
    (2) Dosing and side effects unrelated to etiology of pain

SUGGESTED READING

Reissig JE, Rybarczyk AM: Pharmacologic treatment of opioid-induced sedation in chronic pain. *Ann Pharmacother* 2005;39:727–731.

Section III

DIAGNOSTIC AND THERAPEUTIC INTERVENTIONS FOR CHRONIC PAIN

48 Chemical Neurolysis

1. GENERAL

a. Employed as an adjuvant treatment in providing longer-lasting pain relief to the geriatric patient

b. Works by destroying the nerves that are in contact with the neurolytic solution

c. Frequently used in patients with terminal cancer or certain neuralgias, or when neurolysis by other modalities (e.g., radiofrequency thermocoagulation [RFTC], cryoneurolysis) cannot be readily performed

d. Types of neurolytic blocks for the geriatric patient (various anatomic locations amenable to neurolysis when indications permit) (**Table 48-1**).

e. Prior to a chemical neurolysis, patients must have had successful pain relief after a diagnostic local anesthetic block and no intolerable side effects. Most of the complications are due to the spread of the neurolytic solution to the surrounding anatomic structures (**Table 48-2**).

f. The effects of alcohol-induced neurolysis can last up to a year, whereas phenol takes up to 14 days to cause tissue degeneration and the effects last for up to 14 weeks (albeit less intensely).

TABLE 48–1 Types of Neurolytic Blocks for the Geriatric Patient

Neurolysis of sympathetic chain	Abdominal via splanchnic neurolysis
	Abdominal via celiac plexus neurolysis (abdominal visceral pain)
	Lumbar (extremity sympathetic pain)
	Pelvic via hypogastric plexus neurolysis (pelvic pain)
Neuroaxial neurolysis	Spinal neurolysis
	Epidural neurolysis
Peripheral nerve neurolysis	Head:
	Trigeminal, mandibular, facial glossopharyngeal
	Neck plexuses:
	Cervical, brachial, stellate
	Intercostal

TABLE 48–2 Frequent Side Effects of Neurolytic Blocks (Depending on Location)

• Persistent pain at the site of injection	• Bowel and bladder dysfunction
• Paresthesias	• Motor weakness
• Hyperesthesia	• Deafferentation pain
• Systemic hypotension	• Neuritis

Commonly used neurolytics	Less commonly used neurolytics
• Absolute ethyl alcohol	• Glycerol
• 4%–8% phenol	• Silver nitrate
	• Ammonium sulfate
	• Hypertonic and hypotonic solutions
	• Chlorocresol

2. SYMPATHETIC CHAIN BLOCKS

a. General

   i. Visceral pain associated with cancer may be relieved with oral pharmacologic therapy, which includes combinations of nonsteroidal anti-inflammatory drugs (NSAIDs), opioids, and adjuvant therapy.

   ii. In addition to pharmacologic therapy, neurolytic blocks of the sympathetic axis are also effective in controlling visceral cancer pain and should be considered as important adjuncts to pharmacologic therapy for the relief of severe pain experienced by patients with cancer.

   iii. These blocks rarely eliminate cancer pain because patients frequently experience coexisting somatic and neuropathic pain as well. Therefore, oral pharmacologic therapy must be continued, albeit at lower doses.

   iv. The goals of performing a neurolytic block of the sympathetic axis are to:

   (1) Maximize the analgesic effects of opioid or nonopioid analgesics

   (2) Reduce the dosage of these agents to alleviate side effects

b. Sympathetic chain blocks and their complications

   i. Intrapleural phenol block

   (1) Complications (two categories)

   (a) Traumatic injuries caused by the needle or the catheter

   (b) Those produced by the neurolytic agent injected in the interpleural space

   (2) Pneumothorax may occur in 2% of the patients, and lung injuries have been reported when 5 rigid catheter is used.

   (3) Phrenic nerve palsy resulting in respiratory failure may also occur after this block.

(4) Therefore, bilateral blocks should be avoided.
(5) Systemic effects from drug absorption may also occur because the pleural membranes are highly vascularized.

  ii. Celiac plexus block

    (1) Overview

      (a) Complications associated with celiac plexus blocks ap-
pear to be related to the technique used: retrocrural,
transcrural, and transaortic.

      (b) The incidence of complications from neurolytic celiac
plexus blocks was recently determined by Davis in 2730
patients having blocks performed from 1986 to 1990.

      (c) The overall incidence of major complications (e.g.,
paraplegia, bladder, and bowel dysfunction) was 1 in
683 procedures. However, the report does not describe
which approach or approaches were used to perform
the blocks.

    (2) Complications (with detailed management discussed fur-
ther in deLeon-Casasola) include:

      (a) Orthostatic hypotension
      (b) Backache
      (c) Retroperitoneal hemorrhage
      (d) Diarrhea
      (e) Abdominal aortic dissection
      (f) Paraplegia and transient motor paralysis

  iii. Superior hypogastric block (no complications as per 2000 MD
Anderson Study)

  iv. Ganglion impar block (no complications, limited data)

SUGGESTED READINGS

Davis DD: Incidence of major complications of neurolytic coeliac plexus block. J R
Soc Med 1993;86:264–266.

deLeon-Casasola OA: Critical evaluation of chemical neurolysis of the sympathetic
axis for cancer pain. Cancer Control 2000;7(2):142–148

Hilgier M, Rykowski JJ: One needle transcrural celiac plexus block: Single shot, or
continuous technique, or both. Reg Anesth 1994;19:277–283.

Ischia S, Luzzani A, Ischia A, et al: A new approach to the neurolytic block of the
coeliac plexus: The transaortic technique. Pain 1983;16:333–341.

Jain S, Gupta R: Neurolytic agents in clinical practice. In Waldman S, Winnie A (eds):
Interventional Pain Management. London, WB Saunders, 1996, pp 167–171.

Pellegrino A: Complications of neurolytic blocks. In Ramamurthy S, Rogers JN (eds):
Decision Making in Pain Management. St. Louis, Mosby–Year Book, 1993, p 218.

Plancarte R, Amescua C, Patt RB: Presacral blockade of the ganglion of Walther
(ganglion impar). Anesthesiology 1990;73:A751.

Plancarte R, de Leon-Casasola OA, El-Helaly M, et al: Neurolytic superior hypogastric plexus block for chronic pelvic pain associated with cancer. Reg Anesth
1997;22:562–568.

Raj P, Patt RB: Peripheral neurolysis. In Raj P (ed): Pain Medicine: A Comprehensive
Review. St. Louis, Mosby–Year Book, 1996, pp 188–196.

Singler RC: An improved technique for alcohol neurolysis of the celiac plexus
block. Anesthesiology 1982;56:137–141.

49 Cryoablation

1. GENERAL

a. Best used for a single nerve or site
b. Failure of symptom palliation after successful diagnostic block (30°)
   i. Placebo response
   ii. Nonspecific diagnostic test due to poor needle placement
   iii. Large volume of anesthetic causing diffuse neural blockade
   iv. Systemic absorption of local anesthetic
   v. Technical problems related to generation of the lesion
c. Temporary destruction of the nerve by extreme cold
d. Nerve axon degeneration without damage to surrounding tissue

2. INDICATIONS

a. Analgesia required for weeks to months (2 weeks to 5 months)
b. Especially suitable for well-localized lesions (i.e., neuromas, entrapment neuropathy)

3. CONTRAINDICATIONS

a. Infection
b. Coagulopathy
c. Uncooperative patient
d. Undiagnosed condition
e. Lesioning of a motor nerve

4. PHYSICS

a. The creation of low temperatures by the expansion of a compressed gas (Joule-Thompson Effect), such as nitrous oxide or carbon dioxide
b. The expansion of a compressed gas through a small orifice into a chamber at the top of a probe
c. The probe tip surface is cooled to $-70°$ C to $-80°$ C. Nitrous oxide is most commonly used.
d. Cryoprobes are Teflon coated; incorporate a stimulator to locate the intended nerve and a thermocouple to measure core temperature. Both are located in the tip of the probe.
e. The size of the freeze zone is two to three times the diameter of the probe.

5. HISTOLOGY

a. Exact mechanism of nerve injury is unknown.
b. Wallerian degeneration (axon and myelin sheath degeneration): The endo-, peri-, and ectoneurium remain intact. Axonal regrowth 1 to 2 mm/day.

c. At 0° C, all nerve fibers within the ice ball stop conduction. For prolonged sensory loss, a minimum temperature of –20° C for 1 minute is needed.

d. Regenerating axons are unlikely to form a painful neuroma because there is no external nerve damage and a minimal inflammatory reaction after freezing.

6. TECHNIQUE (PERCUTANEOUS)

a. A small skin wheal is raised with a local anesthetic.

b. Introducers (12-, 14-, and 16-gauge): intravenous catheters

c. A 1.3-mm or 2-mm probe is passed via a catheter introducer toward the target nerve or area.

d. Localization of the nerve is facilitated by the use of the nerve stimulator. For sensory nerves, 50 and 100 Hz at less than 0.5 V; for motor nerves, 2 to 5 Hz.

e. Two or three 2-minute cycles usually suffice.

f. 0.9% saline continuous irrigation at room temperature reduces the risk of skin injury (frostbite).

7. INDICATIONS FOR CRYONEUROLYSIS

a. Postoperative
    i. Postherniorrhaphy: open lesioning of the ilioinguinal nerve
    ii. Post-thoracotomy: intercostal nerve at the site of the lesion and the nerves two levels above and below are cryoablated

b. Chronic pain
    i. Facial pain
        (1) Temporomandibular jaw (TMJ): cryoablation of joint capsule and great auricular nerve
        (2) Trigeminal neuralgia: branches of V1, V2, V3 cryoablated
        (3) Intractable facial pain: malignant disease, posttraumatic, postherpetic
    ii. Thoracic pain
        (1) Thoracotomy scar
        (2) Postherpetic neuralgia
    iii Low-back pain of facet origin: cryoablation of median branch nerve at the pain site and one level above and below the involved facet joint
    iv. Peripheral nerve pain: only for sensory nerves, nerve entrapment, or painful neuroma
    v. Perineal pain: good results (46%) following cryoablation for nerve entrapment postherniorrhaphy
    vi. Sacral pain: rectal pain, coccydynia, and sciatic nerve pain

8. COMPLICATIONS

a. Frostbite at the skin entry site
b. Inadvertent ablation of motor nerve (motor function will return)
c. Infrequent intercostal nerve dysesthesia

SUGGESTED READINGS

Raj P: Pain Medicine: A Comprehensive Review, 2nd ed. St. Louis, Mosby, Inc., 2003.

Wallace M, Statts P: Pain Medicine and Management. New York, McGraw-Hill Companies, 2005.

Warfield C, Bajaa Z: Principles and Practice of Pain Medicine, 2nd ed. New York, McGraw-Hill Companies, 2004.

50 Radiofrequency Lesioning

1. GENERAL

a. The first attempts to use direct current (DC) electricity experimentally were made in the 1870s, and it was introduced into clinical practice in the 1940s.

b. Aranow and Cosman adapted Cushing and Bovie's (1920s) surgical thermocoagulation techniques for generating neural lesions in the 1950s.

c. In contrast to DC generators, radiofrequency generators use continuous high-frequency waves of about 1 MHz.

2. CONVENTIONAL RADIOFREQUENCY TREATMENT, USING A CONSTANT OUTPUT OF HIGH-FREQUENCY ELECTRIC CURRENT

a. Produces controllable tissue destruction surrounding the tip of the treatment cannula

b. When placed at precise anatomic locations, has demonstrated success in reducing a number of different chronic pain states, including chronic neck pain after whiplash injury and trigeminal neuralgia

c. Pulsed radiofrequency utilizes brief "pulses" of high-voltage, radiofrequency range (~300 kHz) electrical current that produce the same voltage fluctuations in the region of treatment that occur during conventional radiofrequency treatment, but without heating to a degree at which tissue coagulates (**Box 50-1**).

BOX 50–1 Lumbar Disk and Ramus Communicans

Trigeminal rhizotomy
Cervical facet denervation
Thoracic facet denervation
Lumbar facet denervation
Dorsal root ganglionotomy
Cervical ganglion rhizotomy

Thoracic ganglion rhizotomy
Lumbar ganglion rhizotomy
Sacral ganglion rhizotomy
Stellate ganglionotomy
Thoracic sympathectomy
Lumbar sympathectomy
Lumbar disk and ramus communicans

3. TECHNIQUE

a. It is critical to control lesion size.
b. The size and consistency of the lesion are governed by four major factors:
    i. Temperature generated
    ii. Rate of thermal equilibrium
    iii. Electrode size and configuration
    iv. Local tissue characteristics

4. COMPLICATIONS

a. Fluoroscopically guided radiofrequency denervation of the lumbar facet joints is associated with a 1.0% incidence of minor complications per lesion site in one study.
    i. Motor weakness
    ii. Sensory loss
    iii. Neuralgia
    iv. Neuropathic pain

SUGGESTED READINGS

Kornick C, Kramarich SS, Lamer TJ, Todd Sitzman B: Complications of lumbar facet radiofrequency denervation. Spine 2004;29:1352–1354.

Masahiko K, Hashizume R, Iwata T, Furuya H et al: Percutaneous radiofrequency lesioning of sensory branches of the obturator and femoral nerves for treatment of hip joint pain, Reg Anesth Pain Med 2001;26(6):576–581.

Richebe P, Rathmell JP, Brennan TJ: Immediate early genes after pulsed radiofrequency treatment: Neurobiology in need of clinical trials. Anesthesiology 2005;102:1–3.

Saberski L, Fitzgerald J, Ahmad M: Cryoneurolysis and radiofrequency lesioning. In Raj PP (ed): Practical Management of Pain, 3rd ed. St. Louis, Mosby, Inc., 2000, pp 753–768.

51 Occipital Nerve Block

1. INDICATIONS

    a. Pain in the occipital region: principally for diagnosis
    b. Occipital neuralgia
    c. Headache: cervicogenic, tension, or vascular
    d. Myofascial pain
    e. Cervical arthritis

2. ANATOMY

    a. Formed by the dorsal rami of the second cervical nerve: provides cutaneous innervation of the posterior scalp
    b. The nerve becomes subcutaneous inferior to the superior nuchal line and medial to the occipital artery.
    c. It may receive a communicating branch from the third cervical nerve as it begins to ascend in the posterior neck.

3. POSITION

    a. The patient is placed in a sitting position with the chin flexed on the chest.

4. PLACEMENT

    a. The most useful landmark is the occipital artery, which is found at a point one-third of the total distance from the external occipital protuberance to the mastoid process on the superior nuchal line.
    b. A 25-gauge, 1- to 1.5-inch needle is inserted medial to the occipital artery at the level of the superior nuchal line; 3 to 5 mL of local anesthetic injected in this area should produce occipital nerve anesthesia.
    c. For a diagnostic block, the dose is limited to 1 to 2 mL to minimize confusion with relief of myofascial pain.
    d. Depot formulations of local anesthetics may provide longer lasting relief.

5. COMPLICATIONS

    a. Intravascular injection is uncommon and systemic toxicity would be a rare occurrence.
    b. In patients who have had suboccipital cranial surgery, caution must be taken to avoid a subcranial injection that may lead to a total spinal anesthetic.

SUGGESTED READINGS

Brown DL: Atlas of Regional Anesthesia, 2nd ed. Philadelphia, WB Saunders Company, 1999, pp 145–146.

1. ANATOMY

a. The stellate (cervicothoracic) ganglion is made up of the lowest cervical ganglion fused with the first thoracic ganglion in 80% of people. The first thoracic ganglion, if not connected, is called the stellate ganglion.

b. The cervicothoracic ganglion is located on or just lateral to the longus colli muscle, which lies just anterior to the transverse processes of the seventh cervical and first thoracic vertebrae.

c. The stellate ganglion is anteromedial to the vertebral artery and medial to the common carotid artery and jugular vein.

d. The vertebral artery enters the vertebral foramen posterior to the anterior tubercle of C6.

2. CLINICAL INDICATIONS

a. Common indications
   i. Acute pain of herpes zoster
   ii. Postherpetic neuralgia
   iii. Chronic regional pain syndrome (CRPS) of the upper extremity, face, neck, and upper thorax
   iv. Frostbite and acute vascular occlusion of the face and upper extremities
   v. Raynaud syndrome
   vi. Sympathetically maintained pain of malignant origin

b. Other indications (based largely on anecdotal cases)
   i. Headaches
   ii. Bell palsy
   iii. Retinal vascular occlusion
   iv. Sinusitis, acute or chronic; Ménière disease
   v. Neck-shoulder-arm syndrome
   vi. Thoracic outlet syndrome
   vii. Angina, myocardial infarction

3. TECHNIQUE

a. Computed tomography (CT) or fluoroscopic guidance dramatically decreases the incidence of complications (i.e., pneumothorax)

b. Classic techniques use C6 or C7 vertebrae as a landmark.
   i. C6 transverse process (Chassaignac tubercle) is identified by palpation or fluoroscopy.
   ii. By using a short 27-gauge beveled needle, with the patient in the supine position and the cervical spine in a neutral position, the junction of the body and transverse process of C6 or C7 is contacted.

iii. The carotid artery is retracted laterally with the sternomastoid to avoid puncture.

iv. After the periosteum is contacted, the needle is withdrawn several millimeters.

v. One milliliter of dye is injected after a negative aspiration for blood and cerebrospinal fluid (CSF).

vi. If no intravascular or intrathecal spread is noted and if there is good spread along the sympathetic ganglia, 0.5 mL of local anesthetic is injected.

vii. After a 2- to 3-minute wait to rule out either intravascular injection (CNS toxicity) or intrathecal injection (spinal analgesia), 2 to 10 mL of local anesthetic is injected.

4. EFFECTS OF STELLATE GANGLION BLOCK

a. Vasodilation
   i. Increased skin temperature: by 2° to 3°
   ii. Possible increase in brain-blood volume
b. L stellate ganglion block: increased heart rate and blood pressure
c. May increase retinal venous blood velocity on blocked side, decreasing intraocular pressure
d. Decrease in tympanic membrane temperature
e. May modulate immune and endocrine systems

5. SIDE EFFECTS

a. Inadvertent block of recurrent laryngeal nerve with associated dysphagia, hoarseness, and a feeling of a lump in the throat
b. Horner syndrome occurs if the superior cervical sympathetic ganglion is also blocked.
   i. Ptosis
   ii. Miosis
   iii. Nasal congestion
   iv. Warmth of the face

6. COMPLICATIONS

a. Injection into the epidural, subdural, or subarachnoid space
b. Pneumothorax
c. Phrenic nerve block leading to difficulty breathing
d. Seizure because of intravascular injection
e. Injury to the esophagus
f. Hematoma
g. Vasovagal attacks

SUGGESTED READINGS

Benzon, et al: Essentials of Pain Medicine and Regional Anesthesia. Philadelphia, Churchill-Livingstone, 2005, pp 851–870.

Wallace M, Statts P: Pain Medicine and Management. New York, McGraw-Hill, 2005, pp 345–346.

53 Gasserian Ganglion Block

1. ANATOMY

   a. The trigeminal ganglion is located at the apex of the petrous temporal bone in the middle cranial fossa near the cavernous sinus.

   b. The ganglion rests in a dural invagination (Meckel cavity) that contains cerebrospinal fluid (CSF).

   c. The trigeminal nerve originates in the brainstem and synapses in
the gasserian ganglion.

   d. The peripheral (midpontine level) branches form the ophthalmic
maxillary and mandibular nerves.

2. INDICATIONS

   a. Diagnostic block to determine whether the source of pain is sympathetic or somatic

   b. Trigeminal neuralgia (most common)

   c. Cancer pain: invasion of orbit, mandible, or maxillary sinus

   d. Intractable cluster headache

   e. Atypical facial pain

3. TECHNIQUE

   a. This procedure must be performed with x-ray or fluoroscopic guidance because of life-threatening side effects (i.e., intra-arterial or
CSF injections).

   b. It is technically difficult.

   c. With the patient in the supine position and the cervical spine extended, a sterile preparation of the face is done, avoiding the eyes.

   d. At 2.5 cm from the corner of the mouth and at the midpupillary
line, local anesthesia is infiltrated into the skin and subcutaneous
tissue.

   e. A 22- or 20-gauge, 10- to 15-cm needle is directed cephalad toward
the medial aspect of the external auditory meatus, passing above
and lateral to the molars.

   f. The needle is advanced until contact is made with the base of the
skull.

   g. The needle is gently repositioned and is walked posteriorly into the
foramen ovale.

   h. Mandibular nerve paresthesia is common. If this occurs, the needle
is redirected until the paresthesia disappears.

   i. The needle stylet is removed after entering the foramen ovale and a
free flow of CSF may be observed.

   j. If no CSF is observed, the needle tip may be anterior to the trigeminal cistern but still within Meckel cave.

k. Contrast medium, 0.1 to 0.4 mL, or the injection of 0.1-mL increments of preservative-free 1% lidocaine and observation of the patient's response may be used for confirmation of needle placement.

l. A negative aspirate of blood or CSF is mandatory before injection. Thermocoagulation and radiofrequency may be the techniques of choice because they avoid the difficulties inherent in chemical neurolysis.

m. Hyperbaric glycerol or phenol (6.5%) in glycerin may be used.

n. Patient should be moved to sitting position with the chin on the chest prior to injection. This favors spread to maxillary and mandibular divisions and spares the ophthalmic division.

o. Absolute alcohol: patient left in supine position.

4. SIDE EFFECTS/COMPLICATIONS

a. Activation of herpes labialis and herpes zoster in 10% of patients

b. Facial and subscleral hematoma

c. Total spinal anesthesia

d. Corneal anesthesia

e. Post procedure dysesthesia and anesthesia dolorosa: 6% of patients; incomplete destruction of the ganglion

f. Weakness of muscles of mastication, Horner syndrome, and facial asymmetry

SUGGESTED READINGS

Raj P: Pain Medicine. A Comprehensive Review, 2nd ed. St. Louis, Mosby, 2003.

Waldman S: Atlas of International Pain Management, 2nd ed. Philadelphia, WB Saunders, 2004.

54 Sphenopalatine Ganglion Block

1. INDICATIONS

   a. Broad applications; in some cases, with little in the literature to support its efficacy

   b. Head and neck cancer

   c. Atypical facial pain, especially if it has a sympathetic component

   d. Successful in a small subset of patients with migraine or cluster headaches

   e. Trigeminal neuralgia: Few case reports support this theory.

2. ANATOMY

   a. It lies in the pterygopalatine fossa

   b. The fossa is posterior to the middle turbinate of the nose and a few millimeters below the lateral nasal mucosa.

   c. The maxillary artery and its branches also are contained within the fossa.

   d. The maxillary nerve is cephalad and slightly lateral to the fossa.

3. PHYSIOLOGY

   a. The ganglion has sensory, motor, and autonomic components.

      i. The sensory fibers from the sphenopalatine ganglion (SPG) block innervate the nasal membranes, soft palate, and parts of the pharynx.

      ii. Postganglionic sympathetic fibers innervate the lacrimal gland and the palatine and nasal mucosa.

      iii. There is no consensus regarding the role of the SPG in the pathogenesis of pain.

4. BLOCKADE

   a. Intranasal topical local anesthetic application

      i. A 3.5-inch cotton-tipped applicator dipped in cocaine or lidocaine is slowly advanced through the nares parallel to the zygomatic arch toward the back of the nasal pharynx.

      ii. A second applicator is advanced slightly superior and posterior to the first.

      iii. The applicators are left in place for 30 to 45 minutes.

      iv. Ipsilateral tearing can be expected.

   b. Greater palatine foramen approach

      i. The foramen is located just medial to the gumline of the third molar. Occasionally, a dimple is identified at the site of the foramen.

    ii. A 120-degree angled dental needle is advanced 2.5 cm through the foramen in a superior and posterior direction. Because the maxillary nerve is just cephalad to the ganglion, a paresthesia may be elicited.

    iii. After a negative aspiration, 2 mL of cocaine or lidocaine is injected.

  c. Infrazygomatic arch approach

    i. This is accomplished with the patient's head in the C-arm.

    ii. When the two pterygopalatine plates are superimposed, they form a vase-like image.

    iii. A curved, blunt-tip needle is inserted under the zygoma, anterior to the ramus of the mandible in a medial cephalad, slightly posterior direction toward the fossa.

      (1) The tip of the needle is advanced until it is adjacent to the lateral nasal mucosa. Once properly placed, 1 to 2 mL of local anesthetic is injected.

    iv. If pain relief is achieved with the preceding blocks, radiofrequency thermocoagulation or electromagnetic field-pulsed radiofrequency lesioning of the SPG can be performed.

    v. The efficacy for SPG block is scant in the current population. It appears to be most efficacious for migraine headaches, atypical facial pain, and sphenopalatine and trigeminal neuralgia.

5. COMPLICATIONS/SIDE EFFECTS

  a. Infection

  b. Epistaxis

  c. Hematoma

  d. Radiofrequency lesioning can cause transient numbness or hypesthesia of the palate, maxilla, or posterior pharynx.

SUGGESTED READINGS

Raj P: Textbook of Regional Anesthesia. Philadelphia, Churchill Livingstone, 2002, pp 223–224.
Waldman W: Interventional Pain Management. Philadelphia, WB Saunders, 1996.

55 Celiac Plexus Block

1. GENERAL

a. The anterolateral horn of the spinal cord is the origin point for the sympathetic innervation of the abdominal viscera.
  i. Preganglionic axons from T5 to T12 join the white communicating rami en route to the sympathetic chain as they exit the spinal cord.
  ii. The axons then pass through the chain to synapses at distal sites, including the celiac, aortic renal, and superior mesenteric ganglia.
  iii. Postganglionic nerves follow along blood vessels to their respective visceral structures.
b. The axons combine to form the greater splanchnic nerve, at T9 and T10; pass through the diaphragm; and end in the celiac plexus.
c. Sympathetic nerves from T10 to T11 and, occasionally, T12 coalesce into the lesser splanchnic nerve and end in either the celiac plexus or aorticorenal ganglion.
d. The celiac plexus is anterior to the aorta, epigastrium, and the crus of the diaphragm.
  i. It wraps around the anterolateral portions of the aorta for several centimeters.
  ii. The plexus is close to the L1 vertebra.
  iii. Fibers within the plexus consist of preganglionic splanchnic nerves, parasympathetic preganglionic nerves from the vagus, some sensory nerves from the phrenic and vagus nerves, and sympathetic postganglionic fibers.
  iv. Nociceptive afferent fibers pass through the celiac plexus, and blockade of these fibers is the goal of the celiac plexus block.
e. These fibers coalesce to form a dense, intertwining network.
  i. The three pairs of ganglia that are formed inside the network are celiac ganglia, superior mesenteric ganglia, and the aortic renal ganglia.
  ii. Postganglionic nerves from these ganglia innervate all of the abdominal viscera with the exception of part of the transverse colon, the left colon, the rectum, and the pelvic viscera.

2. INDICATIONS

a. Multiple abdominal surgeries: can use a corticosteroid preparation added to the local anesthetic solution as an alternative to neurolytic block.
b. Pancreatic cancer or other isolated upper abdominal malignancies: more suited for a neurolytic block.
  i. In addition to pain relief, celiac plexus block also improves gastric motility.

    ii. Complete sympathetic denervation of the gastrointestinal tract allows unopposed parasympathetic activity and increased peristalsis.

    iii. This block is not appropriate for pain from retroperitoneal extension into somatic structures or distant metastases.

  c. Chronic, intractable, abdominal pain of unknown etiology: The celiac plexus block can be attempted after other methods of pain relief have been exhausted and patient has been properly examined and tested for a diagnosis or source of pain.

3. CONTRAINDICATIONS

  a. Patient refusal
  b. Local anesthetic allergy
  c. Severe coagulation disorders
  d. Local infection
  e. Allergy to contrast dye

4. PRONE TECHNIQUE

  a. Obtain informed consent and insert an IV catheter.

    i. Position patient prone with a pillow under the lower abdomen to minimize the lumbar lordosis and allow easier palpation of the spinous processes.

    ii. If positioning is painful to the patient, give premedication through the IV line, but only if the block is not being done for diagnostic performance.

    iii. The block can also be performed with the patient in the lateral position, although this can make needle placement more difficult.

  b. Prep and drape patient in sterile fashion.

    i. Place marks with sterile pen on the following landmarks: spinous processes of T12 and L1 and the inferior border of the 12th rib.

    ii. The T12 spinous process must be correctly identified and marked by following the 12th rib medially and counting cephalad from the L5 spinous process.

  c. The site for needle entry should be marked 7 to 8 cm lateral from the spinous process and immediately inferior to the border of the 12th rib.

    i. Depending on body habitus, use either 20- or 22-gauge needles, 12 to 18 cm long.

    ii. Direct the needle toward the L1 spinous process for block of the celiac plexus.

    iii. Splanchnic nerves are blocked by directing the needle cephalad toward the 11th or 12th thoracic spinous process (**Fig. 55-1**).

  d. Whether the block performed represents a true celiac plexus block or a splanchnic nerve block is determined by the crus of the diaphragm.

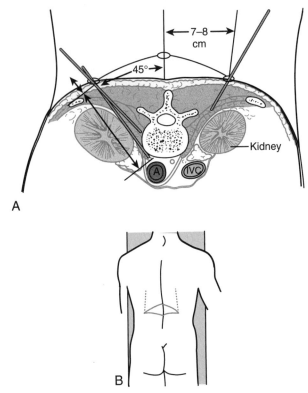

Figure 55–1 A, For a celiac plexus block, the needle is inserted at a 45-degree angle toward the body of L1. The tip slides off the vertebral body anterolaterally and is advanced 1.5 to 2 cm. A, aorta; IVC, inferior vena cava. **B,** Patient positioning and surface landmarks for a celiac plexus block. (From Miller RD, [ed] Miller's Anesthesia, 6th ed. Philadelphia, Elsevier, 2005, p 1712)

      i. If the needle tip is posterior to the crus, the splanchnic nerves will be blocked.

     ii. If the needle tip is anterior and passed transcrurally, the celiac plexus will be blocked.

  e. The amount of sedation required by the patient can be lessened by infiltration with local anesthetics of deep muscular structures and periosteum.

      i. Once the vertebral body has been reached, place a skin marker on the needle 2 to 3 cm from the skin and walk the needle laterally until it just slips from the lateral surface of the vertebral body.

     ii. If adjustments need to be made, make small changes in angle and depth after withdrawing the needle back to the superficial, subcutaneous layer.

f. After passing the lateral aspect of the vertebral body, a "pop" can be felt when the needle passes through the psoas fascia.
   i. The needle then approaches the great vessels and should be advanced slowly.
   ii. On the left will be the aorta and on the right, the inferior vena cava.
g. After proper needle placement, aspirate carefully on both needles before injection.
   i. If blood is found, remove the needle slowly until normal aspiration is achieved.
   ii. On the aortic side, however, pass the needle through the aorta until no blood is seen with aspiration and inject at this location.
h. At first, inject only 2 to 3 mL of a local anesthetic solution containing epinephrine to further diminish chances for either intravascular or intraspinal placement. If results are negative, inject 15 mL of bupivacaine 0.5% with epinephrine 1:200,000 through each needle.

5. ALTERNATIVE TECHNIQUE: ANTERIOR APPROACH

a. An anterior approach to the celiac plexus can be performed by inserting the needle through the abdominal wall at the T12 level.
b. The bowel can be perforated, thus the use of a thin 22-gauge needle is most appropriate.
c. This approach may be beneficial, especially for those patients who cannot lie prone.
d. This procedure is contraindicated in patients with either a large pancreatic mass or other intra-abdominal tumor anterior to the plexus because the needle could possibly puncture these often vascular masses.

6. SIDE EFFECTS AND COMPLICATIONS

a. Hypotension
   i. Secondary to vasodilatation of the large splanchnic bed
   ii. Administer a 500- to 1000-mL IV fluid bolus of lactated Ringer's solution before the block to prevent or minimize the hypotension.
b. Misplacement of needle
   i. Great vessel puncture (most commonly the aorta) results in retroperitoneal hemorrhage.
   ii. Puncture of intervertebral discs repeatedly may cause prolonged back pain.
      (1) Puncture of L1 nerve root can cause paresthesia and painful neuropathies.
      (2) Placement of needle into dural cuff can result in a spinal headache.

    (3) Mistaking the 11th rib for the 12th rib can cause punctur-
ing of the pleural reflection and subpleural place, which
may result in a pneumothorax.

c. Misplacement of infused medicines

  i. Use of epinephrine-containing solutions and aspiration to detect placement of the needle into vessels.

  ii. Local anesthetic infused accidentally into the intrathecal space
can cause a total spinal block.

  iii. Inadvertent injection of alcohol or phenol during neurolytic
block attempts into the intrathecal space is disastrous.

  iv. Medicine that diffuses into the psoas muscle and into the L1
nerve root during attempts at neurolytic blocks will result in
numbness over anterior groin regions and can result in significant motor block if the lumbar plexus is involved.

SUGGESTED READINGS

de Leon-Casasola OA: Sympathetic nerve block. In Raj PP (ed): Practical Management of Pain, 3rd ed. St. Louis, Mosby, Inc., 2000, pp 667–678.

Wedel DJ, Horlocker TT: Nerve blocks. In Miller R (ed): Miller's Anesthesia, 6th ed.
Philadelphia, Elsevier, 2005, pp 1711–1713.

56 Lumbar Facet Block

1. GENERAL

a. The lumbar facet joint in the oblique view has an S-shaped curve.
   i. A thin lucency between the contrast and cortex of adjoined facets outlines the articular cartilage.
   ii. Rupturing of the joint tends to occur at the medial edge of the inferior space.
b. Degenerative arthritis leads to hypertrophy of the facets and cartilage thinning.
   i. The joint space itself is 1 to 2 mL, which becomes smaller after contracture of the space secondary to inflammation, as seen in adhesive capsulitis.
   ii. Synovial proliferation from increased inflammation causes filling defects and lymphatic filling.
c. Facet arthritis and spondylolysis occurring together is a fairly common event.
   i. Communication occurs between a facet joint and an adjacent defective pars interarticularis.
   ii. This relationship was strengthened by studies showing relief of spondylolysis pain with injection at the facet joints.

2. INDICATIONS

a. Focal tenderness over a facet joint
b. Chronic low-back pain with or without radiation but with a normal radiographic evaluation
c. Evidence of disk disease and facet arthritis in the presence of back pain
d. Postlaminectomy syndrome without arachnoiditis or recurrent disk disease

3. CONTRAINDICATIONS

a. Patient refusal
b. Local anesthetic allergy
c. Severe coagulation disorders
d. Local infection
e. Allergy to contrast dye
   i. Facet joint block can be performed without dye or with the use of nonionic contrast, which has a reduced adverse reaction profile.

4. TECHNIQUE: NONRADIOGRAPHIC

a. Not recommended secondary to difficulty of technique without radiographic assistance.
   i. This technique should be used only for lumbar facet joints.
   ii. Place patient in prone position with a pillow placed under the iliac crest on the injured side.
b. Clean the patient's back with sterile preparation.
c. Insert a 22-gauge, 3.5-inch spinal needle perpendicular to the table at an angle of 60 degrees to skin 6 to 8 cm lateral to spinous process midportions.
d. Check for cerebrospinal fluid (CSF) or blood by aspiration on the needle.
e. If no CSF or blood noted, inject 1 to 3 mL of hypertonic saline.
f. If the patient's pain is reproduced, then proceed with injection of 2 to 5 mL of local anesthetic and steroid solution.

5. ALTERNATIVE TECHNIQUE: RADIOGRAPHIC

a. Position patient in the prone position with the affected side elevated by placing a pillow underneath ipsilateral iliac crest. Facet joints can be entered only from a posterior approach in the lumbar and thoracic regions.
b. Flex the hip and knee on the symptomatic side to decrease the lumbar lordosis.
c. Mark the skin where the needles are to be inserted.
d. Prepare and drape the skin in a sterile fashion.
e. Anesthetize the skin and insert a 22-gauge spinal needle vertically toward the facet joint.
f. Care should be taken to pass the tip of the needle directly to the facet joint by observing its tip frequently with fluoroscopy.
g. Sometimes, puncture of the joint capsule can be felt; but, more often, the bone prevents further advance of the needle after entering the joint.
h. When the tip of the needle is superimposed on the facet joint and the needle cannot be advanced any further, the needle tip should be in or very near the facet joint.
i. If injection of multiple joints is needed, inject the most cephalad joint and work caudally.
j. When the needle tip is positioned within the joint, aspirate to ensure there is no return of CSF.
k. Inject the contrast material: Once the needle position is confirmed, 1.5 mL of 0.5% bupivacaine and 20 mg of methylprednisolone acetate are injected into each joint.

6. SIDE EFFECTS AND COMPLICATIONS

a. Allergic reaction: usually an allergy to x-ray contrast or steroid; rarely to local anesthetic

b. Bleeding: rare; bleeding is more common for patients with underlying bleeding disorders.

c. Infection
    i. Minor infections occur in less than 1% to 2% of all injections.
    ii. Severe infections are rare, occurring in 0.1% to 0.01% of injections.

d. Worsening of pain symptoms

e. Discomfort at the point of the injection

f. Nerve or spinal cord damage or paralysis: While very rare, damage can occur from direct trauma from the needle, or, secondarily, from infection, from bleeding resulting in compression, or from injection into an artery causing blockage.

SUGGESTED READINGS

Mooney V, Robertson J: The facet syndrome. Clin Ortho 1976;115:149–156.

Murtagh FR: Computed tomography and fluoroscopy guided anesthesia and steroid injection in facet syndrome. Spine 1988,13(6):686–689.

Neumann M, Raj PP: Facet syndromes and blocks. In Raj PP (ed): Practical Management of Pain, 3rd ed. St. Louis, Mosby, Inc., 2000, pp 745–753.

Pederson HE, Blunck CFJ, Gardiner E: The anatomy of lumbosacral posterior rami and meningeal branches of spinal nerves (sinu-vertebral nerves). J Bone Joint Surg 1956;38A:377–391.

1. GENERAL

a. The medial branches come off the posterior divisions of the lumbar nerves and lie close to the articular processes of the vertebra. These branches then end in the multifidus muscle.
b. The lateral branches supply the sacrospinalis muscle.
   i. The upper three give off cutaneous nerves that pierce the aponeurosis of the latissimus dorsi at the lateral border of the sacrospinalis and descend across the posterior part of the iliac crest to the skin of the buttock, some of their branches running as far as the level of the greater trochanter.
c. The medial branches of the lumbar dorsal rami exit their respective intervertebral foramina, crossing the superior border of the transverse process. The branches then follow along the junction of the transverse process and superior articular process before heading medially to the base of the zygapophyseal joint and under the mamilloaccessory ligament.

2. INDICATIONS

a. Diagnosis of zygapophysial joint pain

3. CONTRAINDICATIONS

a. Patient refusal
b. Local anesthetic allergy
c. Severe coagulation disorders
d. Local infection
e. Allergy to contrast dye

4. TECHNIQUE: NONRADIOGRAPHIC

a. Place the patient in the prone position.
b. Aseptically prepare and drape the patient.
c. Two medial branch blocks are required secondary to the dual innervation of each lumbar facet joint.
   i. Medial branches cross the transverse processes below their origin, as seen with injecting the L3 medial branch at the transverse process of L4 and the L4 medial branch at the transverse process of L5 to block the L4-5 facet joint.
   ii. If the L5-S1 facet joint needs anesthesia, block the L4 medial branch as it passes over the L5 transverse process and the L5 medial branch as it passes across the sacral ala.

d. Using fluoroscopy, identify the transverse process and penetrate the skin using a 22- or 25-gauge, 3.5-inch spinal needle lateral and superior to the target location for L1-L4.
   i. Make contact with the dorsal superior and medial aspects of the base of the transverse process so that the needle top rests against the periosteum.
   ii. Aspirate for cerebrospinal fluid (CSF) or blood before injection.
   iii. Confirm position with contrast injection. Slowly inject (over 30 seconds) 0.5 mL of 0.75% bupivacaine.

e. To inject the L5 medial branch (specifically the L5 dorsal ramus), place patient in the same position.
   i. Maximize exposure between the union of the sacral ala and the superior process of S1 by rotating the C-arm 15 to 20 degrees ipsilateral and obliquely to them.
   ii. Insert a 22- or 25-gauge, 3.5-inch spinal needle directly into the osseous landmarks approximately 2 to 5 cm in an adult until the needle makes contact with the transverse process.

5. SIDE EFFECTS AND COMPLICATIONS

a. Local anesthetic toxicity can occur with large volumes, especially in older or elderly patients.
b. Nerve injury can occur with injection of local anesthetic directly into the nerve.
c. Allergic reaction: usually an allergy to x-ray contrast or steroid; rarely to local anesthetic.
d. Bleeding: a rare complication; bleeding is more common for patients with underlying bleeding disorders.
e. Infection
   i. Minor infections occur in less than 1% to 2% of all injections.
   ii. Severe infections are rare, occurring in 0.1% to 0.01% of injections.
f. Epidural or intrathecal placement of local anesthetic administration. Thus, the use of fluoroscopy with contrast aids in correct placement as well as aspirating for CSF.

SUGGESTED READINGS

Bogduk N, Aprill C, Derby R: Lumbar zygapophyseal joint pain: Diagnostic blocks and therapy. In Wilson DJ (ed): Interventional Radiology of the Musculoskeletal System. London, Edward Arnold, 1995, pp 3-86.

Canale ST: Campbell's Operative Orthopaedics, 10th ed. St. Louis, Mosby, Inc., 2003, p 1975.

Dreyfuss P, Schwarzer AC, Lau P, et al: Specificity of lumbar medial branch and L5 dorsal ramus blocks. A computed tomography study. Spine 1997;22(8):895–902.

58 Lumbar Sympathetic Block

1. GENERAL

a. The lumbar sympathetic chain lies at the anterolateral border of the vertebral bodies.
   i. The lumbar sympathetic chain and ganglia are variable in location, with four sets being more common than five, a result of fusion of the T12 and L1 ganglia.
b. Preganglionic and postganglionic neurons both exist within the lumbar sympathetic chain.
   i. The cell bodies of the preganglionic nerves arise from T11, T12, L1, and L2 and, occasionally, T10 and L3.
   ii. Corresponding anterior spinal nerves carry these axons as they exit the spinal canal, where they join the chain as white communicating rami, and synapse in the appropriate ganglia.
c. Postganglionic axons
   i. Depart the chain as gray communicating rami to become part of the spinal nerves of the lumbar and lumbosacral plexuses
   ii. Or, depart directly to form a diffuse plexus around the iliac and femoral arteries
d. Preganglionic efferent axons, en route to the pelvic viscera, join hypogastric and aortic plexuses.
   i. Afferent, nociceptive fibers in this region accompany the sympathetic fibers and relay pain sensations from the kidney, ureter, bladder, distal portion of transverse colon, left (descending) colon, rectum, prostate, testicle, cervix, and uterus.
e. The anatomic positioning of the lumbar sympathetic chain at the anterolateral border of the vertebral border differs from more cephalad portions of the chain and allows it to be removed from somatic nerves.
   i. The aorta is positioned anteriorly and slightly medial to the chain on the left side.
   ii. The inferior vena cava is more closely approximated to the chain on the right in an anterior plane.
   iii. The psoas muscle is situated posteriorly and lateral to the sympathetic chain.

2. CLINICAL APPLICATIONS

a. Lumbar sympathetic blockade has been used extensively in the treatment of reflex sympathetic dystrophy and causalgia.
   i. Fibers headed for the lower extremity pass through the second and third lumbar ganglia.
   ii. Thus, a sympathetic block placed at this level provides almost complete sympathetic denervation to the lower extremity.

b. Peripheral vascular insufficiency represents the initial indication for lumbar sympathetic block.
   i. Peripheral vascular disease (PVD) continues to be a major reason for sympathetic block, although vascular bypass techniques have partially supplanted use of the sympathetic block.
   ii. Distal disease often responds better to sympathectomy, whereas proximal fixed lesions respond better to surgery.
c. Patients with acute herpes zoster and, possibly, postherpetic neuralgia can benefit from lumbar sympathetic blockade via increased circulation to the vasa nervosum and peripheral structures. This results in decreased inflammation and prevents further neuronal damage.
d. Lumbar block may also be used due to relieve pain from cancer of the lower extremity, gastrointestinal tract distal to the transverse colon, or visceral structures within the pelvis.
e. Neurolysis of the lumbar sympathetic chain can be indicated for recalcitrant reflex sympathetic dystrophy, causalgia, PVD, pelvic malignancies, and deafferentation pain syndromes.
   i. Neurolysis should be considered only after local anesthetic blocks of the lumbar sympathetic chain have documented efficacy but failed to produce long-lasting relief.

3. CONTRAINDICATIONS

a. Patient refusal
b. Local anesthetic allergy
c. Severe coagulation disorders
d. Local infection

4. TECHNIQUE

a. The block is performed while the patient is lying in the prone position with the abdomen resting on a smallish pad.
   i. A Tuohy 18-gauge needle, 12 or 15 cm long, is used.
   ii. The skin is punctured 8 cm lateral to the sagittal plane at the level of spinal processes L2 or L3.
b. The initial angle subtended by the needle is 45 degrees relative to the plane of the skin.
   i. At this angle, some 11 to 12 cm deep, the needle will come up against the bony resistance of the vertebral body, then pull up the needle and increase its angle to make its point go close by the vertebra.
   ii. At 10 cm deep, attach a resistance-free syringe to the needle, and proceed similarly as in epidural space puncture using the method of loss of resistance.

   c. The syringe piston comes up against resistance from the psoas muscle.
- i. Passage through its fascia is followed by a palpable decrease in the resistance to the piston, indicating that the point of the needle has just reached the sympathetic ganglion.
- ii. Ten milliliters of 1% lidocaine injected will induce a complete sympathetic block in the extremity.

5. ALTERNATIVE TECHNIQUE: FLUOROSCOPY

   a. Position the patient prone with one or two pillows placed under the lower abdomen across the anterior iliac crest.
- i. Mark and outline the spinous processes of L2, L3, and L4.
- ii. Check this step further by marking the inferior border of T12 and the posterior iliac crest.
- iii. The midpoint between these two lines, 7 cm from the midline, places the mark at the L2-3 region.

   b. The optimal distance from midline for needle insertion is approximately from 4 to 10 cm.
- i. Distances beyond 8 cm may subject the kidney to possible puncture.
- ii. Distances of 4 to 5 cm, described in the classic approach, do not allow much cross-sectional area of the vertebral body for projection of the advancing needle tip.

   c. Two or three needles have traditionally been placed at the L2, L3, and L4 levels.
- i. Contrast material injected with subsequent x-ray or image intensification has consistently shown good longitudinal spread of solution along the anterolateral border of the vertebral bodies with a single-needle technique.

   d. Advance a 22-gauge, 12- to 18-cm needle slowly until it rests on the vertebral body.
- i. Initially, the needle may be inserted directly toward the vertebral column.
- ii. The angle of the needle with respect to the skin can be as shallow as 45 degrees in thin individuals and somewhat steeper in patients who are more obese.

   e. If the transverse process is bypassed, the bone felt is most likely the vertebral body.
- i. The transverse process should not be confused with the vertebral body whenever shallow bone is encountered.
- ii. Increased adiposity most often exists between skin and transverse process in patients who are obese, making that distance longer and shortening the relative discrepancy between transverse process and vertebral body.

f. Once the vertebral body has been appropriately identified, place a rubber skin marker on the needle 2 to 3 cm from the skin.
   i. Withdraw the needle toward the skin, and redirect it at steeper angle.
   ii. Small-angle changes at the skin are needed secondary to the length of the needle to prevent large changes at the distal end.
   iii. With correct repositioning, the needle will pass just lateral to the vertebral body and rest at the anterolateral border.
   iv. If the needle is placed in the proper location, it should be anterior to the vertebral insertion of the psoas fascia.
g. The aorta and inferior vena cava both lie reasonably close to the sympathetic chain, thus careful aspiration should be done in two planes before injection.
   i. Inadvertent intraspinal placement and intravascular injection can be prevented with test-dose injections of an epinephrine-containing local anesthetic solution.
h. Most preservative-free local anesthetics at commercially prepared concentrations block the sympathetic chain.
i. If a single-needle technique is used, inject 15 mL of volume to ensure proper cephalad and caudal spread of solution.

6. SIDE EFFECTS AND COMPLICATIONS

a. The most common side effect is backache, which results from the placement of the needles through the paravertebral muscles of the back.
b. Intravascular injections of larger volumes of local anesthetics can produce systemic toxicity.
c. Inadvertent subarachnoid injections occur rarely if the needle is mistakenly repositioned from bone into a dural cuff.
d. Not uncommonly, the needle passes through the intervertebral disk.
   i. Any extrusion of disk material would be lateral, away from the spinal canal, and not of any clinical significance.
   ii. Permanent injury is rare.
e. Renal trauma or puncture of a ureter can occur if the needle is inserted more than 7 to 8 cm from the midline.
   i. Injury is minimal unless a neurolytic agent is injected with possible ureteral stricture or extravasation of urine as a result.
f. The genitofemoral nerve or lumbar plexus within the psoas muscle can be accidentally blocked if the needle is placed too far laterally or posteriorly.
   i. This results in numbness or weakness in the groin, anterior thigh, or quadriceps.
   ii. It can also be seen with lateral spread of neurolytic solution from the lumbar sympathetic chain.

SUGGESTED READINGS

de Oliveira R, dos Reis MP, Prado WA: The effects of early or late neurolytic sympathetic plexus block on the management of abdominal or pelvic cancer pain. Pain 2004;110(1-2):400–408.

Fukuda K: Intravenous opioid anesthetics. In Miller R (ed): Miller's Anesthesia, 6th ed. Philadelphia, Elsevier, 2005, pp 379–438.

Price DD, Long S, Wilsey B, et al: Analysis of peak magnitude and duration of analgesia produced by local anesthetics injected into sympathetic ganglia of complex regional pain syndrome patients. Clin J Pain 1998;14(3):216–226.

Rauck R: Sympathetic nerve blocks: Head, neck and trunk. In Raj PP (ed): Practical Management of Pain, 3rd ed. St. Louis, Mosby, Inc., 2000, pp 651–682.

59 Selective Lumbar Nerve Root Block

1. GENERAL

a. The roots of the lumbar plexus emerge from their intervertebral foramina into the fascial plane between the quadratus lumborum muscle posteriorly and the psoas muscle anteriorly.

b. The origin of the lumbosacral plexus is broader than the corresponding brachial plexus in the neck, and the lower sacral roots cannot be easily reached by single injection.

2. INDICATIONS

a. Foraminal stenosis
b. Recess stenosis
c. Far lateral disc protrusions
d. Postoperative epidural adhesions
e. Diagnosing and treating radicular pain/sciatica

3. CONTRAINDICATIONS

a. Patient refusal
b. Local anesthetic allergy
c. Severe coagulation disorders
d. Local infection
e. Allergy to contrast dye

4. TECHNIQUE: RADIOGRAPHIC

a. Place patient in prone position with the injected side elevated at approximately a 30-degree angle.

b. Position patient so there is a perpendicular needle tract toward the safe triangle, a classic injection site underneath the pedicle.

c. The safe triangle is defined by the pedicle superiorly, the lateral border of the vertebral body laterally, and the outer margin of the spinal nerve medially.

c. Prepare and drape the patient in sterile fashion.

d. Apply local anesthetic using 25-gauge needle for skin wheal.

e. Using fluoroscopy, advance a 10-cm, 22-gauge spinal needle to the region of the safe triangle.

f. For the L5 root, tilt the needle in a craniocaudal direction to bypass the iliac wing.

   i. The S1 infiltration of the first sacral nerve root can be performed through the dorsal S1 foramen.

   ii. Confirm needle position by an injection of 0.3 mL of contrast material.

iii. Two milliliters of 0.2% ropivacaine and 40 mg of crystalloid corticosteroid suspension are slowly injected.

5. SIDE EFFECTS AND COMPLICATIONS

a. Allergic reaction: usually an allergy to x-ray contrast or steroid, rarely to local anesthetic
b Bleeding: a rare complication; bleeding is more common for patients with underlying bleeding disorders.
c. Infection
    i. Minor infections occur in less than 1% to 2% of all injections.
    ii. Severe infections are rare, occurring in 0.1% to 0.01% of injections.
d. Technical failure: Inability to insert the needle into the nerve root foramen can occur secondary to obesity, causing poor x-ray pictures, difficulty steering the needle, or severe degree of spondylolisthesis in the lumbar spine.
e. Spinal injection: may occur if the spinal needle enters the intrathecal space in the dural cuff around the nerve root.
f. Nerve injury caused by direct needle trauma.
g. Worsening of the pain: rare complication usually secondary to unknown causes

SUGGESTED READINGS

Christian W, Pfirrmann A, Oberholzer PA, et al: Selective nerve root blocks for the treatment of sciatica: Evaluation of injection site and effectiveness—A study with patients and cadavers. Radiology 2001;221:704–711.
Narozny M, Zanetti M, Boos N: Therapeutic efficacy of selective nerve root blocks in the treatment of lumbar radicular leg pain. Swiss Med Weekly 2001;131:75–80.

60 Selective S1 Nerve Root Block

1. GENERAL

   a. The sacral plexus lies on the back of the pelvis between the piriformis and the pelvic fascia.

      i. In front of it are the hypogastric vessels, the ureter, and the sigmoid colon.

      ii. The superior gluteal vessels run between the lumbosacral trunk and the first sacral nerve, and the inferior gluteal vessels run between the second and third sacral nerves.

   b. The lumbosacral trunk forms the sacral plexus. The anterior division of the fifth and a part of the fourth lumbar nerve appear at the medial margin of the psoas major and join the first sacral nerve.

   c. The nerves from the sacral plexus combine to start forming the sciatic nerve at the lower part of the greater sciatic foramen. The sciatic nerve splits on the posterior thigh into the tibial and common peroneal nerves.

2. INDICATIONS

   a. Foraminal stenosis

   b. Diagnosing and treating radicular pain/sciatica

      i. Patients may have reduced ankle-jerk reflex.

      ii. Symptoms of sciatica originating at this level of the spine may include:

         (1) Pain and/or numbness to the lateral or outer foot

         (2) Weakness that results in difficulty raising the heel off the ground or walking on the tiptoes

3. CONTRAINDICATIONS

   a. Patient refusal

   b. Local anesthetic allergy

   c. Severe coagulation disorders

   d. Local infection

   e. Allergy to contrast dye

4. TECHNIQUE: RADIOGRAPHIC

   a. Place patient in prone position with the injected side elevated at approximately a 30-degree angle.

   b. Prepare and drape the patient in sterile fashion.

   c. Apply local anesthetic using 25-gauge needle for skin wheal.

    d. The S1 infiltration of the first sacral nerve root can be performed through the dorsal S1 foramen.

        i. To perform a selective nerve root block at the level of S1, position the fluoroscopy arm perpendicular to the foramen of S1.

        ii. Insert a 10-cm, 22-gauge spinal needle perpendicular to the surface of the sacrum into the foramen.

        iii. Confirm correct position by image intensifier in two planes and injection of 0.3 mL of contrast material.

        iv. Two milliliters of 0.2% ropivacaine and 40 mg of crystalloid corticosteroid suspension are slowly injected.

5. SIDE EFFECTS AND COMPLICATIONS

    a. Allergic reaction: usually an allergy to x-ray contrast or steroid; rarely to local anesthetic.

    b. Bleeding: a rare complication; bleeding is more common for patients with underlying bleeding disorders.

    c. Infection

        i. Minor infections occur in less than 1% to 2% of all injections.

        ii. Severe infections are rare, occurring in 0.1% to 0.01% of injections.

    d. Technical failure: Inability to insert the needle into the nerve root foramen can occur secondary to obesity, causing poor x-ray pictures, difficulty steering the needle, or severe degree of spondylolisthesis in the lumbar spine.

    e. Spinal injection: may occur if the spinal needle enters the intrathecal space in the dural cuff around the nerve root.

    f. Nerve injury caused by direct needle trauma

    g. Worsening of the pain: rare complication usually secondary to unknown causes

SUGGESTED READINGS

Christian W, Pfirrmann A, Oberholzer PA, et al: Selective nerve root blocks for the treatment of sciatica: Evaluation of injection site and effectiveness—A study with patients and cadavers. Radiology 2001;221:704–711.

Narozny M, Zanetti M, Boos N: Therapeutic efficacy of selective nerve root blocks in the treatment of lumbar radicular leg pain. Swiss Med Weekly 2001;131:75–80.

61 Sacroiliac Joint Block

1. GENERAL

a. The adult sacroiliac joint (SIJ) is auricular and C-shaped.
  i. The short arm of the joint is directed posteromedially and caudally while the long arm is oriented posterolaterally and caudally.
  ii. The size and shape of the SIJ varies among individuals.
b. The SIJ has two hyaline cartilage surfaces joined by fibrocartilage and articular surfaces joined by fibrous tissue.
  i. The SIJ has the features of a synovial joint, such as:
    (1) The presence of synovial fluid.
    (2) Its adjacent bones are connected by ligaments.
    (3) A fibrous capsule surrounds the joint with an inner synovial lining.
    (4) Its surfaces allow motion.
  ii. The anterior articular surface is covered with a thin layer of cartilage and is thicker on the sacrum than on the ilium.
c. SIJ syndrome is a common source of low-back pain.
  i. It can be seen alone or in combination with herniated disk, lateral recess stenosis, or facet syndrome.
  ii. Symptoms include tenderness over the SIJ sulcus, posterior SIJ area, and the muscles adjacent to the SIJ.
d. Lumbosacral flexion and extension may elicit pain, whereas lateral motion only rarely evokes pain in SIJ syndrome.
e. Neurologic findings are usually absent.
f. Fine nerve branches derived exclusively from dorsal rami of spinal nerves S1-S4 provide innervation for the iliosacral joint. These nerves supply the superficial and deep dorsal sacroiliac ligaments as well as the sacrotuberous and sacrospinous ligaments.

2. INDICATIONS

a. SIJ arthritis

3. CONTRAINDICATIONS

a. Patient refusal
b. Local anesthetic allergy
c. Severe coagulation disorders
d. Local infection
e. Allergy to contrast dye

4. TECHNIQUE: RADIOGRAPHIC

a. Cleanse patient with sterile technique; the skin was anesthetized at the site previously marked by visualization under fluoroscopy.

b. Advance a 22-gauge, 3.5- or 5-inch (depending on patient size) spinal needle perpendicularly to the fluoroscopic table.

c. Direct the needle toward the posterior SIJ while keeping the tube in the cephalic direction.

d. Orient the tip of the needle in a cephalic direction.

e. Advance the needle either vertically or angled 10 degrees downward to initially redirect until the needle reaches the joint.

f. Once contact is made with the posterior aspect of the joint, maneuver through the ligaments and capsule into the joint by advancing the needle about 5 to 10 mm, which can usually be done by angling the needle tip slightly laterally to follow the natural curve of the joint.

g. Confirm intra-articular position by injecting 0.2 to 0.5 mL of contrast material.

h. If position is confirmed by the joint outline by contrast, then inject 6 mg (1 mL) of betamethasone sodium phosphate and betamethasone acetate solution and 1 mL of 0.5% bupivacaine hydrochloride.

5. SIDE EFFECTS AND COMPLICATIONS

a. Allergic reaction: usually an allergy to x-ray contrast or steroid; rarely to local anesthetic.

b. Bleeding: a rare complication; bleeding is more common for patients with underlying bleeding disorders.

c. Infection
   i. Minor infections occur in less than 1% to 2% of all injections.
   ii. Severe infections are rare, occurring in 0.1% to 0.01% of injections.

d. Worsening of pain symptoms

e. Discomfort at the point of the injection

f. Nerve or spinal cord damage or paralysis. While very rare, damage can occur from direct trauma from the needle, or secondarily from infection, bleeding resulting in compression, or injection into an artery causing blockage.

SUGGESTED READINGS

Calvillo O, Skaribas I, Turnipseed J: Anatomy and pathophysiology of the sacroiliac joint. Curr Pain Headache Rep 2000;4:356–361.

Grob KR, Neuhuber WL, Kissling RO: Innervation of the sacroiliac joint of the human. Z Rheumatol 1995;54(2):117–122.

Slipman CW, Lipetz JS, Plastaras CT, et al: Fluoroscopically guided therapeutic sacroiliac joint injections for sacroiliac joint syndrome. Am J Physical Med Rehabil 2001;80(6):425–432.

62 | Thoracic Paravertebral Block

1. GENERAL

a. The paravertebral space contains spinal nerves that are contained as small bundles in the adipose tissue of the area. That space lies on either side of the vertebral column as a triangular/wedge shape.

b. The boundaries of this wedge:
   i. Parietal pleura anterolaterally
   ii. Vertebral body
   iii. Intervertebral disk
   iv. Intervertebral foramen medially
   v. Limited by the superior transverse processes posteriorly

c. The spinal nerves in this space are not limited by a thick fascial sheath. Thus, the thoracic paravertebral space is easily anesthetized by injection of local anesthetic.

d. The mechanism of action of the paravertebral block consists of:
   i. Penetration directly into the spinal nerve
   ii. Tracking of the local anesthetic volumes laterally along the intercostal nerve
   iii. Medial expansion throughout the intervertebral foramina.

e. Factors that can affect the level and efficacy of the block are:
   i. Needle advancement inferiorly to transverse process
   ii. Keeping the bevel faced medially
   iii. Large-volume and high-speed injections to overcome mean negative intrathoracic pressures and lack of foraminal stenosis/lateral disc bulging/zygapophysial joint hypertrophy/or epidural fibrosis

2. INDICATIONS

a. Bilateral technique in thoracic surgery and major abdominal vascular surgery
b. Cholecystectomy
c. Cardiac surgery
d. Renal or ureteric surgery
e. Herniorrhaphy
f. Breast surgery (i.e., mastectomy and cosmetic surgery)
g. Treatment of benign or malignant neuralgia in complex regional pain syndromes
h. Hyperhydrosis
i. Rib fractures

3. CONTRAINDICATIONS

a. Patient refusal
b. Local anesthetic allergy

c. Severe coagulation disorders
d. Local infection
e. Allergy to contrast dye. Facet joint block can be performed without dye or with the use of nonionic contrast that has a reduced adverse reaction profile.

4. TECHNIQUE: NONRADIOGRAPHIC

a. The patient can be positioned in the prone, lateral (with blocked side placed superiorly), or sitting position.
b. The patient's back is prepared and draped in sterile fashion.
c. A Touhy needle is advanced perpendicularly to the plane of the patients skin 2 to 3 cm lateral to the spinous process.
d. At a depth of 2 to 5 cm in an adult, the needle will make contact with the transverse process.
e. Re-angle the needle superiorly or inferiorly and advance 1 to 1.5 cm until loss of resistance to air/saline is felt.
f. As the needle passes throughout the superior costotransverse ligament a "click" may be felt on the needle.
   i. Patients may experience paresthesias at this point.
   ii. The dose of local anesthetic required involves a consideration of the number of dermatomes that need to be blocked.
g. No reliable formula has, as yet, been developed; but, typically, in adults, 15 mL will spread over and block at least three dermatomes, and in children, a bolus dose of 0.5 mL·kg will reliably cover at least four dermatomes.

5. ALTERNATIVE TECHNIQUES

a. Using fluoroscopy with contrast injection or continuous monitoring of the needle tip can distinguish paravertebral spaces from intramuscular or intrapleural spaces.
b. Placing paravertebral catheters can be done for longer duration of treatment. The needle is advanced superiorly over the transverse process, which makes feeding the catheter easier.

6. SIDE EFFECTS AND COMPLICATIONS

a. Local anesthetic toxicity can occur with large volumes, especially in older or elderly patients.
b. Nerve injury can occur with injection of local anesthetic directly into the nerve. Use caution if patient complains of severe pain or withdraws from injection.
c. Angling of the needle medially can result in epidural or subarachnoid puncture and total spinal anesthetic. Be careful to always aspirate for blood or cerebrospinal fluid.

d. If the spinal levels are not counted properly and the sensory block occurs below L1, then patients may exhibit quadriceps muscle weakness secondary to femoral nerve block.

e. In younger, muscular patients injection with a large Touhy needle can cause paravertebral muscle pain akin to muscle spasm pain. Injection of local anesthetic into the muscle body before the block occurs (with a 22-gauge needle) can prevent this side effect.

f. Hypotension from spinal injection or intravascular infusion with occasional shock-resistant bradycardia/asystole.

g. Pneumothorax can result from inserting needle too deep and puncturing parietal pleura.

SUGGESTED READINGS

Conacher ID, Kokri M: Postoperative paravertebral blocks for thoracic surgery. A radiological appraisal. Br J Anaesth 1987;59:155–161.

Karmakar MK: Thoracic paravertebral block. Anesthesiology 2001;95:771–780.

Klein SM, Bergh A, Steele SM, et al: Thoracic paravertebral block for breast surgery. Anesth Analg 2000;90:1402–1405.

Richardson J: Paravertebral anesthesia and analgesia. Can J Anesth 2004;51:6, R1–R6.

Thoracic paravertebral block. Available at http://www.nysora.com/techniques/thoracic_paravertebral_block/.

63 Psoas Compartment Block

1. GENERAL

a. Compartment between the psoas major and quadratus lumborum muscles

b. A large volume of injected solution in the compartment anesthetizes the hip and anterolateral thigh.

c. Clinical applications

  i. Psoas compartment block is often used to provide postoperative analgesia for patients undergoing major knee and hip surgery.

  ii. The psoas compartment block offers a single injection rather than three separate needle insertions for anesthesia of the lumbar plexus.

  iii. The technique must be combined with a sciatic block for anesthesia of the entire lower extremity (all areas below the knee).

d. Technique: posterior approach

  i. The patient is placed in the lateral position, with hips flexed and operative extremity uppermost.

  ii. A line is drawn to connect the iliac crests (i.e., intercristal line), identifying the fourth lumbar spine.

  iii. After skin preparation, a skin wheal is raised 3 cm caudad and 5 cm lateral to the midline on the side to be blocked.

  iv. A 21-gauge, 10-cm stimulating needle is then advanced perpendicular to the skin entry site until it contacts the fifth lumbar transverse process.

  v. The needle is redirected cephalad until it slides off the transverse process.

  vi. The lumbar plexus is identified by elicitation of a quadriceps motor response.

  vii. When the needle is in place, 30 mL of solution is injected.

e. Technique: alternative approach

  i. Needle insertion site is the junction of the lateral third and medial two-thirds of a line between the spinous process of L4 and a line parallel to the spinal column passing through the posterior superior iliac spine. (The spinous process of L4 was estimated to be approximately 1 cm cephalad to the upper edge of the iliac crests.).

  ii. The needle is advanced perpendicularly to the skin until contact with the transverse process of L4 is obtained and advanced under the transverse process until quadriceps femoris muscle twitches are elicited.

  iii. Contact must be achieved with the L4 transverse process to establish appropriate needle depth and position.

f. Side effects and complications
    i. The deep needle placement with the posterior (psoas compartment) approach increases the risk of possible epidural, subarachnoid, or intravascular injection.
    ii. Peripheral nerve damage is also a potential risk with this technique (true with all regional techniques).
    iii. Most common side effect of the paravertebral approach to the lumbar plexus is the development of a sympathetic block from extravasation of local anesthetic.
        (1) This unilateral sympathectomy is usually of little clinical consequence, but one of the reasons for choosing a lower extremity block over spinal or epidural blockade is prevention of sympathectomy.
        (2) The advantage of a psoas compartment block is diminished if this effect occurs.

SUGGESTED READINGS

Capdevila X, Macaire P, Dadure C, et al: Continuous psoas compartment block for postoperative analgesia after total hip arthroplasty: New landmarks, technical guidelines, and clinical evaluation Anesth Analg 2002;94:1606–1613.

Chayden D, Nathan H, Chayden M: The psoas compartment block. Anesthesiology 1976;45:95.

1. GENERAL

a. The original approach for steroid deposition until Winnie refined the technique by showing that steroids were more effective when placed at the level of the pathology.

b. Pertinent anatomy
   i. The sacral hiatus is the result of the incomplete fusion of the lower portion of the S4 and entire S5 vertebrae.
   ii. It lies at the most caudal aspect of the sacrum and is covered posteriorly by the sacrococcygeal ligament. This ligament is the point of entry for the performance of this procedure.

c. Indications
   i. Postlaminectomy syndrome: no longer a clear delineation of the epidural space in the lumbar region
   ii. Lumbar spine
   iii. Radiculopathy
   iv. Spinal stenosis
   v. Acute and postherpetic neuralgia
   vi. Vertebral compression fractures
   vii. Coccydynia

d. Contraindications
   i. Patient refusal or uncooperative patient
   ii. Systemic infection or localized infection at the site of needle puncture
   iii. Pilonidal cyst at the base of the spine
   iv. Congenital abnormalities of the dural sac and its contents
   v. Pregnancy

e. Technique
   i. Place the patient in the lateral or prone position with a pillow under the pubis.
   ii. The skin is prepared and draped with use of the sterile technique.
   iii. Locate the posterosuperior iliac spines bilaterally; draw a line connecting them; complete an equilateral triangle in a caudal direction.
   iv. The sacral hiatus lies at the tip of the triangle.
   v. Pierce the sacrococcygeal ligament with a 22-gauge needle at a 45-degree angle. The needle should contact the anterior wall of the sacral canal.
   vi. Withdraw the needle slightly, drop the angle of approach to 20 degrees, and then advance it 1 to 1.5 cm into the canal.
   vii. Before injection of your steroid solution, aspiration should be carried out because a vein or the subarachnoid space can be entered unintentionally (unlikely since the dural sac ends at S2).

f. Complications and side effects
   i. Puncture of the rectum
   ii. Entering a sacral foramina
   iii. Dural puncture
   iv. Infection
   v. Injection into a vein, needle placement in periosteum, marrow of vertebrae
   vi. Subcutaneous injection
   vii. Hematoma, ecchymosis

1. PERTINENT ANATOMY

a. There is a negative cervical epidural pressure that is more pronounced with the patient in the sitting position.
b. Neck flexion moves the cervical enlargement more cephalad resulting in a widening of the epidural space to 3 to 4 mm at C7-T1 (normal, 1.5 to 2 mm).

2. INDICATIONS

a. Cervical radiculopathy
b. Cervicalgia
c. Cervical spondylosis
d. Cervical postlaminectomy syndrome
e. Vertebral compression fractures
f. Upper extremity peripheral neuropathies
g. Postherpetic neuralgia
h. Tension headache

3. CONTRAINDICATIONS

a. Patient refusal or uncooperative patient
b. Drug allergy (local anesthetic)
c. Infection at the site of needle entry
d. Coagulopathy

4. TECHNIQUE

a. Translaminar approach
    i. Fluoroscopic guidance
    ii. Obtain informed consent.
    iii. Achieve anteroposterior view (spinous process is midline to pedicles).
    iv. Sterile preparation and drape with patient in prone position
    v. At the interlaminar foramen, mark skin with Kelly clamp so that the clamp is ipsilateral to the site of pathology, but not more lateral than the lateral margin of the spinous process.
    vi. Infiltrate skin with 1% lidocaine by using a 25-gauge needle.
    vii. A 22-gauge Touhy needle is inserted in a " tunneled view" until it engages the ligamentum flavum. Advance the needle using a lateral fluoroscopic view until the tip is 3 mm posterior to the epidural space.
    viii. Attach a loss-of-resistance syringe (air syringe) to Touhy needle.
    ix. While holding firm pressure on the plunger, advance the needle slowly until a sudden loss of resistance is achieved.

    x. Inject nonionic contrast media (0.2 to 0.5 mL) to confirm epidural spread using lateral fluoroscopic view.

    xi. Confirm adequate contrast media spread to the site of pathology using the anteroposterior fluoroscopic view.

    xii. Inject steroid solution, replace stylet in needle to avoid tracking steroid through the skin, and withdraw the needle.

    xiii. Slowly return patient to sitting position and carefully seat the patient in a wheelchair.

  b. Sitting position

    i. In the sitting position, the cervical spine is flexed and the patient's forehead is placed on a padded sheet in front of him or her.

    ii. The C7-T1 interspace is chosen (because it is the most prominent).

    iii. After the patient's neck is prepared and draped in sterile fashion a skin wheal is made by using 1% lidocaine with a 25-gauge needle.

    iv. Using a 22-gauge Touhy needle, the needle is advanced in an exact perpendicular manner to the floor.

    v. Using either the hanging-drop technique or the loss-of-resistance-to-air technique, the needle is advanced until the epidural space is entered.

    vi. The needle is aspirated (ascertain that the needle is not intravascular or intrathecal) and the medication injected, stylet replaced in the needle, and the needle is removed.

    vii. The patient is gently assisted to a wheelchair.

5. COMPLICATIONS AND SIDE EFFECTS

  a. Intrathecal steroid injection
  b. Arachnoiditis
  c. Meningitis
  d. Hematoma
  e. Infection
  f. Ecchymosis
  g. Spinal cord injury
  h. Injury to nerve roots

66 Thoracic Epidural Approach

1. PERTINENT ANATOMY

a. Ligamentum flavum is not as thick as in the lumbar spine; loss of resistance is less pronounced.
b. There is negative epidural pressure similar to that of the intrapleural pressure.
c. There is an acute downward sloping of the spinous processes, therefore the paramedian approach is widely used.

2. INDICATIONS

a. Chronic pain syndromes
b. Radiculitis
c. Postlaminectomy syndrome
d. Vertebral compression fractures
e. Postherpetic neuralgia

3. CONTRAINDICATIONS

a. Infection at the site of injection
b. Patient refuses or is uncooperative
c. Severe spinal deformity
d. Coagulopathy, untreated bacteremia, or sepsis
e. Severe mitral or aortic stenosis: omit local anesthetic

4. TECHNIQUE

a. Fluoroscopic approach
   i. The patient is positioned prone on the fluoro-table with pillows under the chest to increase thoracic kyphosis.
   ii. Anteroposterior fluoroscopy is performed in a severely cranial-caudad manner. The interlaminar spaces are visualized by the image intensifier in a more caudal direction than the collimator.
   iii. The targeted interlaminar space is visualized, a mark is made, and the skin is infiltrated with 1% lidocaine.
   iv. A Touhy needle is advanced until contact is made with the lamina.
   v. The needle is walked off the lamina, the ligamentum flavum contacted, and the needle is advanced using the loss-of-resistance technique.
   vi. The needle is aspirated to ensure it is not intravascular or intrathecal; 1 mL of dye may be injected to confirm proper placement.

vii. The medication is then injected. The needle is restyletted to avoid a possible epidural cutaneous fistula on removal.

b. Sitting position
i. Patient sits at the edge of the table.
ii. The patient is told to push out the middle of the back in a "scared cat" position, thus making the spinous processes more readily palpable.
iii. The target area is marked, prepared, and draped.
iv. Using the paramedian approach, a point 0.5 inch lateral to the midline at the level of the inferior aspect of the spinous process, a Touhy needle is advanced into the epidural space.
v. The needle is aspirated to ensure that it is not in the intravascular or intrathecal space.
vi. The medication is injected and the needle restyletted to prevent the development of a epidural cutaneous fistula after the needle is removed.

5. COMPLICATIONS

a. Infection
b. Nerve root injury
c. Epidural hematoma
d. Intravascular, subdural, or subarachnoid injection
e. Pleural puncture
f. Postdural puncture headache
g. Ecchymosis of the skin

1. INTRALAMINAR APPROACH

a. Indications
  i. Lumbar radiculopathy
  ii. Spinal or lumbar foraminal spinal stenosis
  iii. Vertebral compression fracture
  iv. Postherpetic neuralgia
  v. Low-back syndrome
b. Contraindications
  i. Pain
  ii. Patient refuses or is uncooperative
  iii. Local anesthetic allergy
  iv. Infection at the site of injection
  v. Coagulopathy
c. Technique: prone position
  i. Patient is positioned in the prone position on the fluoroscopic table.
  ii. An anteroposterior fluoroscopic view is obtained at area of pathology.
  iii. A sterile preparation and draping is done.
  iv. A point is marked above the area of pathology and infiltrated with 1% lidocaine.
  v. A 17-gauge Touhy needle is advanced toward the intralaminar space until it is engaged in ligament.
  vi. The stylet is removed and the needle attached to an air syringe.
  vii. With use of the loss-of-resistance technique, the needle is advanced until either a "giving way" or loss of resistance is felt through the syringe.
  viii. A negative aspiration test is performed and then 1 mL of Omnipaque is instilled to ensure proper needle placement.
  ix. The needle is then injected with the steroid mixture, restyletted, and removed. Restyletting avoids the potential of an epidural cutaneous fistula.
d. Technique: sitting position
  i. The patient is positioned at the edge of the examining table and instructed to push the small of the back out, which allows for greater opening of the intralaminar space.
  ii. The spinous processes are palpated at the area of pathology and a mark is made between them and infiltrated with 1% lidocaine.
  iii. The remainder of the procedure is the same as in the prone position.

e. Complications
   i. Nerve root trauma
   ii. Postdural puncture headache
   iii. Epidural hematoma or abscess
   iv. Intrathecal or intravascular injection of the dye or steroid solution
   v. Backache
   vi. Ecchymosis or infection at the injection site

68 Discography

1. GENERAL
   a. Procedure performed in operating room under sterile conditions
   b. Must have informed consent

2. CONCEPT
   a. Diagnostic procedure for evaluating discogenic segments of the spine
   b. Injection of dye into the nucleus pulposus of the disc may reproduce the patient's pain.

3. INDICATIONS
   a. Axial or radicular pain
   b. Localization of specific intravertebral disk levels prior to surgery
   c. To identify normal disc

4. CONTRAINDICATIONS
   a. Patient refusal
   b. Localized or systemic infection: untreated
   c. Pregnancy
   d. Uncooperative patient
   e. Spinal cord compression with myelopathy
   f. Bleeding diathesis

5. MECHANISM OF ACTION
   a. Intradiscal nociceptive fibers are contained in the annulus fibrosis.
   b. Pressuring the disc stimulates previously sensitized nerve endings causing pain.
   c. If the disc is normal, the patient will feel discomfort.

6. TECHNIQUE
   a. Patient is placed prone on fluoroscopic table.
   b. Sterile preparation and draping.
   c. Fluoroscopic beam: posteroanterior projection to align the margins of the superior and inferior endplates of the vertebral bodies bordering the disc to be tested.
   d. Oblique angulation: Identify a point just lateral to the pedicle where a "bull's eye" approach is used to enter the disc.

e. After piercing the nucleus pulposus, contrast dye is injected fluoro-scopically and the patient's response is noted.
f. Pain or no pain should be determined.
   i. Pain intensity: positive criteria for discography: visual analog scale (VAS) ≥ 6/10 with less than 50 psi intradiscal pressure above opening and less than 3.5 mL of total volume
   ii. Concordance of the pain to the patient's usual experience

7. COMPLICATIONS

a. Discitis
b. Visceral perforation
c. Pneumothorax
d. Neuritis, nerve damage

69 Electrostimulation

1. CONCEPT

a. Based on the "gate control theory of pain" published in 1965
b. Stimulation of large afferent fibers in the dorsal columns closest to the gate, thus preventing the transmission of unusually active small afferent nociceptive fibers
c. Sufficient electrical stimulation is applied, which causes paresthesias covering the pain area without motor effects or discomfort.
d. Impairs vibratory sense but does not affect acute pain

2. INDICATIONS

a. Failed back surgery syndrome: most common
b. Peripheral vascular occlusive disease
c. Segmental injury from spinal cord injury
d. Chronic regional pain syndrome
e. Phantom limb pain
f. Intractable angina
g. Abdominal pain

3. CONTRAINDICATIONS

a. Sepsis
b. Bleeding diathesis
c. Psychological comorbidity
d. Patient refusal
e. Magnetic resonance imaging needs
f. Uncooperative
g. Inability to control device
h. Drug behavior problem
i. Demand cardiac pacemaker

4. TECHNIQUE

a. Must have informed consent; procedure performed in the operating room
b. Trial stimulation
c. Patient is placed prone; a pillow is placed under the costal margin to promote flexion of the spine.
d. Patient is prepared and draped under sterile conditions.
e. Under fluoroscopic guidance, a 15-gauge Touhy needle is inserted in the lumbar area.
f. Epidural space entry is verified and the electrode is inserted through the needle and fluoroscopically guided to the T8-T10 level for lower extremity pain.

g. The electrode is then positioned to the center or either side of the cord to produce electrical stimuli in the area of the predominant pain.
h. The electrode is connected with sterile cables to a battery-powered external testing power source.
i. The parameters of current, frequency, and pulse width are varied so that the patient perceives a pleasant tingling paresthesia covering the area of greatest discomfort.
j. The electrode is sutured into place and externalized to the skin.
k. If, after several days of testing, adequate relief is obtained, a decision is made about whether to permanently implant the system.

5. COMPLICATIONS

a. Cerebrospinal fluid leak
b. Hygroma
c. Infection
d. Subcutaneous pocket malposition
e. Postdural puncture headache
f. Neuritis or nerve root irritation

70 Intradiscal Electrothermal Annuloplasty (IDET)

1. CONCEPT

a. Peripheral parts of the annulus fibrosis contain nociceptive nerves that may become sensitized by chemical and mechanical irritation.
b. Thermal destruction of these sensitized nerves may provide pain relief of discogenic origin.
c. Collagen modification may also play a role in pain relief.
d. Improved disc stability or fissure closure may not occur.

2. SELECTION CRITERIA

a. Constant low-back pain for 6 months or more
b. Failed conservative treatment
c. Concomitant pain reproduced by discogram
d. Less than 30% decrease in disc height
e. No stenosis or instability
f. No evidence of neural compression on magnetic resonance imaging

3. EXCLUSION CRITERIA

a. Prior surgery at symptomatic level
b. Inflammatory arthritis
c. Infection: systemic or localized at procedure site
d. Coagulopathy

4. TECHNIQUE

a. Informed consent obtained.
b. Performed in the operating room under sterile conditions and fluoroscopy.
c. Patient placed prone and prepared and draped.
d. With use of local anesthesia, a thin-walled, 17-gauge needle is placed into the center of the disc.
e. A catheter is passed through the needle and positioned in the posterior portion of the annulus.
f. The coil in the distal 5 cm of the catheter is heated to 90° C for 15 minutes.
g. The patient must be able to report radicular pain; therefore, is only mildly sedated.
h. After heating, intradiscal prophylactic antibiotic is injected.
i. Outcome: 40% of patients have improvement or satisfaction at 1-year follow-up.

5. COMPLICATIONS

a. Discitis
b. Nerve root injury
c. Past treatment for disc degeneration or herniation
d. Increased back pain
e. Osteonecrosis of vertebral body
f. Cauda equina syndrome

71 Vertebroplasty and Kyphoplasty

1. CONCEPT

a. These are conceptually identical procedures, except that kyphoplasty utilizes an inflatable tamp to expand the collapsed vertebral body balloon before the introduction of the mechanical fixation on an injectate (polymethylmethacrylate [PMMA]) is introduced.

b. Prior expansion of the cavity allows infusion of PMMA under lower pressure than vertebroplasty.

2. INDICATIONS

a. Osteoporotic vertebral compression fractures
b. Vertebral angiomas
c. Osteolytic disease
d. Vertebral osteonecrosis

3. CONTRAINDICATIONS

a. Coagulopathy
b. Discitis, osteomyelitis, or sepsis
c. Fracture more than 1 year
d. Significant spinal canal compromise

4. TECHNIQUE

a. Patient is placed in the prone position. The procedure is performed under fluoroscopy or computed tomography scan guidance.

b. An 11-gauge ground marrow needle is directed, under local anesthesia, through a transpedicular approach into the involved vertebrae.

c. Needle depth is assured in lateral fluoroscopic.

d. An intraosseous venogram ensures that the needle tip is not in a blood vessel.

e. The cement is injected under continuous fluoroscopic guidance. It hardens quickly, thus stabilizing the vertebrae.

f. Outcomes: 90% of patients experience pain relief and increased viability at 24 hours postprocedure.

5. COMPLICATIONS

a. Serious complications: 1% to 3%
b. Hemorrhage
c. Rib or posterior element fracture
d. Cement embolization to the lungs or the paravertebral venous plexus
e. Permanent complications: less than 1%
f. Decompression surgery to remove extruded cement or repair of fractured pedicle

72 Nucleoplasty

1. THEORY

a. A method of percutaneous disc decompression that uses radiofrequency energy to ablate nucleus pulposus tissue.
b. The result is a decrease in volume within an enclosed space that leads to a drop in intradiscal pressure, thus reducing the pressure on the nerve roots.

2. PRINCIPLE

a. The intradiscal transmission of energy through a percutaneous electrode excites the surrounding tissues, causing breakage of the molecular bonds of the nucleus pulposus tissue, resulting in the vaporization of disc material into low molecular gases (hydrogen, oxygen, carbon dioxide).
b. The gases exit the percutaneous needle.

3. INDICATIONS

a. Results of magnetic resonance imaging positive for controlled disc herniation
b. Failure of 6 weeks of conservative therapy
c. Discogram-concordant pain
d. Contained disc herniation that is less than 33% of the sagittal diameter of the spinal canal

4. CONTRAINDICATIONS

a. Greater than 1/3 loss of disc height
b. Disc extrusion, free fragment
c. Spinal stenosis or instability
d. Tumor, infection, or fracture of the spine
e. Herniation more than 1/3 sagittal diameter of the spinal canal
f. Complete annular disruption
g. Negative discogram results
h. Obesity

5. TECHNIQUE AND EQUIPMENT

a. The targeted disc is identified and a mark made on the skin.
b. Performed in a similar fashion to intradiscal electrothermal therapy or discography.
c. With the patient in the prone position on the fluoroscopic table, with use of sterile conditions and light sedation, the disc is accessed

by using a posterior-lateral approach with a 17-gauge Crawford needle.

d. The needle is advanced, under fluoroscopic guidance, ventral to the superior articular process to the interface between the annulus fibrosis and the nucleus pulposus.

e. A Perc-D Wand, a 1-mm diameter bipolar instrument connected to a power generator, is advanced into the nucleus pulposus by using the ablation mode.

f. A series of six channels is created within the disc.

g. The disc material escapes in the form of gases (nitrogen, hydrogen, oxygen, carbon dioxide).

h. After the creation of each channel, the wand is withdrawn and the channel is sealed by using the coagulation mode.

i. Approximately 10% of the nucleus pulposus or 1 mL of nuclear material is removed.

j. Complications: similar to those reported after a discogram.

6. OUTCOMES

a. In one study, 45 patients were monitored for up to 6 months.
   i. Two-point reduction in visual analog scale
   ii. Reduced opioid usage
   iii. Increase in patient satisfaction
   iv. Overall success rate: 78%
b. In another study, 30 patients were monitored for 6 months.
   i. Satisfaction rate: 89% with no complications

SUGGESTED READINGS

Raj PP: Pain Medicine: A Comprehensive Review. St. Louis, Mosby Inc., 2003, pp 66–69.

Wallace M, Staats P: Pain Medicine and Management. New York, McGraw-Hill Inc., 2005, 356–359.

73 Implantable Drug Delivery Systems

1. SELECTION CRITERIA

a. Patient acceptance
b. Psychological stability and realistic goals
c. Opioid-tolerant and require long-term opioid therapy
d. Intractable side effects from oral analgesic therapy
e. Intractable spasticity
f. Successful temporary trial in fusion (50% pain reduction)
g. Intractable neuropathic pain after optimal treatment
h. Chronic pain secondary to cancer with a greater than 3-month life expectancy

2. CONTRAINDICATIONS

a. Patient refusal
b. Allergy to the drugs
c. History of frequent septicemia
d. Coagulopathy
e. Less than 3-month life expectancy (relative)

3. TECHNIQUE

a. Patient in lateral position
b. Catheter placement: posterior incision and tunneling of catheter to anterior abdominal wall without repositioning
c. Left or right lateral position depending on whether patient is left- or right-handed
d. Patient is prepared and draped.
e. Two- to three-centimeter incision is made lateral to dorsal spine into subcutaneous fat.
f. By using blunt dissection, a pocket is created in subcutaneous fat.
g. A paramedian approach to the epidural space allows for easier catheter threading.
h. With a 14-gauge Hustal needle, the epidural space is entered by using the loss-of-resistance technique.
i. Ten to 15 mL of saline is injected, dilating the epidural space, which facilitates passage of the catheter.
j. The epidural catheter is passed through the needle to the desired position under fluoroscopic guidance.
k. After needle removal, the catheter is transected 2 to 3 cm beyond the skin edge to allow for easy attachment of the proximal and distal catheter segments.
l. The catheter is secured deep to the fascia.

m. With use of a tunneling tool, the catheter is tunneled subcutaneously around the patient's side and is connected to the pump reservoir.

4. OUTCOMES

a. Varying degrees of success using morphine, hydromorphone, baclofen, clonidine, local anesthetics
b. Decreased incidence of drug side effects
c. Opioid tolerance in some patients

5. COMPLICATIONS

a. Mechanical problems: pump, filter, or implanted device
b. Drug side effects: toxicity- and drug-related side effects
c. Catheter-related injections

74 Deep Brain Stimulation

1. GENERAL

    a. First performed on humans in 1972

2. INDICATIONS

    a. Central pain caused by spinal cord lesions or lower intracranial levels

    b. Pain connected to the spinal thalamic tract

    c. Pain not relieved by spinal cord or peripheral nerve stimulation

    d. Almost always for noncancer pain

    e. Best response: neuropathic, somatic, visceral, and intracranial levels

    f. Phantom or stump pain

    g. Dysesthesias after ablative procedures

    h. Trigeminal neuralgia

    i. Anesthesia dolorosa

3. MECHANISM OF ACTION

    a. Unclear

    b. The system in the thalamus and internal capsule probably does not involve opiates.

4. TECHNIQUE

    a. Under local anesthesia, a burr hole is made 3 cm from the midline in the coronal suture by using computed tomography (CT) or magnetic resonance imaging (MRI) guidance for better localization of the electrode.

5. SITE SELECTION

    a. Type and Severity of pain

    b. Nociceptive pain: Stimulation of the periventricular gray (PVG)/ periaqueductal gray (PAG) provides maximal relief.

    c. Neuropathic pain: Stimulation in and around the thalamus is optimal.

    d. Ablation in and around the internal capsule is preferable because of the small size of the thalamic targets.

    e. Thalamic implantation may cause numbness.

    f. After surgery, a radiofrequency device can be attached that affords the patient independence and mobility.

6. OUTCOMES

a. Deep brain stimulation (DBS) is successful in patients who have cancer with diffuse bone metastasis, brachial or lumbosacral plexopathy, and head and neck cancer pain.

7. COMPLICATIONS

a. Majority due to hardware malfunction
b. Migraine headaches developing in 20% to 25% of patients.

8. TOLERANCE

a. Seems to occur with placement of electrodes in the PVG/PAG regions.
b. Intermittent stimulation and the administration of l-tryptophan for 2 to 3 weeks seems to lessen the occurrence.

9. FUTURE DIRECTIONS

a. More active research is being done on the motor cortex as a possible substitute for DBS.
b. DBS is a late or last option because of difficulty in electrode localization.
c. Performed only by neurosurgeons with a special interest in DBS.

SUGGESTED READING

Coffey R: Deep brain stimulation for chronic pain: Results of two multiunit trials and a structured review. Pain Med 2001;2(3):183–192.

75 | Trigger Point Injections

1. GENERAL

a. Trigger points are discrete, focal, hyperirritable areas located in a taut band of skeletal muscle that produce both a local twitch response and referred pain.

b. Trigger points are classified specifically as active or latent.

   i. An active trigger point causes pain at rest, is tender to palpation, and has a referred pain pattern that is similar to the patient's pain complaints.

   ii. The pain referral is located in a remote part of the body.

   iii. The referral of pain differentiates a trigger point from a tender point.

   iv. A latent trigger point may not cause spontaneous pain, but can cause muscle weakness when palpated.

c. Acute trauma or repetitive microtrauma may lead to trigger points.

d. Microtrauma can occur from immobility, lack of exercise, poor posture, vitamin deficiencies, sleep disturbances, or joint problems.

e. Occupational or recreational activities that produce repetitive stress on a muscle group can cause trigger points.

f. Acute sports injuries, surgical scars, and strains can also cause trigger points.

g. Patients with trigger points usually report decreased range of motion and persistent pain in the extremity involved.

h. This type of pain does not follow a dermatomal or myotomal distribution.

2. TREATMENT

a. Activity and posture modifications are utilized to decrease the stress response.

b. Antidepressants, neuroleptics and nonsteroidal medications are prescribed often.

c. Nonpharmacologic treatment modalities include:

   i. Acupressure

   ii. Ultrasonography

   iii. Application of cold or heat

   iv. Electrical nerve stimulation

   v. Vapo-coolant sprays

   vi. Stretching

   vii. Dry needling

   viii. Local anesthetic injections

d. The vapo-coolant spray and stretch technique involves passively stretching the muscle while simultaneously applying the vapo-coolant spray.

 i. The sudden drop in skin temperature from the spray has an anesthetic effect by blocking both the spinal stretch reflex and pain sensation centrally.

e. Trigger point injections can be performed by either dry needling or by injecting with an anesthetic agent.

 i. A 22-gauge, 1.5-inch needle is adequate.

 ii. A smaller diameter needle may not cause the muscle fiber disruption that is required for a treatment effect and may also get deflected away from the taut muscle by the muscle itself.

 iii. Using a sterile technique, insert the needle 2 cm away from the trigger point, so that the needle can advance into the point at a 25-degree angle to the skin.

 iv. Always withdraw the plunger to ensure no blood vessels were traversed.

 v. If an anesthetic agent is used, inject approximately 0.2 to 0.5 mL of injectate within the taut band.

 vi. Travell recommends stretching the muscles immediately afterward.

 vii. Postinjection pain is common, but the original pain referral should be relieved.

 viii. Reinjection is not recommended until the soreness is resolved.

 ix. Patients are able to return to full activities following the procedure.

3. COMPLICATIONS

a. Vasovagal syncope
b. Infection
c. Pneumothorax
d. Hematoma

4. CONTRAINDICATIONS

a. Anticoagulants
b. Bleeding disorders
c. Infection
d. Allergy to anesthetic
e. Acute muscle trauma

SUGGESTED READINGS

McPartland JM: Travell trigger points: Molecular and osteopathic perspectives. J Am Osteopath Assoc 2004;104:244–249.

Mense S, Simons DG: Muscle Pain: Understanding its Nature, Diagnosis, and Treatment. Philadelphia, Lippincott Williams & Wilkins, 2001.

76 Acupuncture

1. HISTORY

a. During the first few centuries in China, acupuncture began to supplant magicoreligious healing beliefs.

b. Needle-like therapy using bamboo or bone needles to open abscesses contributed to its development.

c. Heat stimulation at precise regions of the body (clearly similar to acupuncture channels) may have preceded needling of acupuncture sites.

d. Bloodletting, at what would later be described as acupuncture points, is another possible origin.

e. "Inner Classic of the Yellow Empire," an East Asian medical text, from the first century B.C., contained acupuncture as one of the key therapies.

2. THEORY: TRADITIONAL CHINESE

a. Based on two opposing forces, the yin and the yang, and the dynamic interaction of people and nature. Health is maintained as long as the forces are in balance.

b. Qi (pronounced "chee") is the concept of energy that flows through different channels (meridians) on the inside and the surface of the body. Each meridian is continuous on its course and is the same on either side of the body.

c. Each meridian is either yin or yang in its nature and is associated with one of the body's internal organs (i.e., the liver channel or meridian).

d. The meridians emerge at the body surface at well-described areas called acupuncture points.

e. There are 361 classic acupuncture points among the 12 paired and 2 unpaired meridians.

3. POSSIBLE MECHANISM

a. Acupuncture activates sensory endings in muscle fibers that, in turn, send signals to the spinal cord and brain.

b. These signals lead to the release of endorphins and enkephalins into the cerebrospinal fluid that block afferent pathways. This, however, does not explain the long-lasting effects of acupuncture seen in many patients.

4. INDICATIONS

a. Recent clinical studies have shown that there may be efficacy in the treatment of acute herpetic neuralgia, bone pain from metastasis, osteoarthritis of the knee, low-back pain, and radicular pain.

b. Initially, in this country, acupuncture was recommended for dental pain, nausea, and vomiting.

5. CONTRAINDICATIONS

a. Patient refusal
b. Pregnancy (relative): avoid points known to induce labor.
c. Bleeding diathesis, anticoagulant drugs (relative): minor bruising
d. Caution in patient with pacemaker: electromagnetic interference
e. May mask symptoms of an acute medical process (i.e., appendicitis)

6. ADVERSE EVENTS

a. Tiredness (8.2%)
b. Drowsiness (2.8%)
c. Worsening of symptoms (2.8%)
d. Dizziness, faintness, nausea, headache, and chest pain (>1%)

7. POINT SELECTION

a. Local points: lie over, on, or in close proximity to the involved area
b. Adjacent points: lie near the affected area
c. Distal points: most often used, points between the elbows and fingers and knees and toes
d. Point combinations/prescription of points
   i. Combining points from the left and right side of the body, front and back, upper and lower body
   ii. Classic or modern prescription

8. WHERE SHOULD THE NEEDLES BE INSERTED?

a. Precise site is specific to each patient.
b. Acupuncture points are felt as depressions between the surface muscular divisions.
c. An acupuncture point is found at a fixed distance of body inches, or Cun, described as equivalent to the greatest width of the distal phalanx of the patient's thumb, from a body landmark (i.e., skin crease or bony prominence).
d. Needle tender points in the affected area.
e. Seventy percent of acupuncture points can be found in the same area as commonly described trigger points.

9. TREATMENT METHOD

a. Insertion of an acupuncture needle to a depth of 0.5 to 8 cm, depending on body location (30- to 32-gauge, personal preference).

b. The angle of needle penetration, the time it is left in place, and whether heat is applied or it is twisted do not seem to be supported by good evidence.

c. Point selection is governed by the constitutional symptoms or pattern of pain presented by the patient.

10. TRAINING INFORMATION FOR PHYSICIANS

a. Contact your state's licensing board (usually 100 to 300 hours of CME credits).

b. Payment
   i. Medicare denies coverage pending proof of scientific efficacy.
   ii. Health maintenance organizations, workmen's compensation vary with regard to coverage on a state-to-state basis.

SELECTED READINGS

Deadman P, Baker K, Al-Khafaj M, et al: A Manual of Acupuncture. East Sussex, England, Journal of Chinese Medicine Publications, 1998.

Helms JM: Acupuncture Energetics. Berkeley, CA, Medical Acupuncture Publishers, 1995.

Mann F: Reinventing Acupuncture. Boston, Butterworth-Heinemann, 2000.

77 Transcutaneous Electrical Nerve Stimulation

1. GENERAL

a. Transcutaneous electrical nerve stimulation (TENS) is a procedure that provides low-voltage electrical pulses to the nervous system by passing electricity through the skin via electrodes.

b. Although the literature on how TENS works is controversial, it is widely accepted that it is an effective treatment for pain.

c. Several theories postulate that TENS stimulates the sensory A fibers with high-frequency stimulation, which closes the "gate" to the transmission of pain in the central nervous system (CNS).

d. TENS allows for pain control without the adverse systemic effects of pain medication.

e. The most frequently utilized mode of stimulation for acute pain is termed the conventional or high-frequency and short-pulse-width mode.

   i. Acts by stimulating AC fibers, which conduct faster than C fibers and block pain. Treatment duration for quick analgesia is 1 to 20 minutes; for short duration analgesia, 30 to 120 minutes.

   ii. Treatment is daily, or several times a day, depending on response and duration of analgesia.

f. The most frequently utilized mode of stimulation for chronic pain is termed low-rate TENS.

   i. Has a slower analgesic effect to help chronic pain more effectively

   ii. Acts by stimulating C fibers and indirectly the hypothalamus

   iii. Endorphins are released from the pituitary and bind to opiate receptors in the brain to produce an analgesic effect.

   iv. Treatment time is 30 to 45 minutes for shorter-duration analgesia and 2 to 6 hours for longer duration.

   v. Treatment is usually one time per day.

g. The intensity of stimulation is increased to the patient's perception of strong paresthesias without muscle contraction.

h. The placebo effect is approximately 30%, which is similar to most medications.

2. INDICATIONS

a. Acute pain
b. Chronic pain
c. Phantom limb pain
d. Postoperative pain
e. Ischemic pain
f. Raynaud's disease

g. Postherpetic pain
h. Osteoarthritis
i. Neuropathic pain
j. Rheumatoid arthritis

3. PRECAUTIONS

a. Anterior neck pain
b. Cardiac disease
c. Epilepsy
d. Over eyes
e. Mucosal surfaces
f. Stroke
g. CNS disorders
h. Incompetent patients
i. Children
j. Wounds

4. CONTRAINDICATIONS

a. Cardiac pacer
b. Over carotid sinuses
c. Pregnant uterus
d. Over pharyngeal area

SUGGESTED READINGS

Nelson RM, Currier DP: Clinical Electrotherapy, 2nd ed. Norwalk, Conn. Appleton & Lange, 1991.
Walsh D: TENS: Clinical Application and Related Theory. New York, Churchill Livingstone Publications, 1997.

78 Therapeutic Heat

1. GENERAL

a. Superficial heat causes an increase in skin and subcutaneous tissue temperature.

b. Examples include hot packs, paraffin wax, fluidotherapy, and infrared light.

c. The goal of heating is to raise the tissue temperature to a therapeutic level without adverse responses.

d. The greatest degree of temperature elevation occurs within 0.5 cm from the skin surface.

e. Muscle temperatures at depths of 1 to 2 cm will require 15 to 30 minutes of heat exposure.

f. Superficial heat can raise the intra-articular temperatures within joints.

g. Adipose tissue insulates against heat; therefore, areas of increased adipose tissue will insulate deeper structures from having an effect from superficial heat.

h. Heat causes both analgesia and relaxation, which are helpful in chronic conditions.

i. Other physiologic effects include:
   i. Increased nerve conduction velocity
   ii. Increased local sweating
   iii. Increased oxygen and nutrient supply at the cellular level
   iv. Increased clearing of metabolites
   v. Increased phagocytosis

j. Heat may cause edema acutely or clear chronic edema.

k. Treatment time is 15 to 30 minutes at 43° C to 45° C.

l. Hot packs or electric heating pads should lie on top of the patient.
   i. The patient should not lie on the pads because this can cause secondary burns or erythema ab igne.

m. Heating is an adjunct, not a cure for any of the indications for which it is used.

2. INDICATIONS

a. Pain and stiffness

b. Muscle spasm

c. Postherpetic neuralgia

d. Collagen vascular diseases

e. Provision of greater extensibility of soft tissue

f. Arthritis

g. Superficial thrombophlebitis

h. Chronic inflammation

3. CONTRAINDICATIONS

   a. Arterial insufficiency
   b. Impaired sensation
   c. Malignancy
   d. Acute inflammation
   e. Infection
   f. Scar tissue
   g. Poor thermal regulation

SUGGESTED READINGS

Hayes K: Manual for Physical Agents, 4th ed. Norwalk, Conn. Appleton & Lange. 1992.

Michlovitz S: Thermal Agents in Rehabilitation, 3rd ed. Philadelphia, F.A. Davis, 1996.

79 Therapeutic Cold

1. GENERAL

   a. Therapeutic cold, or cryotherapy, is a broad term that incorporates ice packs, ice massage, ice immersion, cold whirlpool, and vapo-coolant spray.
   b. Cryotherapy lowers the temperature of the skin and subcutaneous tissue by removing heat from the body by conduction or evaporation.
   c. Conduction is the most common method of cooling and occurs by placing ice packs on the skin or by immersing a body part in cold water.
   d. The extent of the temperature change is proportional to:
      i. The temperature difference between objects
      ii. The time of exposure
      iii. The conductivity of the tissue being cooled
      iv. The type of cooling method
   e. Evaporation cools the skin by applying a liquid to tissue that is colder than the skin temperature itself.
   f. Vapocoolant sprays such as Fluori-Methane are sprayed in a fine stream to drop the skin temperature to 15° C with minimal changes to subcutaneous tissue or muscle temperatures.

2. INDICATIONS

   a. Acute pain. Occurs by several methods:
      i. Slowing nerve conduction velocities
      ii. Anesthetizing the area
      iii. Acting as a counterirritant
   b. Inflammation: applicable during acute stages of sprains and strains
   c. Spasm: reduces spasm; other modalities may now be more effective
   d. Spasticity: occurs with upper motor neuron diseases, reduced for 1 hour
   e. Burns: reduces pain associated with skin sensitivities

3. CONTRAINDICATIONS

   a. Cold urticaria
   b. Cryoglobulinemia
   c. Raynaud phenomenon
   d. Paroxysmal cold hemoglobinuria
   e. Areas of compromised circulation

4. PRECAUTIONS

a. Hypertensive patient: a transient rise in blood pressure can occur
b. Hypersensitivity to cold
c. Thermoregulatory disorders: elderly or very young
d. Arterial insufficiency
e. Over wounds
f. Impaired sensation or cognition

SUGGESTED READINGS

Hayes K: Manual for Physical Agents, 4th ed. Norwalk, Conn. Appleton and Lange, 1992.

Michlovitz S: Thermal Agents in Rehabilitation, 3rd ed. Philadelphia, F.A. Davis Company, 1996.

1. BIOFEEDBACK

a. Electromyographic biofeedback is used to assist the patient in developing voluntary control in neuromuscular relaxation or muscle reeducation after injury.

b. The goal is to train the patient to perceive changes without the use of measuring devices.

c. The most commonly used instruments include those that record peripheral skin temperatures, indicating the extent of vasoconstriction and vasodilatation.

d. Utilizes electronic instruments to measure, process, and feedback reinforcing information by using auditory and visual signals.

e. Allows the patient to make small changes in performance that are immediately noted and rewarded so that large changes can subsequently occur.

f. Measures the electrical activity produced by the depolarization of a muscle fiber as an indication of muscle contraction.

g. Indications
   i. Muscle guarding
   ii. Pain
   iii. Spasticity
   iv. Spinal cord injury

2. MASSAGE

a. Mechanical stimulation of tissue by rhythmically applied pressure and stretching.

b. Pressure compresses soft tissue and distorts nerve endings.

c. Stretching applies tension to soft tissue.

d. Classical types include stroking, compression, percussion, and friction.

e. Has a reflexive effect on cardiovascular system.
   i. Improves circulation back to the heart.
   ii. Stimulates tissue release of histamine and acetylcholine.
   iii. Decreases blood pressure by dilating capillaries.
   iv. Temporarily decrease stroke volume and heart rate.
   v. Stimulate the parasympathetic system, causing decreased respirations.

f. The endorphins that are secondarily released help block pain transmission.

g. Increases blood platelet counts.

h. Indications
   i. Myofascial pain system
   ii. Lymphedema

      iii. Relaxation
      iv. Scar tissue release
  i. Contraindications
      i. Malignancy
      ii. Cellulitis
      iii. Lymphangitis
      iv. Recent bleeding
      v. Deep venous thrombosis

3. TRACTION

a. Causes an increase in vertebral separation, which subsequently decreases the pressure on the discs and articular cartilage of the facet joints.
b. Increases synovial fluid exchange, causing a release of pain-generating metabolites from the discs and facet joints.
c. By reducing the pressure on pain-sensitive structures, pain is secondarily reduced.
d. Cervical traction involves 25 to 50 pounds of pressure
e. Lumbar traction involves 50 to 100 pounds of pressure.
f. Duration of treatment is approximately 20 minutes.
g. Traction applied with intermittent forces is beneficial for foraminal narrowing and assists with disc herniations.
h. Traction applied with continuous force is an effective way to stretch muscles and, therefore, is used primarily with muscle spasm.
i. Indications
    i. Cervical or lumbar muscle spasm
    ii. Cervical or lumbar back pain
    iii. Nerve root dysfunction
    iv. Disc bulging
j. Contraindications
    i. Osteoporosis
    ii. Infection
    iii. Malignancy
    iv. Pregnancy
    v. Congenital spinal deformity
    vi. Ligamentous instability
    vii. Restrictive lung disease
    viii. Active peptic ulcer disease

4. THERAPEUTIC ULTRASOUND

a. Uses sound waves with frequency greater than 20,000 Hz.
b. Can cause temperature elevations in tissues to depths of 8 cm.
c. Converted to heat at the bone-muscle interface.
d. Absorbed and attenuated more in bone, followed by tendon, skin, muscle, and fat.

e. Phonophoresis: technique that uses ultrasound to deliver medication, such as anti-inflammatory drugs and local analgesics, through the skin to the underlying tissue.

f. The techniques utilized are either direct or indirect.

g. The direct technique is the most common type of application. The applicator is moved slowly over a 4-inch area in a circular or back-and-forth motion.

h. The indirect technique is used for uneven surfaces. The applicator and body part are placed in a container of degassed water.

i. Indications
   i. Contractures
   ii. Chronic arthritis
   iii. Bursitis
   iv. Tendonitis
   v. Sprains
   vi. Neuromas
   vii. Musculoskeletal pain

j. Contraindications
   i. Cardiac pacers
   ii. Pregnancy
   iii. Tumors
   iv. Thrombophlebitis
   v. Infected areas
   vi. Epiphysis of growing bones
   vii. Cardiac disease
   viii. Over eyes
   ix. Laminectomies
   x. Impaired circulation

k. Precautions
   i. Unhealed fracture sites
   ii. Over tendon or ligament repairs
   iii. Osteoporosis
   iv. Plastic implants
   v. Metal implants

SUGGESTED READINGS

Cameron M: Physical Agents in Rehabilitation. Philadelphia, W.B. Saunders, 1999.

Hayes K: Manual for Physical Agents, 4th ed. Norwalk, Conn. Appleton & Lange, 1992.

Prentice W: Therapeutic Modalities for Allied Health Professionals, 2nd ed. New York, McGraw-Hill, 2002.

Salvo S: Massage Therapy: Principles and Practice. Philadelphia, WB Saunders, 1999.

Tan JC: Practical Manual of Physical Medicine and Rehabilitation. St. Louis, Mosby-Year Book Inc., 1998.

Section IV

EDUCATIONAL AND
PSYCHOLOGICAL MANAGEMENT

81 Patient Education

1. PATIENT EDUCATION IS DIRECTLY PROPORTIONAL TO COMPLIANCE

a. Poor compliance leads to poor outcomes.
   i. Increased hospitalizations
   ii. Increased health care costs
   iii. Decreased quality of life
b. Compliance is correlated with better patient outcomes.
   i. Increased patient satisfaction
   ii. Improved patient health

2. EDUCATIONAL GOALS

a. Increase patient knowledge about illness
   i. Diagnosis
   ii. Risk factors
   iii. Treatment options
   iv. Prognosis
b. Increase understanding of preventive measures
   i. Lifestyle modification
   ii. Medication regimens
c. Treatment of psychosocial aspects of disease
   i. Anxiety
   ii. Depression
   iii. Isolation

3. POSITIVE PATIENT-PHYSICIAN INTERACTION

a. Helpful educator
   i. Cordial physician and staff
   ii. Patient must understand diagnosis
   iii. Patient must understand illness
b. Patient compliance
   i. Health belief model: Patients don't start therapy because they believe there will be no benefit.
   ii. Patients stop their medication because of side effects or complications with dosing.

   c. Educational environment
      i. Neutral atmosphere
      ii. Demonstrated to improve quality of life

4. OBSTACLES TO EFFECTIVE COMMUNICATION

   a. Illiteracy
      i. At the public hospital, 26% of patients couldn't understand their appointment cards.
      ii. At the same location, 35% of English-speaking patients couldn't understand the health care literature.
   b. Elderly patients
      i. Cognitive deficits
      ii. Increased medications
      iii. Physical limitations

5. EVIDENCED-BASED DATA

   a. Patients treated for rheumatoid arthritis
      i. Randomized to the education group, there was 86% compliance at 12 weeks versus the nonintervention group that had 64% compliance.
      ii. In the education group, only 2 patients stopped the medication because of side effects, but in the nonintervention group 12 patients withdrew from the study.
   b. Patients treated for depression
      i. Counseled patients were compliant 63% versus uncounseled patients who were only 39% compliant.
   c. Written and audio material
      i. Providing patients with written and audio material led to a significant increase in compliance.
      ii. At 6 months, the group with written and audio material had an increase in compliance from 15% to 19%.
      iii. The group without the material had a decrease in compliance of 22%.

SUGGESTED READING

Gold DT, McClung B: Approaches to patient education: Emphasizing the long-term value of compliance and persistence. Am J Med 2006;119(4A):32s–37s.

82 Behavioral Therapy in Pain Management

1. OBJECTIVES

a. Teach more adaptive coping skills
b. Treat comorbid anxiety and mood disorders
c. Promote adherence to treatment and rehabilitation
d. Develop a sense of control over the pain disorder
e. Improve quality of life
f. Diminish the sick role and promote independence
g. Increase sources of support

2. TYPES OF PSYCHOTHERAPIES

a. Behavioral therapy
   i. Relaxation techniques: to decrease the intensity of the perception of pain
      (1) Tension and relaxation of isolated muscle groups to gain awareness of presence of muscle tension
      (2) Mental imagery and diverting attention to a neutral pleasant stimuli as a distraction from pain
      (3) Awareness of body sensations and use of imagery to transform their perception, e.g., pain by warmth
      (4) Diaphragmatic breathing
   ii. Operant conditioning: to avoid maladaptive behaviors
      (1) Avoid "as needed" medications
      (2) Positively reinforce independent behavior and rehabilitation
      (3) Negatively reinforce the sick, dependent, and disable role
   iii. Psychoeducation: to get patient involved in treatment plan and gain understanding about the perception of pain
   iv. Hypnosis
   v. Biofeedback: to gain awareness of bodily sensations such as muscle tension with use of objective measures, such as electromyograms.
b. Cognitive behavioral therapy (cognitive restructuring)
   i. Identify, monitor, and modify cognitive distortions integrated with the pain perception that can increase the intensity of the perception of pain
      (1) For example, catastrophizing "Nothing will ever help me" by "This is a difficult moment that I will be able to handle and there is treatment for it that can help me"
   ii. Problem-solving techniques
c. Spiritual therapy: as a source of support and to regain hope

SUGGESTED READINGS

Haythornthwaite JA, Heinberg LJ: Psychological interventions for chronic pain. In Benzon HT, et al (eds): Essentials of Pain Medicine and Regional Anesthesia, 2nd ed. Philadelphia, Elsevier 2005, pp 209–211.

Thomas EM, Weiss SM: Nonpharmacological interventions with chronic cancer pain in adults. Cancer Control 2000;7(2):157–164.

83 | Group Therapies

1. INTRODUCTORY

a. Treatment outcome is probably the same as that for individual therapy.
b. Cost effective (approximately half as much) for the patient and time efficient for the therapist.
c. Interaction among participants is important because chronic sufferers often feel misunderstood and isolated.
d. Members tend to be supportive and may share similar circumstances.

2. GROUP DYNAMICS

a. Ideally, 5 to 7 patients, which allows time for individual expression.
b. Would consider individual therapy for a potentially disruptive patient.
c. Women are more receptive (than men) to group therapy, seek treatment more often, and tend to have more chronic pain problems.
d. Group members tend to have similar cultural and socioeconomic backgrounds.

3. COMMON ISSUES AMONG CHRONIC PAIN SUFFERERS

a. They feel threatened by their pain condition (something is seriously wrong with me).
b. They have a sense of desperation.
c. The patients tend to deal with overly negative and distorted automatic thoughts: an example of catastrophic thinking.
d. They believe that doctors are supposed to be able to help you and that they are unable to help themselves.

4. THERAPEUTIC APPROACH

a. Assessment questionnaire, 166 items: evaluates cognitive function
   i. Homework assignments
      (1) Done between sessions
         (a) The sufferer endeavors to identify stressors that increase pain and those that don't.
         (b) The therapist attempts to work through these issues with the patient and encourages group participation.

    ii. Goals of therapy

        (1) To have the group members begin to understand the importance of their automatic thoughts and pain-related beliefs.

        (2) Stress–pain connection: Stress increases pain, managing it decreases it.

        (3) How we feel about pain and respond to it is shaped by our judgments and thoughts.

            (a) The teacher's emphasis is on the clients taking more responsibility for their pain through self-management behaviors.

            (b) Clients are in doubt about how to decouple the thought and emotion.

            (c) By learning how to accept their pain, it is possible that one's life will be more satisfying despite the pain, and that one will not equate disability with pain.

    iii. Take-home messages

        (1) "I have pain but it doesn't rule my life."

        (2) It is hoped that clients will begin to view themselves as a well person with pain rather than a disabled sufferer.

5. AVAILABLE RESOURCES

    a. American Psychiatric Association: www.psych.org
    b. National Institute of Mental Health: www.nimh.nih.gov
    c. National Mental Health Association: www.nmha.org

SUGGESTED READING

Thorn B, Kuhajda M: Group cognitive therapy for chronic pain. J Clin Psychol 2006;62:1355–1366.

84 Family Management

1. RESPONSE OF FAMILY MEMBERS TO CHRONIC PAIN

a. Supportive; encourages the chronic pain sufferer to remain socially active and to be as functional as possible. This approach may lessen the pain problem.

b. However, the family unit may reinforce the pain behavior, in which case the pain problem escalates.

c. The effects on the partners of chronic pain sufferers

    i. Coping strategies tend to be ineffective. The problem worsens and this adversely affects the family unit, which then may become dysfunctional.

    ii. The marital relationship

        (1) The chronic pain sufferer tends to become dependent; he or she may no longer fulfill their role in the home, which interferes in the partner's household activities, causing conflict.

        (2) The partner's feelings toward the pain sufferer may have changed resulting in a decrease or absence of sexual activity.

    iii. The effect on the children

        (1) Decreased parenteral tolerance of childhood behavior.

        (2) The child may mimic the sufferer's behavior in an attempt to get attention.

        (3) The shared responsibility for care of the children is altered.

    iv. Social contacts

        (1) As the sufferer becomes more withdrawn, social contacts lessen, resulting in the loss of friends.

        (2) Family members begin distancing themselves from the sufferer as they tire of his or her negativity.

2. FAMILY THERAPY: A BRANCH OF PSYCHOTHERAPY

a. Family members must be involved at the start of pain treatment programs.

b. An attempt is made to help organize the family coping in the best possible way.

c. Family therapy is oriented on the "here and now" and views the whole family as the patient.

d. The emphasis is on communication, not introspection.

e. Typically, a course of family therapy is five or six sessions.

3. AVAILABLE RESOURCES

    a. American Family Therapy Academy: www.afta.org.

    b. American Association for Marriage and Family Therapy: www.aamft.org.

SUGGESTED READINGS

Bonica J: The Management of Pain. Vol. 2, 2nd ed. Philadelphia, Lea & Febiger, 1990, pp 1753–1756.

Snelling J: The effect of chronic pain on the family unit. J Adv Nurs 1994;19:543–551.

85 Aggression

1. GENERAL

a. Pathophysiology: Aggression is behavior that is intended to threaten or inflict physical injury on another person or organism.
b. Functions of anger
   i. Painful emotions
   ii. Painful physical sensations
   iii. Frustrated desires
   iv. Perceived threat
c. Causes of anger
   i. Inferential distortions: emotional reasoning, filtering, etc., lead people into misinterpreting the facts
   ii. Expectations held as demands: the presence of a deeply rooted belief that the world or one's circumstances "have to" or "need to be" a certain way
   iii. Discomfort tolerance: perceived threats to well-being
   iv. Global rating of other people: labeling
d. Key strategies for assessing anger associated with pain
   i. Listen
   ii. Attend not only to what is said, but how it is said
   iii. Offer encouragement
   iv. Identify mistaken beliefs and fears
   v. Try to correct misunderstandings
   vi. Above all, do not get angry yourself
e. Key strategies for anger management
   i. Relaxation
   ii. Cognitive restructuring
   iii. Problem solving
   iv. Communication
   v. Physical exercise
   vi. Changing your environment
f. Resources
   i. American Psychological Association
     (1) 1-800-374-2721
     (2) TDD/TYY 202-336-6123
   ii. American Psychiatric Association: www.psych.org

SUGGESTED READINGS

American Journal of Psychiatry: www.psychiatryonline.org
Bruehl S, Chung OY, Burns JW: Anger expression and pain: An overview of findings and possible mechanisms. J Behav Med 2006;29:593–606.

86 Suicide

1. GENERAL

a. Suicide is the eighth leading cause of death in the United States.

2. RISK FACTORS

a. Gender
   i. Men are more likely to commit suicide, with a rate of occurrence of 18.5 per 100,000 population.
   ii. Men are more likely to attempt suicide in much more violent ways.
   iii. The rate for women was 4.1 occurrences per 100,000 population.
b. Age
   i. Suicide rate increases with age.
   ii. There are two major peaks of incidence among adolescents and young adults with the rate of teenage suicides increasing dramatically.
   iii. People over the age of 65 years have the highest rate of suicide.
   iv. Married people are less likely to commit suicide. Thus, isolated individuals, divorced, widowed people are at higher risk.
c. Ethnicity
   i. In the United States, the majority of suicides occur in whites.
   ii. Studies in 1995 showed the following suicide rates:
      (1) For white men, it was 19.7/100,000 population.
      (2) For black men, it was 12.4/100,000 population.
      (3) For Hispanic men, it was 12.3/100,000 population.
      (4) Native-American men had the highest rate at 20.1/100,000 population.
d. Religion
   i. Protestants have, in the past, had a higher suicide rate than Catholics or Jews.
e. Geography
   i. Western states have the highest suicide rates.
   ii. Rural areas tend to have higher suicide rates per capita than urban areas.
f. Season
   i. Most suicides occur in spring, with the month of May having the most.
   ii. Regions with long dark winters have high suicide rates (i.e., Scandinavia, Alaska, etc.) as do people suffering from seasonal affective disorders.
g. Profession
   i. Police and public safety officers are at high risk secondary to work hours, exposure to violent/gruesome situations, availability of guns, alcohol usage, and high divorce rate.

ii. Doctors, especially those dealing with terminally ill patients, are at high risk.
    (1) In the United States, the equivalent of an entire medical school class commits suicide among all medical fields put together every year.
iii. Dentists also commit suicide at a high rate.

h. Financial/cultural level
   i. Economic depressions increase the risk as do areas with high poverty and crime.
   ii. Certain cultures view suicide as more acceptable than others. For example, historically, the Japanese have viewed suicide as an honorable death in certain situations.

3. CERTAIN ACTIVITIES MAY BE LINKED WITH COMMITTING SUICIDE

a. Selling large property (house, car, etc.)
b. Visiting friends and family members unexpectedly
c. Making a will
d. Buying a gun, hose, or rope
e. Writing suicide notes
f. Visiting a primary care physician
   i. Many patients contemplating suicide visit their primary care physician within 3 weeks before they commit suicide, yet do not divulge they are going to commit suicide.
   ii. Thus, the doctor must carefully interview and examine their patient and be observant for changes in personality or affect.

4. CHARACTERISTICS OF SUICIDAL INDIVIDUALS

a. Preoccupation with death
b. Isolated or withdrawing from social areas
c. No major links to friends or family
d. Emotionally distant
e. Lack of humor and difficulty concentrating: often seem to be "in their own world" and have propensity toward anhedonia.
f. Dwell on the past and lack of hope for the future
g. Feelings of helplessness

5. COEXISTING ILLNESSES

a. Depression
b. Schizophrenia
c. Anxiety disorders
d. Posttraumatic stress disorders (PTSDs)
e. Substance abuse
f. Delirium

g. Dementia
h. Genetic predisposition to suicide
i. Acquired immunodeficiency syndrome
j. Gastrointestinal cancers
k. Head injury
l. Epilepsy
m. Temporal lobe epilepsy
n. Huntington chorea
o. Klinefelter syndrome
p. Multiple sclerosis
q. Porphyria
r. Delirium tremens
s. Cushing disease
t. Renal failure on hemodialysis
u. Peptic ulcer disease
v. Spinal cord injuries

6. THERAPY

a. Medications
    i. Lithium decreased the rate of suicide seven fold in patients with bipolar disorder.
    ii. When dosed correctly for suicidal depression, antidepressants can be quite effective, but it has been estimated that only 8% to 25% of patients on antidepressants are adequately treated.
b. Perform a minimental examination to make sure underlying diagnoses/problems are not being missed and that the patient shows competency.
c. Meet the patient's family to evaluate patient's support system.
d. Thoroughly interview the patient and determine whether:
    i. The patient has had previous suicide attempts
    ii. The patient is medically stable, not under the influence of any drug/intoxication
    iii. The patient has no available firearms
    iv. The underlying mental illness is being treated
    v. The patient has an adequate support system
    vi. The physician trusts that the patient will follow his or her recommendations.

SUGGESTED READINGS

Buzan RD, Butt L: Suicide: Risk factors and management. In Jacobson JL (ed): Psychiatric Secrets, 2nd ed. Philadelphia, Hanley and Belfus, 2001.
Silverman MM, Maris RW: Suicide Prevention: Toward the Year 2000. New York, Guilford Press, 1995.
Soreff S. Suicide. Available at: http://www.emedicine.com/cgibin/foxweb.exe/checkreg@/em/checkreg?http://www.emedicine.com/med/topic3004.htm September 28, 2006.

87 Depression

1. DEMOGRAPHICS

    a. In 1996, Banks and Kerns systematically reviewed 14 studies using Diagnostic and Statistical Manual of Mental Disorders (DSM) criteria for diagnosing depression in patients with chronic pain and found the prevalence of depression to be between 30 and 54.

    b. This is approximately double that of the general population, which, according to the National Comorbidity Study, is 15%.

    c. In 1997, Fishbain et al. reviewed 40 studies directly associated with the relationship between depression and chronic pain. The overwhelming majority supported the hypothesis that depression is a consequence of the chronic pain state.

    d. Studies suggest that both a familial predisposition to depression and a previous personal history of a depressive episode increases the likelihood of developing major depression after experiencing chronic pain.

2. DIAGNOSIS

    a. To diagnose a major depressive episode, at least five of the following criteria must be present during the same 2-week period.

    b. Symptoms must result in a deterioration of function.

    c. At least one of the symptoms must be either depressed mood or a loss of interest or pleasure.

    d. Symptoms
        i. Depressed mood most of the day and nearly every day
        ii. Markedly diminished interest or pleasure in almost all daily activities
        iii. Significant unintentional weight loss or gain
        iv. Insomnia or hypersomnia nearly every day
        v. Psychomotor agitation or retardation that is observable by others
        vi. Fatigue or loss of energy almost every day
        vii. Feelings of worthlessness or excessive or inappropriate guilt
        viii. Diminished ability to think or concentrate
        ix. Recurrent thoughts of death or suicidal ideation
            (1) Cognitive-affective symptoms are weighted more heavily in patients with chronic pain.

    e. These symptoms must not be due to another psychiatric disorder or to a general medical condition (i.e., hypothyroidism).
        i. Major depression in the context of chronic pain is a comorbid condition.
        ii. Therefore, even when pain is treated successfully, major depression will need to be treated simultaneously.

   iii. However, research has established that treating pain without treating depression, or vice versa, will lead to a worse outcome than if both are treated together.

   iv. In general, if a patient meets criteria for depression in the context of chronic pain, even if subthreshold depression (less than 5 of the 9 criteria above), it merits treatment.

   v. There is significant "criterion contamination" when attempting to diagnose depression in the chronic pain population.

   vi. Sleep disturbance, motor retardation, loss of energy, changes in appetite and weight, and other somatic symptoms are common symptoms in chronic pain without depression, and cognition is often affected by chronic pain treatment modalities, particularly by centrally active medications.

   vii. Thus, in chronic pain, specific attention should be paid to the cognitive-affective symptoms of mood and anhedonia (criteria 1, 2, 7, 8, and 9 above)** and if either no. i or no. ii is present, and there are a total of 3 of the cognitive-affective criteria (1, 2, 7, 8, or 9) that persist more than a few weeks, treatment should be considered because even untreated minor depression worsens the outcome of pain treatment.

   viii. Clinical clues that a patient is experiencing a depressive episode in the context of pain management are:

     (1) Relatively rapid increase in medication needs

     (2) Increase in doctor-patient interactions

     (3) Increase in interactions with office personnel

     (4) New plateau in efficacy of analgesics

     (5) Missed appointments

     (6) Lack of participation in or dropping out of other treatment, such as physical therapy or group therapy

  f. When patients exhibit such signs, a focused repeat history and physical should be performed to ferret out the etiology. Pseudoaddiction and diversion must be considered as well as the psychiatric spectrum of disease (see Chapter 90).

3. TREATMENT

  a. Studies have shown that dual-acting agents are more active than selective norepinephrine reuptake inhibitors (NRIs), which are more active than selective serotonin reuptake inhibitors (SSRIs).

  b. This finding, combined with the commonly held belief that serotonin-norepinephrine reuptake inhibitors (SNRIs) have a decreased time to remission of depressive symptoms, make them the first-line agent in treatment.

  c. For maximum combined depression/analgesic efficacy, these agents (Duloxetine, Venlafaxine) should be titrated to their maximum tolerated doses. These medications should not be stopped abruptly.

      i. Recommended dosing
- (1) Duloxetine 30 mg PO every morning for 1 week and then increase to 60 mg PO every morning. If no response after 4 weeks, increase to 90 mg, and then if no response, to 120 mg.
- (2) Venlafaxine SR 37.5 mg for 1 week, then increase to 75 mg for 2 weeks, then to 112.5 for 2 weeks, and so on up to 300 mg.

d. SSRIs are first-line agents in the treatment of a major depressive episode. They may be better tolerated than NRI agents and may be more appropriate when used in the context of a complicated pain regimen.
- i. These agents (fluoxetine, escitalopram, paroxetine, etc.) are frequently underdosed and should be maximized as side-effect profile allows. These agents are dosed in the morning. Fluoxetine has a long half-life.
- ii. Recommended dosing
  - (1) Zoloft 25 mg PO every morning, titrate by 25 mg weekly until goal dosage of 150 to 200 mg PO every morning is reached.

e. Atypical antidepressants (mirtazapine, bupropion) have a role in treating specific symptoms and in augmentation of other antidepressants.
- i. No atypical antidepressant, alone, has been shown to have analgesic properties, so they are not suggested as monotherapy.
- ii. Consider psychiatric consultation.
- iii. Bupropion is the antidepressant of choice for many patients with pain because it tends not to cause sexual side effects or weight gain. Sustained-release bupropion, taken twice daily, is used because it lowers the risk of seizures.
- iv. Recommended dosing
  - (1) Buproprion SR 100 mg in morning for 1 week, 100 mg twice daily for 3 weeks, and increase to 150 mg SR twice daily if needed.

f. Tricyclic antidepressants (TCAs) may also act as analgesics in managing neuropathic pain states.
- i. Dosing, however, is quite different for these entities.
- ii. Side effects (sedation, dry mouth, urinary retention), particularly with the first generation TCAs (e.g., amitriptyline, doxepin, imipramine) limit their use as a primary antidepressant, especially in the elderly.
- iii. These agents (nortriptyline, amitriptyline) should be used for their analgesic and sedative properties and, subsequently, dosed at bedtime.
- iv. Recommended dosing
  - (1) Nortriptyline 10 mg PO at bedtime. Titrate, as tolerated, to a dose of 50 mg PO at bedtime.

(2) Desipramine 25 mg PO at bedtime. Titrate, as tolerated, to a dose of 75 to 100 mg PO at bedtime.

g. Mood stabilizers and antipsychotics are not first-line agents in the treatment of depression.

  i. They may, however, be useful in treating specific symptoms associated with the syndrome.

  ii. Mood lability, agitation, and impulse control can be huge problems in chronic pain treatment and these agents can help with symptom reduction.

  iii. These medications should be utilized in conjunction with psychiatric referral.

  iv. Recommended dosing

    (1) Seroquel 25 mg PO at bedtime. Titrate, as tolerated and required, to a dose of 100 mg PO at bedtime. If symptoms persist, consider referral.

h. Nonpharmacologic treatments should not be discounted.

i. Exercise, as the pain allows, has been shown to improve mood and perceived quality of life.

j. Psychotherapy has been shown to be as effective as antidepressant therapy.

k. Structural and functional brain changes have been demonstrated by positron emission tomography and functional magnetic resonance imaging.

l. In addition, the combination of psychotherapy and antidepressants has been shown to be more effective than either alone.

m. Modern psychotherapy is often goal-specific and time-limited. Referral for these services is recommended.

4. GOALS/REFERRAL

a. The practitioner should not be satisfied with anything less than a partial remission (defined as a 50% reduction in symptoms) at 6 to 8 weeks after initiation of therapy.

b. Partial remission requires dose increase or augmentation, either pharmacologic or psychotherapeutic.

c. If full remission is achieved, therapy should be continued for at least 6 months. Thirty percent of patients will remit with any given SSRI at 8 weeks in the primary care setting.

d. Previous episodes predict recurrence: three episodes yield a 90% likelihood of a fourth. Multiple previous episodes dictate indefinite antidepressant therapy.

e. If full remission is not achieved within 3 months, psychiatric referral is required.

1. DEMOGRAPHICS/BASIC INFORMATION

a. Acute pain almost always causes fear or anxiety.

b. Once safety is assured, fear may recede, but anxiety about pain control and pain recurrence may remain.

c. Anxiety in this context may increase pain and also cause the patient to behave inappropriately, interfering with treatment.

d. Controlling acute anxiety with education and short-term use of benzodiazepines and, in certain cases, with neuroleptics may help the patient cooperate with the remainder of treatment.

e. Studies in the chronic pain population using a structured Diagnostic and Statistical Manual of Mental Disorders (DSM) clinical interview, such as the severe combined immune deficiency (SCID), place the overall prevalence of anxiety disorders between 16% and 29%, close to that of the general population.

f. Patients with chronic pain often worry about many things.
    i. Job performance
    ii. Disability
    iii. Finances
    iv. Family activities
    v. Sexual performance

g. Patient may feel threatened by pain and its consequences.

h. Despite the frequent preexistence of anxiety disorder, its influence on chronic pain should not be minimized.
    i. The increased muscle tension that anxiety produces adds significantly to pain perception.
    ii. Anxiety activates sympathetic outflow, increasing ectopic firing in neuropathic pain conditions and lowering the threshold for nociceptor activation by noxious stimulation.
    iii. Fear of reinjury upon movement, in the extreme called kinesophobia, may promote avoidance of physical activity and deconditioning, leading to musculoskeletal pain conditions.
    iv. Avoidant behaviors may be reinforced by others in the household. As a result, patients may lose their household role, experiencing diminished self-efficacy and other dysphoric cognitions, and increasing risk for major depression.
    v. Patients who are anxiety-sensitive may misinterpret the meaning of sensations associated with their chronic pain. For instance, myofascial pain may be misconstrued as cancer recurrence.

2. DIAGNOSIS

a. The Diagnostic and Statistical Manual of Mental Disorders, Fourth Edition, Text Revision (DSM-IV-TR) lists the following anxiety disorders:
    i. Panic disorder with or without agoraphobia
    ii. Agoraphobia without history of panic disorder

     iii. Specific and social phobias

     iv. Obsessive-compulsive disorder

     v. Posttraumatic stress disorder

     vi. Acute stress disorder

     vii. Generalized anxiety disorder

     viii. Anxiety disorder due to general medical condition

     ix. Substance-induced anxiety disorders

     x. Anxiety disorders not otherwise classified

b. It is easy to see how these disorders can complicate a pain disorder and vice versa. It is best to ask a few screening questions that do not cast a pejorative light on the patient.

     i. Chronic pain causes lots of problems for people and, therefore, naturally is very stressful, often causing anxiety, fear, and worries.

     ii. It is important for me to know about this because stress can influence the success of your treatment.

     iii. Have you been experiencing any anxiety, excessive worries or fears, or behaving in a way that is unusual or problematic?

     iv. How do you handle it (them)?

     v. Is this affecting your life or your ability to manage or cope with your pain?

c. You can then, if you wish, ask more specific questions as listed below, or you may decide to refer to a mental health specialist.

     i. The following table lists the DSM-IV-TR diagnostic criteria for anxiety disorders along with initial screening questions that may help a clinician discover, diagnose, and treat a patient with a chronic anxiety disorder.

     ii. For the sake of completeness, all the anxiety disorders have been listed.

     iii. For the sake of clarity, criteria and questions have been modified to relate specifically to the pain medicine practitioner (**Table 88-1**).

d. When diagnosing an anxiety disorder, it is important to rule out iatrogenic causes.

     i. Patients on short-acting medications, for pain or anxiety, can experience acute psychiatric and physical withdrawal symptoms that approximate anxiety disorders.

     ii. Once a diagnosis is made and other causes are ruled out, treatment is merited.

3. TREATMENT

a. In general, the symptoms of anxiety disorders can be difficult to extinguish. The immediate goal is to reduce suffering while long-term strategies are put in play.

b. The standard treatment for anxiety disorders is the selective serotonin reuptake inhibitor (SSRI) class. Doses should be maximized unless side effects prohibit this.

TABLE 88–1 Anxiety-related Interview Questions

Diagnosis	Interview Questions

Panic disorder without agoraphobia (300.1)
A. Both 1 and 2
  1. Recurrent unexpected panic attacks (see below)
  2. At least one of the attacks has been followed by a month or more of the following:
    • Persistent concerns about having another attack
    • Worry about the implications of the attack or its consequences
    • A significant change in behavior related to the attacks
 	
A-1. Discrete panic attacks during which at least 4 of the following symptoms developed abruptly and reached a peak within 10 minutes:
• Sensation of shortness of breath or smothering
• Feeling dizzy, unsteady, light-headed or faint
• Palpitations, pounding heart, or accelerated heart rate
• Trembling or shaking
• Sweating
• Feeling of choking
• Nausea or abdominal distress
• Depersonalization or derealization
• Numbness or tingling sensations (paraesthesias)
• Chills or hot flashes
• Chest pain or discomfort
• Fear of dying
• Fear of losing control or going crazy
 	
B. Absence of agoraphobia
C. Not due to direct physiologic effects of a substance or general medical condition
D. Not accounted for by another disorder, such as social phobia, specific phobia, obsessive-compulsive disorder, PTSD, or separation anxiety disorder
	Do you ever have panic attacks?
	Do you ever get attacks where you suddenly feel terrified or like you are about to die?
	Do you ever suddenly feel overwhelmed to the point where you become physically ill?
	Do you ever feel afraid to go out of the house because you are worried about becoming overwhelmed or having an attack in front of people?
	Are you a chronic worrier?

(continued)

Diagnosis	Interview Questions
Panic disorder with agoraphobia (300.21) Fear of being in places or situations from which escape might be difficult or embarrassing or in which help might not be available in the event of a panic attack. As a result, restricted activity.	

Generalized anxiety disorder (300.02)
A. Excessive anxiety and worry occurring more days than not for at least 6 months
B. The person finds it difficult to control the worry.
C. Associated with at least 3 of the following 6 symptoms (some symptoms present most days for the past 6 months)
  • Difficulty concentrating or mind going blank
  • Muscle tension
  • Irritability
  • Sleep disturbance
  • Restlessness or feeling keyed up and on edge
  • Being easily fatigued
 	
D. Not caused by another Axis I psychiatric disorder
E. Causing significant distress or impairment in social, occupational, and other important areas of functioning
F. Not due to the direct physiologic effect of a substance or general medical condition, or exclusively during mood disorder, psychotic disorder, or pervasive developmental disorder
	Do you worry about things you really can't control?
	When you worry, do you get physically ill or uncomfortable?

Obsessive-compulsive disorder (300.3) A. Obsessions or compulsions	

Diagnosis	Interview Questions
Obsessions: recurrent and persistent thoughts, impulses, or images that are intrusive and inappropriate and cause distress; not simply excessive worries about real life problems that person attempts to ignore or suppress. The person recognizes that the obsessions are the product of his/her mind.	Do you worry excessively about: • Being dirty or contaminated with germs? • Doing certain things exactly the same way? Is it hard to stop thinking about something over and over (obsessive thought)?
Compulsions: repetitive behaviors that a person feels driven to perform in response to an obsession. The behavior is aimed at preventing or reducing distress or preventing some dreaded event or situation, but is not realistic.	Do you feel like you have to do certain things over and over again, such as: • Wash your hands, shower • Count or check things • Say certain words Is it hard to keep yourself from doing something over and over (compulsive behavior)?

B. At some point the person recognizes that obsessions or compulsions are excessive or unreasonable.

C. Obsessions and compulsions cause marked distress, are time-consuming or significantly interfere with the person's normal routine, occupational functioning, or usual social activities or relationships.

D. Not restricted to association with another Axis I Disorder

E. Not due to the direct physiologic effects of a substance or general medical condition

Anxiety disorder due to general medical condition (293.89)

A. Prominent anxiety, panic attacks, or obsessions or compulsions

B. The direct physiologic consequence of a general medical condition — i.e., pheochromocytoma

C. Not better accounted for by another mental condition — i.e., psychosis with persecutory delusions

(*continued*)

Diagnosis	Interview Questions
D. Causes clinically significant distress or impairment in social, occupational, or other important areas of functioning	
Substance-induced anxiety disorder	
A. Prominent anxiety, panic attacks, or obsessions or compulsions	
B. Evidence for either:	i.e., methylphenidate use
• Symptoms developed during or within 1 month of substance intoxication or withdrawal	
• Medication is directly related to the disturbance	
C. Not accounted for by another anxiety disorder	
Posttraumatic stress disorder (PTSD) (309.81)	
A. The person has been exposed to a traumatic event in which both of the following were present:	Have you ever been in a situation where you, or someone close to you, was almost killed, injured, or threatened in a way that caused you to feel terrified or extremely emotional?
• The person experienced, witnessed, or was confronted with an event or events that involved actual or threatened death or serious injury, or a threat to the physical integrity of self or others.	Some experiences to ask about: • Sexual trauma • Combat experience • Witnessing death and destruction • Physical assaults
• The person's response involved intense fear, helplessness, or horror.	Do you feel like you've never quite gotten over (traumatic event)? Did you ever feel back to normal after you experienced (traumatic event)? Do you have dreams or disturbing thoughts about (traumatic event)?

Diagnosis	Interview Questions
B. The traumatic event is persistently reexperienced in one (or more) of the following ways: • Recurrent and intrusive distressing recollections of the event, including images, thoughts, or perceptions. • Recurrent distressing dreams of the event. • Acting or feeling as if the traumatic event were recurring. Intense psychological distress at exposure to internal or external cues that symbolize or resemble an aspect of the traumatic event. • Physiologic reactivity on exposure to internal or external cues that symbolize or resemble an aspect of the traumatic event. • Persistent avoidance of stimuli associated with the trauma and numbing of general responsiveness (not present before trauma), as indicated by three (or more) of the following: efforts to avoid thoughts, feelings, or conversations associated with the trauma. • Efforts to avoid activities, places, or people that arouse recollections of the trauma. • Inability to recall an important aspect of the trauma. Markedly diminished interest or participation in significant activities	
C. Persistent symptoms of increased arousal as indicated by two (or more) of the following: • Difficulty falling or staying asleep • Irritability or outbursts of anger • Difficulty concentrating • Hypervigilance • Exaggerated startle response	

(*continued*)

Diagnosis	Interview Questions

D. Duration of the disturbance is more than 1 month
E. The disturbance causes clinically significant distress or impairment in social, occupational, or other important areas of functioning.

Acute stress disorder (308.3)

Exposure to a traumatic event with both:

A. The person experienced, witnessed, or was confronted (with) an event with actual or threatened death or serious injury or threat to physical integrity.

B. During or after the event, three or more of the following:

- A sense of numbing, detachment, or absence of emotional responsiveness; a reduction in awareness of surroundings (in a daze)
- Marked avoidance of stimuli that arouse recollection of the trauma
- Marked anxiety or increased arousal
- Causes clinically significant distress or impairment in social, occupational, or other important areas of functioning
- Lasts for a minimum of 2 days and a maximum of 4 weeks and occurs within 4 weeks of event
- Not due to the direct physiologic effects of a substance or general medical condition

Have any previous surgeries or treatment modalities caused you physical injury of disability?
Would previous bad experiences change your decision-making in pain-management?

Do you think these feelings are commensurate with your past experiences or out of the ordinary?

Phobic disorder
Specific phobia (300.29)

A. Marked and persistent fear that is unreasonable, cued by the presence or anticipation of a specific object or situation

Are there any specific things like needles, anesthesia, or physical exams that make you very nervous?
Do you think your fear is more than normal?
If you were faced with it right now, do you think you could handle it?

Diagnosis	Interview Questions
B. Exposure to the phobic stimulus almost invariably provokes an immediate anxiety response	
C. Person recognizes fear is excessive or unreasonable	
D. The phobic situation is avoided or endured with intense anxiety or distress	
E. Significantly interferes with person's normal routine, occupational functioning, or social activities and relationships, or there is marked distress about having the phobia	
F. In individual younger than 18 years, duration of at least 6 months	
G. Not accounted for by another disorder	

Social anxiety disorder (300.23)

Diagnosis	Interview Questions
A. Marked and persistent fear of one or more social or performance situations in which person is exposed to unfamiliar people or by possible scrutiny by others.	Are there any social situations that make you very nervous? When you are in this situation, do you get physically ill or afraid you are being criticized or judged? Does this happen every time you are in this situation?
B. Exposure to specific stimulus almost invariably provokes anxiety.	
C. Person recognizes fear is excessive or unreasonable.	
D. The feared situations are avoided or endured with intense anxiety or distress.	
E. Significantly interferes with person's normal routine (social activities, relationships) or causes marked distress about having the fear	
F. If younger than 18 years, duration is more than 6 months	
G. Not due to physiologic effects of a substance or general medical condition	
H. The fear is not due to an associated general medical or mental condition.	

    i. Recommended dosing: sertraline (Zoloft) 25 mg PO every morning for 1 week. Increase dose by 25 mg weekly until a target dose of 150 to 200 mg is reached and symptoms are controlled.

c. As with depression, serotonin-norepinephrine reuptake inhibitor (SNRI) would be preferred in patients that have a chronic pain comorbidity. However, SNRIs often cause transient anxiety until the central nervous system (CNS) equilibrates.

    i. Recommended dosing: duloxetine 30 mg PO every morning for 1 week, then increase to target dose of 60 mg PO every morning. A benzodiazepine may be used, as necessary, to cover transient anxiety (see below).

d. Benzodiazepines are a necessary evil in the treatment of anxiety disorders – evil, because, if not monitored closely, they can cause a difficult-to-treat psychological and physical dependency and worsen the anxiety and pain; necessary, because they treat acute anxiety very effectively until other treatments, that are indicated for longer term, take effect.

    i. They can be used briefly to great effect for anxiety associated with acute pain. Their use should be closely monitored and, as with opiates, longer-acting agents are preferred.

    ii. Even in a diagnosis of panic disorder, the symptoms usually remit before even the quickest benzodiazepine can take effect. More often, what is being treated in panic disorder is the fear of having another attack.

    iii. Short-term benzodiazepines (alprazolam [Xanax], lorazepam [Ativan]) have significant abuse and diversion potential and should be used only as a last resort in the chronic phase of an illness, or to have on hand as safety.

    iv. Recommended dosing: lorazepam 0.5 to 1.0 mg PO every 6 hours, as needed, for no more than 2 weeks

    v. Long-acting benzodiazepines (clonazepam [Klonopin], diazepam [Valium]) play a significant role in the initial treatment of anxiety disorders.

    vi. They cause an immediate, significant symptom reduction and increase compliance with primary treatments (SSRI, SNRI) that can take up to 8 weeks to exert full effect after being titrated to the appropriate dose. When this time has elapsed, slow benzodiazepine reduction should be attempted.

    vii. Recommended dosing: clonazepam 0.5 to 1 mg PO twice daily for up to 8 weeks, with subsequent taper of 0.5 mg PO weekly

e. A growing literature supports the use of low-dose atypical antipsychotics (quetiapine, risperidone) in place of benzodiazepines for acute anxiety mediation.

    i. They are effective in reducing symptoms and have significantly reduced abuse potential.

    ii. Dose-limiting side effects include somnolence and orthostasis. Long-term side effects include weight gain and considerable increases in hemoglobin A1c.

    iii. This author suggests them as a first-line, short-term agent for anxiety reduction. If need for them persists long-term, psychiatric referral may be merited.

    iv. Recommended dosing: quetiapine 25 mg PO at bedtime with 12.5 mg PO three times daily as needed. After one week, give the total daily dose at bedtime with supplemental doses during the day as needed. Continue to monitor.

4. EXPECTATIONS/REFERRAL

a. As with depression, the minimum acceptable response is partial remission (50% reduction in symptom severity) at 8 weeks.

b. At this point, the regimen should be reviewed with antidepressant maximized and benzodiazepines/antipsychotics appropriately mediating anxiety.

c. General compliance and possible benzodiazepine misuse should also be queried. If full remission is not present at 16 to 20 weeks, psychiatric referral should be initiated.

89 Addiction

1. PATHOPHYSIOLOGY

a. Addiction is a primary, chronic, neurobiologic disease, with genetic, psychosocial, and environmental factors influencing its development and manifestations.
b. It is characterized by behaviors that include one or more of the following:
   i. Impaired control over drug use
   ii. Compulsive use
   iii. Continued use despite harm
   iv. Craving

2. EPIDEMIOLOGY

a. It is estimated that up to 1 in 3 people suffer from at least one type of addiction.
b. The latest estimate for the costs to society of illicit drug abuse alone is $181 billion (2002). When combined with alcohol and tobacco costs, they exceed $500 billion including health care, criminal justice, and lost productivity.
c. One of every $12 of the nation's personal health care expenditures is spent on prevention, diagnosis, and treatment of people suffering from addictive diseases.
d. In 2004, approximately 22.5 million Americans 12 years or older needed treatment for substance (alcohol or illicit drug) abuse and addiction. Of these, only 3.8 million people received it.

3. TREATMENT AND PREVENTION

a. There is compelling evidence indicating that adequate prevention and treatment can reduce addiction rates.
b. No single treatment is appropriate for all individuals.
c. Treatment needs to be readily available.
d. Effective treatment attends to multiple needs of the individual, not just his or her drug addiction.
e. Remaining in treatment for an adequate time is critical for treatment effectiveness.
f. Counseling and other behavioral therapies are critical components of virtually all effective treatments for addiction.
g. For certain types of disorders, medications are an important element of treatment, especially when combined with counseling and other behavioral therapies.
h. Treatment does not need to be voluntary to be effective.

    i. Possible drug use during treatment must be monitored continuously.

    j. Psychotherapy
        i. Family therapy
        ii. Individual therapy
        iii. Group therapy

    k. Pharmacotherapy
        i. Anxiolytics
        ii. Opiate replacement therapy
        iii. Negative reinforcement medications

    l. Other
        i. Acupuncture
        ii. Hypnotherapy
        iii. Criminal justice therapy

4. AVAILABLE RESOURCES

    a. The American Society of Addiction Medicine: www.asam.org
    b. National Institute of Drug Abuse: www.nida.nih.gov
    c. Addiction hotlines
        i. Addiction Help Line: 1 (800) 516-2571
        ii. Alcoholics Anonymous: www.alcoholics-anonymous.org/
        iii. Narcotics Anonymous: www.na.org

SUGGESTED READINGS

The National Treatment Improvement Evaluation Study (NTIES): Highlights. DHHS Publication No. (SMA) 97–3159. Rockville, Md.

U.S. Department of Health and Human Services, Substance Abuse and Mental Health Services Administration, Center for Substance Abuse Treatment, Office of Evaluation, Scientific Analysis and Synthesis, 1997, pp 241–242.

1. BACKGROUND

a. In recent decades, use of opioids for both chronic cancer pain and noncancer pain has been increasing.
b. Several types of opioid misuse include:
   i. Individuals who use opioids prescribed for pain to treat other symptoms such as depression, anxiety, or sleep disturbance
   ii. Patients who are physically dependent on opioids who continue to use opioids beyond the resolution of pain to avoid withdrawal symptoms
   iii. Recreational users who seek euphoric effects, which poses a significant personal risk
   iv. Individuals who divert opioids to share with others or for financial gain, which poses a significant public health risk
c. Although chronic pain and addiction are disorders that frequently occur together, it remains unclear whether substance abuse occurs at a higher rate in patients with chronic pain than in the general population (incidence, ~3%-19%). Nevertheless, opioids should not be denied to patients for fear of potential addiction, even when they have a prior history of substance abuse.
d. Careful supervision and monitoring of opioid therapy helps to reduce opioid misuse and diversion.

2. DEFINITIONS

a. Addiction: aberrant use of a specific psychoactive substance in a manner characterized by loss of control, compulsive use, preoccupation, and continued use despite harm.
b. Dependence
   i. Psychological dependence: need for a specific psychoactive substance either for its positive effects or to avoid negative psychological or physical affects associated with its withdrawal.
   ii. Physical dependence: a physiologic state of adaptation to a specific psychoactive substance characterized by the emergence of a withdrawal syndrome during abstinence, which may be relieved in total or in part by readministration of the substance.
c. Substance abuse: use of psychoactive substance in a manner outside of sociocultural conventions.
d. Tolerance: state in which an increased dosage of a psychoactive substance is needed to produce a desired effect.
e. Pseudo-addiction: patients with chronic pain who may exhibit drug-seeking behavior because their pain is undermedicated. Increasing doses of opioids and improvement in pain control usually eliminate the drug-seeking behavior.

3. DIAGNOSIS

a. Overwhelming focus on opiate issues during clinic visits that impedes progress with other issues regarding the patient's pain

b. Pattern of early refills, escalating use in the absence of acute change in the patient's medical condition

c. Multiple calls or visits to obtain opiates, early refills, steals or tampers with prescriptions

d. Lost, stolen, or spilled medications

e. Supplemental sources of opiates, including multiple providers, emergency room visits, friends and relatives, or illegal sources

f. Use of opioids for purposes other than pain

g. Deterioration in activities of daily living

h. Medical history and physical examination stigmata of abuse or obvious signs of intoxication

i. Positive laboratory markers of possible intravenous drug use (HIV, hepatitis)

j. Discordant urine toxicology screening

SUGGESTED READINGS

American Academy of Pain Medicine, The American Pain Society, and the American Society of Addiction Medicine. Definitions related to the use opioids for the treatment of pain: A consensus document. Chevy Chase, Md, ASAM, 2001.

Chabal C, Erjavec MK, Jacobson L, et al: Prescription opioid abuse in chronic pain patients: Clinical criteria, incidence, and predictors. Clin J Pain 1997;13:150–155.

Fishbain DA, Rosomoff HL, Rosomoff RS: Drug abuse, dependence, and addiction in chronic pain patients. Clin J Pain 1992;8(2):877–885.

91 Detoxification

1. PATHOPHYSIOLOGY

   a. Detoxification is form of drug rehabilitation used to treat alcoholism or other drug addiction.

      i. The process involves abstinence to clear the drug from the body, accompanied by social and environmental support during the associated physiologic and psychological changes.

2. ACUPUNCTURE DETOXIFICATION

   a. Acupuncture detoxification provides an Eastern tradition, which embraces a systemic/holistic perspective that is an adjunctive treatment for addiction to drugs and/or alcohol through stimulating points on the external ear.

3. TREATMENT AND PREVENTION

   a. Detoxification can be said to have three immediate goals:

      i. Provide a safe withdrawal from alcohol or other drug(s) of dependence and enable the patient to become free of nonprescription medications.

      ii. Provide a withdrawal that is humane and that protects the patient's dignity.

      iii. Prepare the patient for ongoing treatment of his or her dependence.

   b. Some detoxification procedures are specific to particular drugs of dependence, but others are based on general principles of treatment and are not drug-specific.

   c. Initial medical assessment should include evaluation of predicted withdrawal severity and medical or psychiatric comorbidity.

   d. The severity of a given patient's withdrawal cannot always be predicted with accuracy.

   e. The initial medical assessment should facilitate selection of an appropriate level of care for detoxification

   f. Every means possible should be used to ameliorate the patient's withdrawal signs and symptoms.

   g. Medication should not be the only component of treatment. Psychological support is extremely important in reducing the patient's distress during detoxification.

   h. The plan of care for detoxification should be individualized.

4. PHARMACOLOGIC MANAGEMENT

a. Two general strategies for pharmacologic management of withdrawal:
  i. Suppression of withdrawal by a cross-tolerant medication
  ii. Decreasing signs and symptoms of withdrawal by alteration of another neuropharmacologic process

5. AVAILABLE RESOURCES

a. National Acupuncture Detoxification Association: www.acudetox.com
b. The American Society of Addiction Medicine: www.asam.org
c. National Institute of Drug Abuse: www.nida.nih.gov
d. Addiction hotlines
  i. Addiction Help Line: 1 (800) 516-2571
  ii. Alcoholics Anonymous: www.alcoholics-anonymous.org
  iii. Narcotics Anonymous: www.na.org

SUGGESTED READINGS

Alling FA: Detoxification and treatment of acute sequelae. In JH Lowinson, P Ruiz, and RB Millman (eds): Substance Abuse: A Comprehensive Textbook 2e. Baltimore, Md, Lippincott Willliams & Wilkins, 1992, pp 402–415.

American Psychiatric Association. Diagnostic and Statistical Manual of Mental Disorders, Fourth Edition. Washington, DC, American Psychiatric Association, 1994.

Otto KC. Acupuncture in the treatment of substance abuse. Acupuncture Today 2001;2(8). Available at: http://www.acupuncturetoday.com/mpacms/at/article.php?id=27724.

Section V

CLINICAL PAIN SYNDROMES

92 Tension Headache

1. PRESENTATION

a. Most common type, but rarely presents to physician self-limited
b. Pressure or tightness around the head
   i. Often extends back from the forehead to the posterior neck
c. Waxes and wanes
d. No nausea, vomiting, bruxism, fever, recent trauma
e. Photophobia or phonophobia may be present

2. PATHOPHYSIOLOGY

a. Both central and peripheral mechanism
b. May share a common biochemical etiology with migraine
   i. Norepinephrine and serotonin implicated
c. Muscle contraction causing vasoconstriction and ischemia no longer thought to play a role

3. DIAGNOSTIC CRITERIA

a. Lasts hours or may be continuous
b. At least two of the following:
   i. Bilateral
   ii. Tightening, nonpulsating quality
   iii. Moderate or mild intensity
   iv. Not aggravated by physical activity
c. Has both of the following:
   i. Only one of: phonophobia, photophobia, or mild nausea
   ii. Neither moderate nor severe nausea or vomiting
d. Subtypes
   i. Infrequent episodic tension-type headache (TTH): headache less than 1 day per month
   ii. Frequent episodic TTH: episodes 1 to 14 days per month
   iii. Chronic TTH: headache more than 15 days per month

4. TREATMENT

a. For mild to moderate episodes:
   i. Acetaminophen: 1000 mg
   ii. Aspirin: 500 to 1000 mg

    iii. Nonsteroidal anti-inflammatory drugs (NSAIDs)
- (1) Ibuprofen: 200 to 400 mg
- (2) Naproxen: 275 to 550 mg

b. Prevention of chronic TTH
- i. Amitriptyline: 10 to 75 mg daily
- ii. Nonpharmacologic therapies
  - (1) Relaxation training
  - (2) Cognitive behavioral therapy
  - (3) Electromyographic biofeedback
- iii. Selective serotonin reuptake inhibitors (SSRIs) have not been shown to have an effect.

93 Cervicogenic Headache

1. CLINICAL PRESENTATION

a. Pain perceived in the head but the source lies in the neck
b. Prevalence: 0.4% to 4.6%; more common in females
c. Mean age of 43 years
d. Begins in the neck and spreads anteriorly to ipsilateral orbital, temporal, or frontal areas
e. Movement or external pressure on the neck precipitates the pain
f. Moderate intensity, nonthrobbing nature
g. Infrequent nausea, vomiting photo/phonophobia
h. Head or neck trauma is common in history

2. PATHOPHYSIOLOGY

a. Common pathway of cervical and trigeminal afferents input to neurons of the dorsal horn of the upper three segments of the spinal cord

3. DIAGNOSIS

a. Depends on clinical and laboratory evidence
b. Head pain referred from the neck, fulfilling the following:
   i. Clinical, radiologic, or laboratory evidence of a lesion within the cervical spine or soft tissues of the neck
   ii. At least one of the following:
      (1) Source of pain in the neck as demonstrated by clinical signs
      (2) Abolition of headache by diagnostic block including greater occipital or lesser occipital nerve block or facet block at C2-C3
      (3) Pain resolving within 3 months of successful treatment of the underlying lesion

4. TREATMENT

a. Medications are not usually effective as the sole treatment.
   i. Nonsteroidal anti-inflammatory drugs (NSAIDs) and muscle relaxants have been used for acute treatment and prevention.
b. Physical therapy plays an important role.
   i. Neck stretching and cervical manipulation
c. Feedback, relaxation techniques, and cognitive-behavioral therapy are also helpful.

1. CLINICAL PRESENTATION

a. One-year prevalence of 12% (18% in women, 6% in men)
b. Peak at 22 to 55 years
c. Seventy-two percent of all patients first present to primary care specialist.
d. Variability in presentation between patients and even between attacks in the same patient
e. Two main types: migraine with aura and migraine without aura
   i. Migraine with aura
      (1) Only 15% to 20% have aura
      (2) Becomes more common as patient ages
      (3) Aura usually precedes headache and lasts 0.5 to 1 hour
      (4) Headache worsens as aura recedes
f. Common features of migraine
   i. Nausea, which usually worsens with headache
   ii. Vomiting, which is typically only seen in childhood
   iii. Photo- and phonophobia are present
   iv. Patient has abnormal sensitivity to sensory stimuli
      (1) Patient will have desire to lie motionless in a dark, quiet room
   v. Pain is moderate to severe and throbbing in quality.
   vi. May be unilateral temporal, coronal, or occipital; it may also change laterality.
   vii. Duration of untreated is 4 to 72 hours

2. PATHOPHYSIOLOGY

a. A primary brain disorder with secondary involvement of meningeal blood vessels
b. The generator of migraines is thought to be in the upper brainstem, most likely nuclei that modulate craniovascular pain afferents.
c. The attack begins with trigeminal neuron release of substance P, a calcitonin gene-related peptide, and neurokinin A.
   i. Neurogenic inflammation, meningeal blood vessel dilatation, and plasma protein extravasation follow.
      (1) Serotonin released from trigeminal nerve endings mediates at least some of these.
d. There is also most likely a central process that results in the cutaneous allodynia experienced by patients.
e. The aura is associated with reduced cerebral activity and oligemia spreading in a wave-like fashion from the occipital area forward.

3. DIAGNOSIS

a. Migraine with aura

   i. At least five attacks fulfilling the following:

     (1) Untreated attacks lasting 4 to 72 hours

     (2) At least two of the following:

       (a) Unilateral

       (b) Pulsating

       (c) Moderate to severe pain intensity

       (d) Aggravated by or causing the avoidance of routine physical activity

   ii. Not attributed to any other disorder

b. Migraine without aura

   i. At least two attacks fulfilling 1, 2, and 3:

     (1) No motor weakness and aura consisting of at least one of:

       (a) Fully reversible visual symptoms that include positive (flickering lights, spots, or lines) and/or negative features (loss of vision)

       (b) Fully reversible sensory symptoms that include positive features (pins and needles) and/or negative features (numbness)

       (c) Fully reversible dysphasic speech disturbance

     (2) At least two of the following are present:

       (a) Homonymous visual symptoms and/or unilateral sensory symptoms

       (b) At least one aura symptom develops gradually over 5 or more minutes and/or different aura symptoms occur in succession over 5 or more minutes.

       (c) Each symptoms lasts from 5 to 60 minutes.

     (3) Headache fulfilling headache without aura

   ii. Not attributed to any other disorder

4. TREATMENT

a. Acute treatment

   i. Triptans are the mainstay for treatment

     (1) 5-HT 1B1D agonists

   ii. Nonspecific pain medications

     (1) Nonsteroidal anti-inflammatory drugs (NSAIDs), acetaminophen, aspirin, and opiates rarely

   iii. Antiemetic drugs

     (1) Promethazine, prochlorperazine, chlorpromazine, or metoclopramide

   iv. Ergot derivatives

     (1) These have been mostly supplanted by the triptans but are still useful in prolonged attacks or in high recurrence rates.

5. PREVENTION

a. Indications for acute treatment include headache that significantly interferes with daily routine despite acute treatment; failure of, contraindications to, or adverse reactions to acute medications.

b. β-adrenergic blockers
   i. Propranolol: 80 to 240 mg day
   ii. Metoprolol: 100 to 200 mg day

c. Antidepressants
   i. Amitriptyline: 10 to 75 mg day
   ii. Fluoxetine: 10 to 80 mg day

d. Anticonvulsants
   i. Topiramate: 100 to 400 mg day

e. Calcium channel blockers
   i. Verapamil: 160 to 320 mg day

f. Nonpharmacologic therapies, including biofeedback, relaxation training, and cognitive-behavioral therapy.

95 Cluster Headache

1. PRESENTATION

a. Rare compared with migraine
   i. Affects 0.1% to 0.9 % of the population
b. Greater incidence in males than in females
c. First attack most likely occurs in individuals in their 20s.
d. Cyclical, can occur the same time of day or the same time of year
   i. Remission period may last several weeks to several years
      (1) Positron emission tomography (PET) scans have implicated the hypothalamic gray area ipsilateral to the pain.
e. Pain begins quickly and reaches maximal levels within minutes.
f. Pain is usually unilateral in the periorbital, temporal, or frontal areas.
g. Can last from 15 minutes to 2 hours
h. Ipsilateral symptoms of autonomic dysfunction, rhinorrhea, or congestion; lacrimation or conjunctival injection; miosis or ptosis
i. Hot-poker pain description

2. PATHOPHYSIOLOGY

a. Activation of ipsilateral posterior ventral hypothalamus on PET scanning
b. Vasodilatation is solely extracerebral in contrast to migraines.
c. Trigeminovascular system is most likely the final common pathway.

3. DIAGNOSIS

a. At least five attacks fulfilling b to d
b. Severe or very severe unilateral orbital, supraorbital, or temporal pain that lasts 15 to 180 minutes if untreated
c. Headache has at least one of the following:
   i. Ipsilateral conjunctival injection or lacrimation
   ii. Ipsilateral nasal congestion or rhinorrhea
   iii. Ipsilateral eyelid edema
   iv. Ipsilateral forehead or facial sweating
   v. Ipsilateral miosis or ptosis
   vi. Sense of restlessness or agitation
d. Attacks have a frequency of every other day up to eight per day.
e. Not attributable any other disorder

4. TREATMENT

  a. Abortive treatments
   i.   100% oxygen via face mask for up to 15 minutes
   ii. Lidocaine 4% drops in ipsilateral nostril
   iii. Olanzapine: 2.5 to 10 mg PO at onset
   iv. Sumatriptan: 6 mg SC
   v.   Dihydroergotamine: 1 mg IM, IV, SC at onset; may repeat hourly for up to 3 mg
   vi. Zolmitriptan: 2.5 to 10 mg at onset, up to 10 mg/day and 30 mg/week
  b. Preventative treatments
   i.   Prednisone: 60 mg/day with a gradual taper over 3 weeks
   ii. Ergotamine: 2 mg PO per day, but cannot be given with triptans
   iii. Verapamil: 240 to 720 mg/day with monitoring by electrocardiogram
   iv. Topiramate: 15 to 125 mg/day
   v.   Melatonin: 10 mg/day

96 Postdural Puncture Headache

1. CLINICAL PRESENTATION

a. Onset is within 3 days of procedure in 90% of cases.
  i. Onset is within the first 48 hours in 66% of cases.
  ii. Rarely between 5 and 14 days
  iii. Rarely immediately following
b. Location is predominantly over frontal and occipital areas
  i. Frequently radiates to neck and shoulders.
c. Pain is severe
d. Exacerbated by movement and changing to an upright posture
e. Relieved by lying down
f. Hallmark is worsening on changing from lying to standing
g. Associated symptoms: nausea, vomiting, tinnitus, vertigo, and diplopia

2. PATHOPHYSIOLOGY

a. Dural puncture secondary to diagnostic spinal tap or accidental dural puncture from epidural anesthesia
b. Loss of cerebrospinal fluid (CSF) leads to intracranial hypotension.
c. Magnetic resonance imaging (MRI) can demonstrate sagging of the intracranial structures and meningeal enhancement.
  i. The enhancement is attributed to the vasodilatation of thin-walled vessels in response to the hypotension.
  ii. Two possible mechanisms:
    (1) Low pressure leads to traction on intracranial structures in the upright position.
    (2) Monro-Kellie hypothesis states that the sum of the volumes of the brain, CSF, and blood must remain constant.
      (a) The venodilation would then be responsible for the headache.
d. Seventy-two percent resolve within 7 days; 85% resolve within 6 weeks.

3. DIAGNOSIS

a. A history of accidental or deliberate dural puncture is necessary.
b. Tests
  i. MRI with findings as described above
  ii. Lumbar puncture with low CSF pressure
c. Major intracranial pathology must be excluded.
d. The presence of a severe postural headache is necessary.

4. TREATMENT

a. Epidural blood patch (EBP) is the standard.
  i. Must rule out infection in the back or bloodstream and coagulopathy
  ii. 88% to 96% initial efficacy
  iii. Headache may still recur in up to 50% of patients.
    (1) Repeat of EBP does not decrease efficacy rates.
    (2) In recurrent headache, it is necessary to reevaluate for other possible causes.
b. Temporizing treatments can include:
  i. Caffeine: 300 to 500 mg PO or IV twice daily
  ii. Tight abdominal binder
  iii. Keeping the patient lying flat

97 Spontaneous Intracranial Hypotension

1. CLINICAL PRESENTATION

  a. The headache is usually generalized.
   i. May be frontal, occipital, or nuchal
  b. Not relieved by analgesics
  c. Aggravated by upright position, vigorous movement, jugular compression, Valsalva maneuver
  d. Visual symptoms have been reported, including diplopia, scotoma, and blurred vision
  e. Auditory and vestibular symptoms are present similar to postdural puncture headache (PDPH)

2. PATHOPHYSIOLOGY

  a. Leak of cerebrospinal fluid (CSF) from unidentified cause
  b. Three proposed mechanisms
   i. Occult tear
    (1) This can occur after the dura has been subject to complex motion as in racquet sports.
    (2) Tarlov cysts may predispose patients to leaks.
    (3) Spinal arachnoid diverticula are more common in patients with Marfan syndrome and this may predispose them to tears.
   ii. Decreased production is an unlikely cause.
   iii. CSF overabsorption is also an unlikely cause.
   iv. The specific pathophysiology producing pain is likely the same as in PDPH.

3. DIAGNOSIS

  a. Magnetic resonance imaging (MRI) findings are similar to PDPH.
  b. Computed tomography (CT)-myelogram will show extravasation of the CSF into the paraspinal soft tissue.
  c. Radionuclide cisternography
   i. Primary use is to show location of CSF leak
   ii. Would show abnormally rapid bladder presence of dye in states of CSF overabsorption
   iii. In a theoretical case of decreased production, it would show abnormally slow ascent.

4. TREATMENT

  a. Epidural blood patch (EBP) is the initial therapy after location of leak is identified.
   i. One study reported a success rate of 36% with the initial EBP, 33% for a second, and 50% in patients receiving four or more.
  b. Surgical closure of leak may be necessary for recurrent leaks.

98 Trigeminal Neuralgia

1. PATHOPHYSIOLOGY

a. Trigeminal neuralgia most commonly occurs from arterial compression of the nerve at the skull base (an ecstatic basilar artery is most commonly the culprit). Trigeminal neuralgia also occurs in the absence of any structural abnormality.

2. DIFFERENTIAL DIAGNOSIS

a. Postherpetic neuralgia
b. Glossopharyngeal neuritis
c. Chronic sinusitis
d. Temporomandibular joint (TMJ)
e. Atypical facial pain
f. Posttraumatic neuralgia
g. Cluster headache
h. Multiple sclerosis (MS)

3. CLINICAL ISSUES

a. Presentation
   i. Repetitive, brief attacks of sharp, severe, stabbing pain in the distribution of one or more divisions of the fifth cranial nerve (trigeminal nerve).
   ii. Most episodes last several seconds, but can occur many times a day.
b. General points
   i. Pain is generally localized in the second or third (lower) divisions of the nerve, most commonly at the corner of the mouth and lateral aspect of the nose.
   ii. Triggers are small areas of the face that precipitate an attack when touched.
   iii. Triggers can be light touch, heat, cold, and wind.
   iv. Magnetic resonance imaging (MRI) of brain with and without contrast is needed to rule out tumor, MS, vascular malformation, infection, etc.
c. Natural history
   i. Usually occurs in patients older than 50 years and has either a progressive or fluctuating course over many years.
   ii. Spontaneous remissions lasting many months and even years can occur.

4. TREATMENT

a. Microvascular decompression, radiosurgery for trigeminal neuralgia due to arterial compression

b. Medical treatment: carbamazepine, gabapentin, baclofen, phenytoin, valproic acid
   i. Should be tried for at least 2 weeks for response.
   ii. Carbamazepine and valproic acid should be started at half the recommended dose and titrated up over 2 to 3 weeks.

c. Tricyclic antidepressant and nonsteroidal anti-inflammatory drugs when other treatment fails.

99 Temporomandibular Disorders

1. PATHOPHYSIOLOGY

   a. Temporomandibular disorders (TMDs) encompasses a variety of different disorders that may present with pain, limited jaw opening, and crepitus (joint noise).

   b. TMD now comprises the following:

      i. Internal derangements

      ii. Degenerative joint disease (DJD)

      iii. Myofascial pain

2. IMAGING FINDINGS

   a. DJD of the temporomandibular joint (TMJ) produces a characteristic radiographic appearance as the affected condyle becomes flattened and osteophytes form on the anterior border.

3. DIFFERENTIAL DIAGNOSIS

   a. Atypical facial pain

   b. Sinusitis

   c. Temporal arteritis

   d. Otitis media/externa

   e. Trigeminal neuralgia

   f. Tension headache

   g. Postherpetic neuralgia

   h. Posttraumatic neuralgia

4. CLINICAL ISSUES

   a. Presentation

      i. TMD typically presents with pain, limited jaw movement (opening), and crepitus.

      ii. Precipitating events found in less than half of TMJ sufferers; usually some form of trauma (biting on a hard object, blunt trauma to the face or chin, or opening the jaw too wide or long).

   b. General points

      i. TMD that spontaneously originates without a trigger is more likely to be associated with emotional or psychological factors.

      ii. Internal derangement characterized by anterior and medial displacement of the articular disk. The disk will reduce upon opening of the mouth and displace again upon closing.

      iii. DJD is characterized by crepitus and pain on jaw movement. Painful stage usually lasts less than a year and can be managed effectively with nonsteroidal anti-inflammatory drugs (NSAIDs).

      iv. Most patients with TMD suffer from a combination of muscle and joint pain (60%-70%)

  c. Natural history

      i. Poorly understood

5. TREATMENT

a. Similar to the treatment of tension headache, with NSAIDs and physical therapy the mainstay.

b. Biofeedback, trigger point injection efficacy unknown

c. Benzodiazepines can be helpful for myofascial pain, but are addictive

d. Tricyclic antidepressants useful for chronic pain, with selective serotonin reuptake inhibitors for those who cannot tolerate tricyclics.

e. Surgical options include arthrocentesis, arthroscopic joint surgery, and open joint surgery.

100 Atypical Facial Pain

1. PATHOPHYSIOLOGY

a. Unknown, although psychiatric pathology is found in 60% to 70% of sufferers

2. DIFFERENTIAL DIAGNOSIS

a. Temporomandibular joint (TMJ)
b. Trigeminal neuralgia
c. Posttraumatic neuralgia
d. Postherpetic neuralgia
e. Cluster headache
f. Tension headache

3. CLINICAL ISSUES

a. Presentation
   i. Chronic burning or aching pain without focal findings or any triggers (unlike trigeminal neuralgia, which is stabbing, localized, and triggered pain).
b. General points
   i. Severity of atypical facial pain fluctuates but is rarely absent.
   ii. Pain is typically located in the face and rarely involves the head or scalp (unlike cluster or tension headaches.)
   iii. Masticator muscle spasm rare
   iv. Women between 30 and 50 years typically affected
c. Natural history
   i. Spontaneous remissions rare, despite medical therapy

4. TREATMENT

a. Atypical facial pain is managed with antidepressants, typically amitriptyline

5. PROGNOSIS

a. Poor

101 Herpes Zoster

1. PATHOPHYSIOLOGY

a. Varicella-zoster virus (VZV) infects the trigeminal nerve in childhood as chickenpox and remains dormant in the ganglia for decades.

b. Trigeminal herpes zoster can reactivate many decades later in the form of herpetic skin eruptions in the distribution of the trigeminal nerve branches.

c. Herpes zoster most frequently affects the thoracic region, but lesions in the trigeminal distribution are almost as common. Eruptions or pain usually precipitated by trauma or stress in the setting of a weakened immune system.

d. Postherpetic neuralgia occurs when the pain persists 2 months after the initial eruption of vesicles or onset of pain.

2. DIFFERENTIAL DIAGNOSIS

a. Atypical facial pain
b. Temporomandibular joint (TMJ)
c. Posttraumatic neuralgia
d. Trigeminal neuralgia
e. Glossopharyngeal neuralgia
f. Sinusitis

3. CLINICAL ISSUES

a. Presentation
   i. Trigeminal herpes zoster presents as skin eruptions in one or more distributions of the trigeminal nerve.
   ii. The acute infection causes severe burning, itching, and stabbing pain. Secondary infection can occur and worsen the pain.
b. Natural history
   i. The vesicles or skin lesions usually resolve with or without medical therapy over a period of 1 to 2 months.

4. TREATMENT

a. The acute phase of herpes zoster is treated with antivirals such as acyclovir or valacyclovir.
   i. Steroids in the form of a rapid taper can also be used over a several week period.
   ii. Opiates or nonsteroidal anti-inflammatory drugs (NSAIDs) may be needed for pain relief.

b. Postherpetic neuralgia is poorly treated with the above medications and may require anticonvulsants such as Neurontin, tricyclic antidepressants, or baclofen to control the often shooting/stabbing pain.

5. PROGNOSIS

a. Most patients will recover spontaneously within 1 to 2 months.
b. Older or severely immunocompromised patients are less likely to experience a quick or complete resolution of symptoms.

SUGGESTED READINGS

Broussard JS Jr: Derangement, osteoarthritis, and rheumatoid arthritis of the temporomandibular joint: Implications, diagnosis, and management. Dent Clin North Am 2005;49(2):327–342.

Finkel A: Headache and facial pain. In Bailey BJ (ed): Head and Neck Surgery Otolaryngology, 2nd ed. Philadelphia, Lippincott Williams & Wilkins, 2006, pp 247–263.

Nurmikko TJ, Eldridge PR: Trigeminal neuralgia: Pathophysiology, diagnosis and current treatment. Br J Anaesth 2001;87(1):117–132.

1. SHARP AND LOCALIZED SOMATIC PAIN

a. Usually insidious and persistent in nature and lasting for hours to days

b. Can be positional and exacerbated by chest wall movement

2. WORKUP OF MUSCULOSKELETAL CHEST PAIN

a. Initial workup must focus on differentiating potential life-threatening visceral pathology from musculoskeletal origin.
   i. Cardiac or pulmonary chest pain can present with distinct symptoms including chest tightness, radiation to arms or neck, numbness, exertional dyspnea, cough, chills, and fever.

b. History
   i. Description of time course of illness and exacerbating features
   ii. Constant vs. intermittent pain symptoms or pain symptoms related to chest wall movement
   iii. Pain in the neck, shoulder, or thoracic spine may cause referred pain to the chest wall.
   iv. Chronic pain in multiple locations with fatigue and sleeping pattern changes is suggestive of fibromyalgia.
   v. Ankylosing spondylitis frequently involves the chest wall and may present with chronic lower back pain, skin lesions (psoriasis), and ocular changes (uveitis, conjunctivitis, photophobia).
   vi. Rheumatoid arthritis may predispose patients to sternoclavicular joint pain.

c. Physical examination
   i. First, direct attention to ruling out abnormalities of the lungs, heart, and upper abdomen.
   ii. The most important diagnostic feature of chest wall syndromes is chest wall tenderness that consistently reproduces the pain. This may be elicited with palpation or with movement.
   iii. Assess mobility of the cervical spine, shoulders, thoracic spine, and chest wall expansion with deep breathing.
      (1) Assess for any areas of localized joint swelling.
      (2) Also examine mobility of the lumbar spine to possibly suggest a spondyloarthropathy.
   iv. Thoracic spine malignancy causing point tenderness must be differentiated from costovertebral joint arthritis, which usually occurs with chest wall expansion.
   v. A generally normal musculoskeletal examination, except for the presence of multiple "tender points," may be suggestive of fibromyalgia.

d. Laboratory and radiological studies
   i. Should be used primarily to evaluate cardiac, pulmonary, or abdominal sources of pain.
   ii. Studies should be patient-specific based on history and physical examination.
      (1) Rheumatic disease may be assessed with erythrocyte sedimentation rate (ESR) or rheumatoid factor (RF) laboratory tests.
      (2) HLA-B27 antigen assays may be needed in diagnosis of ankylosing spondylitis.
      (3) Bone lesions may be assessed on plain films.
      (4) Spine magnetic resonance imaging (MRI) is indicated if radicular symptoms are present or if thoracic spine malignancy is suspected.
      (5) Computed tomography (CT) and MRI may also aid in determining the extent of soft tissue involvement.
   iii. Bone scan scintigraphy may show uptake implying localized inflammatory processes with many musculoskeletal syndromes, after trauma, or with tumors.

3. MAJOR CAUSES OF MUSCULOSKELETAL CHEST PAIN

a. Isolated musculoskeletal chest pain syndromes:
   i. Costosternal syndromes (costochondritis)
      (1) Presents with single or multiple areas of tenderness that reproduce the pain.
      (2) The upper costal cartilages at the costochondral or costosternal junctions are commonly noted to be tender.
      (3) There is usually minimal swelling.
      (4) Disease is usually self-limiting with occasional relapses.
      (5) Treatment is with nonsteroidal anti-inflammatory drugs (NSAIDs) and rest, and recovery is commonly spontaneous.
      (6) Posterior chest wall syndromes (costovertebral pain) are similar in function and treatment unless caused by herniated disc disease.
   ii. Tietze's syndrome
      (1) Usually young adults will present with benign, painful localized swelling of the costosternal, sternoclavicular, or costochondral joints.
      (2) Excessive coughing has been described in some patients to exacerbate the process.
      (3) Treatment with NSAIDs and local steroid injections may improve acute symptoms with pain subsiding within a few weeks.
   iii. Sternalis syndrome and xiphoidalgia
      (1) Rare syndromes that localize discomfort to the sternum or xiphoid process, respectively.

(2) Symptoms are aggravated by compression, coughing, and eating of large meals.

(3) Typically, they are self-limiting and treatment is usually NSAIDs and rest. Reports of steroid/local anesthetic injections have shown them to be useful.

iv. Spontaneous sternoclavicular subluxation

(1) Exclusively occurs in women in 5th to 6th decade of life where there is spontaneous, atraumatic, subluxation of the sternoclavicular joint.

(2) Usually occurs on dominant side and supportive (nonoperative) therapy is generally recommended.

b. Rheumatic diseases

i. Rheumatoid arthritis: can manifest as sternoclavicular joint disease and may be noted radiographically.

ii. Ankylosing spondylitis

(1) May manifest initially in up to 18% of patients as thoracic spine and chest wall pain.

(2) Pain results from an autoimmune inflammatory disease state affecting the thoracic joints.

iii. Psoriatic arthritis: 5% to 10% of patients with psoriasis may develop chest wall arthritis.

iv. Polychondritis: systemic inflammation of cartilage including ears, nasal cavity, respiratory tract, costochondral, and manubriosternal areas.

v. Fibromyalgia

(1) Common tenderness points noted on lower back, neck, shoulders, and hips.

(2) Diffuse musculoskeletal pain is accompanied by fatigue and sleeping pattern changes.

c. Systemic diseases

i. Stress fractures

(1) High suspicion in cases of trauma or patients with significant osteoporosis or rheumatoid arthritis.

(2) Radiographic evidence may be needed.

ii. Neoplasms: chest wall invasion or thoracic spine malignancy

iii. Sickle cell disease: acute chest syndrome with pulmonary infarction

4. TREATMENTS FOR MUSCULOSKELETAL CHEST PAIN USUALLY INCLUDE A COMBINATION OF PHARMACOLOGIC AND NONPHARMACOLOGIC THERAPY

a. Pharmacologic therapy includes:

i. NSAIDs

ii. Muscle relaxants

iii. Antidepressants

      iv. Anticonvulsants
      v. Topical local anesthetic agents or steroids
      vi. Local steroid and/or local anesthetic injections
      vii. Disease modifying antirheumatic drugs (DMARDs)
      viii. Opioid analgesics
  b. Nonpharmacologic therapy includes:
      i. Psychiatric evaluation
      ii. Physical therapy measures
      iii. Patient education

1. GENERAL

a. Chronic abdominal pain is usually defined as visceral abdominal pain that has been present for at least 3 to 6 months that can be continuous or discontinuous in nature and can be functional or organic in pathology.

b. Workup of chronic abdominal pain

   i. Differentiate benign functional pathology (i.e., irritable bowel syndrome [IBS]) from stable organic pathology (i.e., chronic pancreatitis, ulcerative colitis, etc.) from possible unstable organic pathology requiring immediate evaluation and treatment (i.e., peptic ulcer disease, gastrointestinal (GI) or hepatic cancer, subacute peritonitis, partial small bowel or large bowel obstruction, etc.)

   ii. History

   (1) Description of time course of illness

   (2) Constant vs. intermittent pain symptoms or pain symptoms related to bowel movements

   (3) Other GI manifestations, such as a change in bowel habits, chronic diarrhea, bloody stools, nausea or vomiting, or dyspepsia, may be related to inflammatory bowel disease or other organic pathology.

   (4) Excessive alcohol intake or recurrent gallstones should point toward potential chronic pancreatitis.

   (5) Emotional or psychological stressors that relate to pain symptoms

   (6) Lower abdominal pain in women is discussed under "Pelvic Pain."

   iii. Physical examination

   (1) Weight loss, unstable vital signs, or signs of dehydration or malnutrition may be suggestive of organic pathology.

   (2) Pain on superficial and deep palpation

   (3) Enlarged liver or spleen, distension and signs of bowel obstruction, ascites, abdominal masses, signs of peritonitis are all suggestive of acute organic pathology.

   (4) Continuous pain worsened with flexion of the abdomen suggests chronic abdominal wall pain possibly related to herpes zoster, thoracic nerve radiculopathy, or anterior cutaneous nerve entrapment syndrome.

   iv. Laboratory data and other studies

   (1) Complete blood count (CBC), chemistry with calcium, liver function tests (LFTs) with lipase

   (2) Possible need for electron spin resonance (ESR), C-reactive protein, and/or immunoglobulin (Ig) A endomysial or transglutaminase antibody tests to differentiate acute organic disease or celiac sprue.

(3) If organic pathology is suggested, then further appropriate studies may be required, including computed tomography (CT) scan or abdominal ultrasonography (U/S), colonoscopy and/or esophagogastroduodenoscopy (EGD), thyroid function tests (TFTs), and stool cultures/ova/parasite analysis.
  c. Differential diagnosis of chronic abdominal pain
    i. Functional disorders
      (1) IBS
      (2) Functional dyspepsia
    ii. Organic GI disorders
      (1) Inflammatory bowel disease (ulcerative colitis, Crohn disease)
      (2) Chronic pancreatitis
      (3) Chronic constipation
      (4) Absorption diseases (celiac sprue, lactose intolerance)
      (5) Peptic ulcer disease
    iii. Gynecologic/pelvic disorders: see "Pelvic Pain"
    iv. Musculoskeletal
      (1) Poor posture/body mechanics
      (2) Lumbar or thoracic disk disease
      (3) Herpes zoster
      (4) Abdominal wall hernia or muscle strain
    v. Psychiatric/psychosocial
      (1) Sexual abuse

SUGGESTED READINGS

Holland-Hall C, Brown R: Evaluation of the adolescent with chronic abdominal pain. J Pediatr Adolesc Gynecol 2004;17:23–27.

Penner R, Majumdar S: Diagnostic approach to abdominal pain in adults. Adult Primary Care and Internal Medicine. Available at: http://www.uptodate.com/physicians/adult_primary_care_toclist.asp. September 2006.

  d. Chronic pancreatitis
    i. Background and clinical presentation
      (1) Chronic pancreatitis typically presents as chronic persistent abdominal pain with intermittent flares. It is characteristically accompanied by pancreatic insufficiency, malabsorption, and steatorrhea.
      (2) Causes range from chronic alcohol abuse, recurrent gallstone disease, hypercalcemia, hyperlipidemia to genetic, and idiopathic factors.
      (3) Peak presentation is between 35 and 55 years.
      (4) Classically, pain is epigastric and radiates to the back.
      (5) Pain may be postprandial or constant.
      (6) May present with nausea/vomiting, weight loss, electrolyte disturbances, or exocrine and/or endocrine failure.
      (7) Overt diabetes mellitus usually occurs late.
      (8) Chronic pancreatitis is described to sometimes "burn out" over a very variable period from months to years, which may lead to persistent pain relief.

ii. Diagnosis
   (1) Thorough history and physical examination should be performed.
   (2) Results of diagnostic and imaging studies may be normal.
   (3) Differential diagnosis includes pancreatic cancer, lymphoma, pancreatic endocrine tumors, peptic ulcer disease, gallstones, IBS, and a variety of other rare conditions.
   (4) Laboratory studies
      (a) Lipase and amylase may be elevated but have no prognostic significance.
      (b) CBC and electrolytes may be normal. Calcium and glucose levels may be elevated.
      (c) LFTs and bilirubin may be elevated potentially because of obstruction.
      (d) Fecal Sudan stain is diagnostic for steatorrhea. Fecal elastase may be a sensitive marker for early pancreatic insufficiency.
   (5) Imaging findings
      (a) Abdominal x-rays: calcium deposits in pancreatic duct in 30% of patients
      (b) Endoscopic retrograde cholangiopancreatography (ERCP): The test of choice for diagnosis may reveal a dilated, tortuous main duct with proteinaceous or calcified plugs.
      (c) Endoscopic U/S: requires a skilled gastroenterologist and may show stones or dilated pancreatic duct.
      (d) CT scan: useful in differentiating other acute pathology from chronic inflammation
      (e) Magnetic resonance cholangiopancreatography (MRCP)
      (f) Multiple pancreatic function tests: most sensitive is the secretin stimulation test to determine bicarbonate-rich pancreatic fluid production
iii. Treatment
   (1) Dietary and lifestyle modification: Cessation of alcohol is imperative. Small meals that are low in fat will decrease pancreatic demand.
   (2) Pancreatic enzyme supplementation: (lipase, protease, amylase) unlikely to help alcoholic pancreatitis but is useful for early disease and idiopathic disease.
   (3) Acid suppression: H2 receptor blockers and proton pump inhibitors
   (4) Octreotide: incomplete evidence
   (5) Analgesics
      (a) Should be considered after lifestyle modification and enzyme supplementation have failed.
      (b) Opioid addiction is fairly common.

- (c) A short course of opioids with tricyclic antidepressants (TCAs) and nonsteroidal analgesics may be enough to break the cycle of pain, but usually escalating opioid regimens are required.
- (d) Longer-acting medications such as MS Contin or Fentanyl patches are more effective than short-acting agents.
- (6) Celiac nerve block with either alcohol or steroids provides variable pain relief duration but has been shown to be very effective in the pancreatic cancer subpopulation.
- (7) Endoscopic therapy: Decompression of a dilated and obstructed pancreatic duct by a skilled endoscopist may relieve ductal hypertension and pain.
- (8) Surgery
  - (a) Decompression, resection, or denervation procedures may be performed.
  - (b) A decompression or drainage operation may be performed if a dilated main pancreatic duct is present.
  - (c) Subtotal pancreatic resections have shown better pain relief, but usually leave the patient as a diabetic and with significant exocrine dysfunction.
  - (d) Denervation procedures interrupt the nerve fibers in the celiac ganglion and splanchnic nerves and can be accomplished through open or thoracoscopic techniques.

SUGGESTED READINGS

Ammann RW, Muellhaupt B: The natural history of pain in alcoholic chronic pancreatitis. Gastroenterology 1999;116:1132–1140.

Dimagno E: Toward understanding (and management) of painful chronic pancreatitis. Gastroenterology 1999;116:1252–1257.

Dite P, Ruzicka M, Zboril V: A prospective, randomized trial comparing endoscopic with surgical therapy for chronic pancreatitis. Endoscopy 2003;35:553–558.

Freedman S: AGA technical review: Treatment of pain in chronic pancreatitis. Gastroenterology 1998;115:765–776.

Freedman S: Treatment of chronic pancreatitis. Available at: www.UpToDate.com. 2005.

Mergener K, Baillie J: Chronic pancreatitis. Lancet 1997;350:1379.

- e. Ulcerative colitis (UC)
  - i. Background and clinical presentation
    - (1) UC is an inflammatory bowel disease characterized by recurrent episodes of inflammation involving and limited to the mucosa of the large colon and almost invariably involving the rectum.
    - (2) Men and women are affected equally, and peak incidence is between 15 and 30 years, with a second peak between 60 and 80 years. Ten percent to 25% of affected patients have a first-degree relative with either Crohn disease or UC.
    - (3) Mild disease (proctitis) may present with intermittent crampy abdominal pain, tenesmus, and periods of

constipation similar to IBS but will be accompanied by rectal bleeding and bloody stools.

(4) Moderate and severe disease (pancolitis) may present with severe abdominal pain, profuse bleeding, fever, malnutrition, hypoalbuminemia, and weight loss. Very severe disease can lead to transluminal inflammation and bowel perforation.

(5) Major local complications of UC include massive hemorrhage, fulminant colitis and toxic megacolon, intestinal perforation or stricture, and the development of colon cancer.

(6) Extraintestinal manifestations include:

  (a) Peripheral arthritis involving the knees, ankles, elbows, and wrists occurs in 10% to 20% of patients, with possible progression to axial arthritis mimicking ankylosing spondylitis.

  (b) Nonspecific elevation of alanine aminotransferase

  (c) Three percent to 5% of patients with UC develop primary sclerosing cholangitis (PSC), a progressive fibrosis and scarring of the bile ducts, potentially requiring liver transplantation for treatment.

  (d) Skin manifestations may be present such as erythema nodosum (most common) and pyoderma gangrenosum (uncommon).

  (e) Eye involvement with uveitis and episcleritis

  (f) Lung disease, ranging from mild to severe, decreases in diffusion capacity

  (g) Autoimmune hemolytic anemia

  (h) Hypercoagulable state with potential for deep venous thrombosis formation

(7) General time course of UC is typically seen as intermittent exacerbations alternating with periods of remission.

  (a) Mild disease is usually managed conservatively and is benign.

  (b) Moderate to severe disease needs aggressive medical management and, possibly, surgical intervention.

(8) Differential diagnosis may include Crohn disease, infectious colitis (*Salmonella, Shigella, Escherichia coli, Clostridium*, etc.), radiation colitis, ischemic colitis, and medication-related colitis.

ii. Diagnosis

(1) Complete history and physical examination should reveal characteristic symptoms and signs. A thorough abdominal and rectal examination should be performed.

(2) Sigmoidoscopy or colonoscopy

  (a) Typical endoscopic appearance of inflamed, erythematous, ulcerated mucosa is seen with loss of usual vascular markings.

    (b) Biopsy will reveal crypt abscesses and atrophy of glands.

  (3) Ultrasound: noninvasive approach at diagnosis but not as reliable as direct visualization.

  (4) Barium enema: rarely used and should be avoided if toxic megacolon is suspected.

iii. Treatment

  (1) Management of IBD may require life-long treatment and depends on the severity of the disease.

  (2) Mild disease

    (a) Mainstay of treatment is still enema or suppository therapy.

      (i) 5-Aminosalicylic acid (5-ASA) or hydrocortisone enemas are used.

      (ii) Patients may require foam preparations if they are unable to use an enema.

    (b) Maintenance therapy may not be needed in mild disease to preserve remission.

    (c) Steroid side effects can still occur with enema therapy due to systemic absorption.

    (d) Symptomatic therapy with antispasmodics or antidiarrheal agents may be necessary.

      (i) Opioids are not recommended and should be used sparingly.

      (ii) Disease remission should provide pain relief.

  (3) Moderate to severe disease

    (a) Usually will require oral therapy.

    (b) Sulfasalazine is an anti-inflammatory and immunosuppressant drug taken orally and is broken down into 5-ASA and sulfapyridine. Usually takes 4 to 6 weeks for control; may also be used for maintenance of remission.

    (c) 5-Aminosalicylates (mesalamine) are associated with fewer side effects than sulfasalazine and can be given in much higher doses.

    (d) Oral corticosteroids (prednisone) are highly effective but cause multiple side effects and require gradual tapering of therapy before discontinuation.

    (e) Immunomodulatory therapy (6-mercaptopurine, azathioprine) may be considered for refractory disease or steroid-dependent patients.

    (f) Hospitalization is recommended for cases of pancolitis or severe proctitis for intravenous fluid therapy, electrolyte replacement, bowel rest, and parenteral nutrition. Intravenous steroids (hydrocortisone, methylprednisolone) and intravenous cyclosporine may be required to induce remission.

(4) Surgery
    (a) Consider if no improvement with medical management or if surgical abdomen develops for bowel perforation or toxic megacolon.
    (b) Total colectomy is advised if premalignant or malignant changes are present. Stool drainage procedure can be performed (ileostomy) or a small bowel reservoir can be fashioned with potential of maintaining continence.

SUGGESTED READINGS

Cohen R, Woseth D, Thisted R: A meta analysis and overview of the literature on treatment options for left-sided ulcerative colitis and ulcerative proctitis. Am J Gastroenterol 2000;95:1263–1276.

Kornbluth A, Sachar D: Ulcerative colitis practice guidelines in adults. Am J Gastroenterol 2004;99:1371–1385.

Stein R, Hanauer S: Medical therapy for inflammatory bowel disease. Gastroenterol Clin N Am 1999;28:297–321.

f. IBS
  i. Background and clinical presentation
    (1) IBS is characterized by chronic, variable, crampy abdominal pain with enhanced visceral perception and altered bowel reactivity to feeding and environmental/psychological stimuli, resulting in intermittent diarrhea and/or constipation and persisting for at least 3 months.
    (2) It is the most commonly diagnosed GI condition with a prevalence of 10% to 15% in North America with a 2:1 female predominance.
    (3) IBS does NOT usually present with unstable vital signs, bloody stools, malnutrition or anorexia, electrolyte disturbances, weight loss, or sleep disturbances. These clinical signs and symptoms should prompt investigation toward organic pathology.
    (4) Presenting signs and symptoms
      (a) Altered bowel habits: intermittent diarrhea with or without mucus, and/or intermittent constipation. May relate to environmental or psychological stressors.
      (b) Abdominal bloating or increased flatulence/belching
      (c) Gastroesophageal reflux disease (GERD), dysphagia, early satiety, and nausea are all common findings.
      (d) Impaired sexual function, dysmenorrhea, dyspareunia
  ii. Diagnosis
    (1) There is no biological disease marker, radiological finding, or true diagnostic study.
    (2) Exclude organic causes in a cost-effective manner.
    (3) Identify positive symptoms consistent with condition.

iii. Treatment
  (1) Develop an effective patient-physician relationship and provide reassurance and education about the illness.
  (2) Dietary modifications (altering fiber, caffeine, tobacco, lactose intake) and lifestyle modifications that remove emotional stressors.
  (3) Medications are reserved for severe disease impacting normal lifestyle.
    (a) Antispasmodics/anticholinergics
    (b) Loperamide, diphenoxylate, cholestyramine
    (c) Laxatives: milk of magnesia, sorbitol, polyethylene glycol
    (d) Current research in 5-HT3/5-HT4 receptor antagonists
    (e) Antidepressants: TCAs (amitriptyline, imipramine), selective serotonin reuptake inhibitors (SSRIs) (fluoxetine, paroxetine)
  (4) Psychological treatment for severe symptoms or failure with medications

SUGGESTED READINGS

Brandt L, Bjorkman D, Fennerty M, et al: Systematic review on the management of irritable bowel syndrome in North America. Am J Gastroenterol 2002;97:S7–S26.

Chun A, Desautels S, Wald A: Clinical manifestations and diagnosis of irritable bowel syndrome. In Rose BD (ed). Waltham, MA: UpToDate, 2005.

Drossman D, Camilleri M, Mayer E, et al: AGA technical review: Irritable bowel syndrome. Gastroenterology 2002;123:2108–2131.

Drossman D, Whitehead W, Camilleri M: Irritable bowel syndrome: A technical review for practice guideline development. Gastroenterology 1997;112:2120–2137.

Hammer J, Talley N: Diagnostic criteria for the irritable bowel syndrome. Am J Med 1999;107:5S–11S.

Saito Y, Locke G, Talley N: A comparison of the Rome and Manning criteria for case identification in epidemiological investigations of irritable bowel syndrome. Am J Gastroenterol 2000;95:2816–2824.

1. CHRONIC PELVIC PAIN

   a. Nonmenstrual pain located below the umbilicus persisting for at least 6 months, resulting in functional disability or requiring therapy.

2. EVALUATION OF THE PATIENT WITH CHRONIC PELVIC PAIN

   a. History
      i. Description and temporal relation of pain to menses, stressful events
      ii. Presence of coexisting pain (headache, backache)
      iii. Menstrual history
      iv. Obstetric history
      v. Presence of dyspareunia
      vi. Work and leisure habits
      vii. Problems involving other organ systems (urinary tact, gastrointestinal [GI] tract)
      viii. Previous pelvic and abdominal infections
      ix. Response to previous medical/surgical therapy
      x. Previous operations or diagnostic procedures
      xi. Screening for domestic violence, substance abuse, sexual abuse, depression
   b. Physical examination
      i. Thorough abdominal, bimanual, pelvic and rectal examination
      ii. Evaluation for the presence of masses, surgical scars, or hernias
   c. Laboratory analysis
      i. Complete blood count (CBC), C-reactive protein, erythrocyte sedimentation rate (ESR), venereal disease research laboratory (VDRL), urinary analysis and culture, cultures for gonococcal infection (GC)/Chlamydia, wet mount, Papanicolaou (Pap) smear
   d. Imaging
      i. Ultrasound, computed tomography (CT) scan, magnetic resonance imaging (MRI)
   e. GI and genitourinary (GU) tract evaluations (colonoscopy, cystoscopy) as indicated
   f. Psychiatric evaluation
   g. Laparoscopy (particularly for chronic pelvic inflammatory disease [PID] and endometriosis)

3. INTERSTITIAL CYSTITIS (IC)

   a. Clinical presentation
      i. Syndrome characterized by urinary symptoms (urgency, frequency, feeling of incomplete voiding, nocturia) in the

presence of pelvic or bladder pain which is due to noninfectious causes

ii. Progressive disease that can become associated with more recurrent and more debilitating bouts of symptoms

iii. Coexisting depression often present

iv. Pelvic pain is often relieved by voiding

v. Female (10:1) and white predominance

b. Pathophysiology

i. Etiology is unclear, but many theories exist; the true cause is likely multifactorial.

ii. Associated with a disruption in the protective barrier at the urothelial surface (glycosaminoglycan layer), which allows irritants found in the urine (particularly potassium) to activate nerves and muscle in the underlying tissue, leading to pain and inflammation

iii. Neural sensory upregulation in bladder

iv. Mast cell degranulation, defect in uroepithelium repair mechanisms, and the increased presence of inflammatory mediators (substance P and kallikrein) believed to also potentially play a role

c. Diagnosis

i. No universally accepted diagnostic criteria, therefore diagnosis is usually clinical

ii. Symptoms in the absence of other identifiable causes (most commonly urinary tract infection [UTI])

iii. Physical examination may reveal suprapubic tenderness and pain on manual palpation of the anterior vaginal wall

iv. Intravesical potassium sensitivity test (PST) tests for abnormal urethral permeability, which is supportive of the diagnosis of IC. It is positive in 80% of patients with IC and only 4% of controls.

(1) A solution of 40 mL of sterile water is instilled into the patient's bladder over 2 minutes. After 5 minutes, the patient is asked to rate pain/urgency (increasing scale of 0-5) and then the solution is drained.

(2) Next, a solution of 40 mL of KCl (40 mEq/100 mL) is instilled into the patient's bladder over 2 minutes. After 5 minutes, the patient is again asked to rate pain/urgency (increasing scale of 0-5).

(3) The bladder is then drained and irrigated with sterile water.

(4) A positive test is noted if the patient has assigned a pain or urgency score of at least two points above zero for the solution of amaranthus caudatus lectin (ACL) and reports that the KCl solution provoked more severe symptoms.

(5) A positive PST provides evidence for the diagnosis of IC.

v. Cystoscopy can reveal bladder mucosa petechiae and glomerulations (submucosal hemorrhages) or a classic Hunner ulceration in advanced disease.

      (1) Mucosal biopsies may be taken to rule out other disease entities, but there are no pathologic histologic features of IC.

  vi. Urodynamic testing may show decreased functional capacity and increased sensory urgency, but it is neither sensitive nor specific enough to be recommended for the diagnosis of IC.

d. Treatment

  i. Dietary: avoidance of potassium-rich foods and spicy foods

  ii. Stress and anxiety reduction

  iii. Pentosan polysulfate sodium

      (1) Heparinoid drug, which is thought to aid in the repair of injured uroepithelium, can be administered in oral formulation or intravesically as an adjunct in more serious cases.

      (2) Treatment duration of a minimum of 1 year for mild cases and 2 years for severe cases before an accurate assessment of therapy benefit can be derived.

  iv. Other oral therapies include gabapentin, tricyclic antidepressants (TCAs), and selective serotonin reuptake inhibitors (SSRIs) to inhibit neural activation.

  v. Antihistamines, azathioprine, and corticosteroids have also been used with variable success rates.

  vi. Dimethylsulfoxide

      (1) Intravesical instillations of 50 mL every 2 weeks for 6 to 8 weeks followed by 50 mL every 2 weeks for 3 to 12 months

      (2) Symptom relief in 50% of patients

      (3) Teratogenic, therefore should be avoided in pregnancy

  vii. Interventional therapy includes acupuncture, hydrodistention of the bladder, cystectomy and urinary diversion, and transelectric nerve stimulation.

4. PELVIC INFLAMMATORY DISEASE (PID)

a. Clinical presentation

  i. Defined as an acute infection of the upper genital tract structures in females that is precipitated by a sexually transmitted agent

  ii. Lower bilateral abdominal pain and dyspareunia in majority of cases

  iii. New vaginal discharge, UTI symptomatology, abnormal uterine bleeding may also be associated

  iv. Most frequent gynecologic cause for emergency room visits

  v. Most common cause of chronic pelvic pain in patient populations with a high prevalence of sexually transmitted diseases (STDs)

  vi. Risk factors: previous history of PID, promiscuous lifestyle, age younger than 35 years, African American race, nonbarrier contraception, smoking, cervical instrumentation

    vii. Fitz-Hugh-Curtis syndrome: focal perihepatitis, which occurs in 5% to 10% of patients with PID

  b. Pathophysiology

    i. Scarring and the formation of adhesions contribute to the long-term sequelae of PID, which include increased risk of ectopic pregnancy, increased infertility rates, and chronic pelvic pain.

    ii. Most common cause is *Chlamydia trachomatis* followed by *Neisseria gonorrhoeae*. Other implicated organisms include *Gardnerella vaginalis, Bacteroides, Ureaplasma, Streptococcus agalactiae*

  c. Diagnosis

    i. Physical examination

      (1) Diffuse lower abdominal tenderness; +/– rebound

      (2) Fever

      (3) Purulent endocervical discharge or tenderness

      (4) Uterine and adnexal tenderness

    ii. Laboratory analysis

      (1) Urinalysis with urine pregnancy test: used to rule out UTI and pregnancy, respectively, as causes for pain

      (2) Wet mount: The appearance of white blood cells (WBCs) and Gram (–) intracellular diplococci is more suspicious for PID.

      (3) Elevated C-reactive protein and ESR

      (4) Cultures for GC and Chlamydia, which, if present, increase the risk for PID

    iii. Imaging

      (1) Ultrasound: thickened fluid-filled oviducts and free pelvic fluid

      (2) Laparoscopy: gross salpingitis, abnormal fimbriae, purulent exudates or cul-de-sac fluid

  d. Treatment

    i. All patients should be counseled on benefits of safe sexual practices in addition to obtaining further testing for other STDs such as HIV, human papilloma virus (HPV), hepatitis C virus (HCV), and syphilis.

    ii. With regard to the acute infection, depending on the patient clinical picture, some will require admission to the hospital but others can be treated with outpatient antibiotics.

    iii. Chronic pelvic pain

      (1) Ovulation suppression with oral contraceptives

      (2) TCAs or SSRIs

      (3) Adhesiolysis

      (4) Surgical removal of affected pelvic organs

5. VULVODYNIA

  a. Clinical presentation

    i. Vulvodynia is pain in the vulvar area occurring in the absence of a specific, relevant infectious, inflammatory, neoplastic, or neurologic disorder.

ii. Pain may be precipitated by contact that is either sexual or non-sexual.

iii. Variable symptoms: constant or episodic, unilateral or bilateral, may replicate UTI symptoms or chronic yeast infection.

iv. Pain usually starts at the inner thigh and moves toward the vestibule.

v. Two major pain patterns exist.

(1) Vulvar vestibulitis syndrome: Pain localized strictly to the vestibule of the vulva that requires contact or pressure to illicit discomfort. Most common in premenopausal women.

(2) Dysesthetic vulvodynia: Pain, which may occur spontaneously in the absence of pressure or friction, is not limited to the vestibule.

b. Pathophysiology

i. Can result from long-term tissue damage (nociceptive) or from peripheral nerve injury (neuropathic pain)

ii. Pudendal nerve injury, manifestation of postherpetic neuralgia, referred pain from pelvic orthopedic injury, referred pain from vertebral column disease (ruptured disc, spinal stenosis, spinal arthropathies) have also been implicated as potential etiologies.

c. Diagnosis

i. Diagnosis of exclusion

ii. Infectious causes of vulvar pain and skin diseases (namely, lichen planus) must first be ruled out.

d. Treatment

i. Lubrication during sexual activity

ii. Topical estrogen

iii. TCAs for neuropathic pain and coexisting depression

iv. Gabapentin for neuropathic pain

v. Topical local anesthetics (e.g., eutectic mixture of local anesthetics [EMLA] cream)

vi. Trigger point injections with steroid/local anesthetics

vii. Acupuncture

viii. Pelvic floor evaluation and rehabilitation, if indicated

ix. Interferon alpha (INF-alpha) local injection

x. Vestibulectomy

6. ENDOMETRIOSIS

a. Definition: endometrial glands and stroma outside the endometrial cavity and uterine musculature

b. Clinical presentation

i. Affects 7% of women of childbearing age

ii. Most common cause of chronic pelvic pain in patient populations with a low prevalence of STDs

iii. Common presentations: pain (50%), infertility (25%), pain and infertility (25%), ovarian endometrioma (<5%)

    iv. Pain does not correlate with disease severity; 30% of those with endometriosis do not have pain.
  c. Pathophysiology
    i. Multiple theories, but most popular are retrograde menstruation though the fallopian tubes, metaplasia, hematogenous and lymphatic spread, or direct placement in the wound
  d. Diagnosis
    i. Diagnostic laparoscopy only definitive test
    ii. Physical examination may reveal cervical stenosis, uterosacral ligament abnormalities (nodularity or focal tenderness), and lateral displacement of the cervix caused by asymmetric endometriotic involvement of one uterosacral ligament.
  e. Treatment
    i. Expectant management useful for women with minimal disease and perimenopausal women
    ii. Initial medical therapy consists of at least a 3-month trial of nonsteroidal anti-inflammatory drugs (NSAIDs) and oral contraceptives.
    iii. Treatment for more advanced disease includes danazol, progestins, or gonadotropin-releasing hormone (GnRH) analogs.
    iv. Danazol:
      (1) This 19-nortestosterone derivative with progestin-like effects acts by direct inhibition of endometriotic implant growth and direct inhibition of ovarian enzymes needed for estrogen production.
      (2) This induced amenorrhea causes endometrial atrophy within the uterus and in ectopic locations.
    v. Progestins (Provera, Depo-Provera): cause initial decidualization, eventual atrophy of endometriotic tissue, and amenorrhea
    vi. GnRH analogs: induce pituitary downregulation and a hypoestrogenic state that leads to amenorrhea
    vii. Surgical therapy for patients with severe and debilitating endometriosis that hasn't responded to medical treatment
      (1) Laser ablation of endometriosis lesions
      (2) Laparoscopic uterosacral nerve ablation
      (3) Presacral neurectomy

7. OVARIAN DISEASE

  a. Ovarian pain impulses are transmitted via the hypogastric plexus and celiac plexus along sympathetic afferent fibers and enter the central nervous system (CNS) at T10.
  b. Ovarian pain is frequently referred to the anterior thighs because of the somatic afferent fibers.
  c. Differential diagnosis of ovarian pain includes carcinoma, infection, ruptured ovarian follicle, ovarian torsion, ruptured ectopic

pregnancy, acute twisted ovarian cyst, and ovarian remnant syndrome.
d. Treatment
   i. Surgical management for ectopic pregnancies, ovarian torsion, malignancy
   ii. NSAIDS, antidepressants, injection therapy
   iii. Transcutaneous electrical nerve stimulation (TENS), acupuncture, and physical therapy as possible adjuncts

8. UTERINE FIBROID DISEASE

a. Also referred to as leiomyomas, myomas, fibroids
b. Most common benign neoplasm of the female reproductive tract
c. Present in one-third of women of reproductive age
d. Clinical presentation
   i. Most commonly presents with abnormal uterine bleeding
   ii. Other presentations: infertility, pelvic pain, symptoms such as urinary frequency related to the presence of large tumors
   iii. Factors associated with increased risk of fibroid development:
      (1) African American race
      (2) Early exposure to oral contraceptive pills
      (3) Nulliparity
      (4) Family history
   iv. Tend to be less symptomatic in nonpregnant women
   v. Pregnant patients with fibroids are at increased risk of miscarriage, postpartum bleeding, premature labor, and obstructed labor.
   vi. Fibroids often regress in size at menopause.
e. Pathophysiology
   i. Fibroids arise from a single progenitor myocyte and result from excessive cell growth and genetic mutation.
   ii. Estrogen and progesterone exposure enhance fibroid growth.
   iii. Fibroids can outgrow their blood supply.
   iv. Pedunculated fibroids can undergo torsion and result in acute or chronic pelvic pain.
   v. Fibroids may hemorrhage, ulcerate, undergo degeneration, or have malignant conversion to leiomyosarcomas.
f. Diagnosis
   i. Irregularly shaped uterus and masses may be felt on bimanual exam
   ii. Anemia from menorrhagia may be present on laboratory analysis
   iii. Transvaginal uterine ultrasound
   iv. Hysteroscopy or hysterosalpingography
   v. MRI: useful in evaluating intramural and submucosal myomas
g. Treatment
   i. Small asymptomatic myomas should be conservatively managed with biannual examinations.

ii. NSAIDs in combination with oral contraceptive pills are useful for pain control and regulation of menses.

iii. Surgical options include myomectomy, endometrial ablation, and myolysis for women of reproductive age or hysterectomy for definitive therapy.

iv. For patients who will undergo surgical resection, GnRH agonist therapy, such as depot leuprolide 3.75 mg IM monthly for 2 to 3 months, can be given preoperatively to significantly reduce tumor size and, thus, decrease surgical complication.

v. Uterine artery embolization is an investigational technique for women with a single large fibroid tumor

9. MYOFASCIAL PAIN

a. Clinical presentation
   i. Patients complain of focal hyperirritable anatomic areas (trigger points) that may limit activity.
   ii. A myofascial trigger point is a discrete painful area located within a taut band of skeletal muscle or associated fascia that, on compression, reproduces a characteristic discomfort and referral pattern.
   iii. Pain is often described as aching or burning.
b. Pathophysiology
   i. Myalgia results from continuous habitual muscular contraction that may be exacerbated by stress.
   ii. Sustained vasoconstriction of myofascial tissues may result in metabolic waste accumulation and release of nociceptive chemicals that lead to local sensitization of pain fibers.
   iii. Neuromuscular junction and endplate dysfunction may lead to the excessive muscle fiber activation, predisposing them to fatigue and resultant myalgia.
   iv. Previous surgery, minor trauma, sports that produce chronic pelvic stimulation, unusual sexual activities, and recurrent infections all predispose patients to the development of trigger points.
c. Diagnosis
   i. Fifteen percent of patients with chronic pelvic pain meet diagnostic criteria for myofascial pain syndrome.
   ii. Based on clinical findings, but imaging can be used to rule out other potential etiologies of pain.
   iii. The back and abdomen are common locations of trigger points in patients with pelvic myofascial pain syndrome.
d. Treatment
   i. Multimodal therapy
   ii. NSAIDs, muscle relaxants
   iii. Trigger point injections (local anesthetics/steroids)
   iv. Topical anesthetic medications
   v. Massage therapy, "myofascial releases"
   vi. Electrical neuromodulation

10. COCCYDYNIA

a. Clinical presentation

   i. Pain in the area of the coccyx (tailbone) is called coccydynia or coccygodynia.

   ii. Five times more common in women than men

     (1) Coccyx larger in women

     (2) More posterior location of sacrum and coccyx

     (3) Characteristics of the ischial tuberosities that leave a woman's coccyx more exposed and susceptible to trauma both in common situations (sitting position) and during childbirth

     (4) Pain during or after sitting, the level of pain depending on how long you sit

     (5) Acute pain while moving from sitting to standing

     (6) Pain caused by sitting on a soft, but not a hard surface

     (7) Deep ache around the coccyx

     (8) Sensitivity to finger pressure on the tip or edges of the coccyx

     (9) Shooting pains down the leg

     (10) Pain during bowel movements, and sometimes before

     (11) Pain during sexual intercourse, either in men or women

     (12) Development of pericoccygeal soft tissues

     (13) Pelvic floor muscle spasms

     (14) Referred pain from lumbar pathology

     (15) Arachnoiditis of the lower sacral nerve roots

     (16) Local posttraumatic lesions

     (17) Somatization

b. Pathophysiology

   i. In 70% of cases, source is coccygeal disks or joints.

   ii. Coccydynia can ensue after falls, childbirth, repetitive strain, or surgery.

   iii. First and second coccygeal segments are mobile.

     (1) More than 25 to 30 degrees considered hypermobile

     (2) Normal coccygeal mobility 30 degrees anteriorly, 1 cm laterally

   iv. Posterior luxation is a common feature if body mass index (BMI) is greater than 27.4 in women and 29.4 in men.

   v. Straight vs. curved coccyx

   vi. Two cases of avascular necrosis (AVN) of coccyx

     (1) Women: Rule out anal elevator syndrome (careful inspection of pelvic floor muscles and ligaments).

c. Diagnosis

   i. Physical examination

   ii. X-ray

   iii. MRI

d. Treatment

   i. Conservative treatment:

     (1) Rest, NSAIDs, warm-water baths

    ii. Manipulation of coccyx: internal and external

       (1) Works best on patients without unstable coccyx

   iii. Corticosteroid/ local injections

       (1) In joint space

       (2) Around coccyx

   iv. Blocks

       (1) Caudal

       (2) Ganglion impar

    v. Dry needling, acupuncture

   vi. Sacral nerve root stimulation, TENS

  vii. Surgical removal of coccyx

 viii. Dorsal root ganglio (DRG) lesioning of S5

   ix. Superior hypogastric nerve block

SUGGESTED READINGS

Alvarez D, Rockwell PG: Trigger points: Diagnosis and management. Am Family Physician 2002;65(4):653–660.

Edwards L: New concepts in vulvodynia. Am J Obstet Gynecol 2003;189(3): S24–S30.

Epperly A, Viera AJ: Pelvic inflammatory disease. Clin Family Pract 2005;7: 67–78.

Lifford K, Barbieri RL: Diagnosis and management of chronic pelvic pain. Urol Clin N Am. 2002;29(3):637–647.

Mahutte N: Medical management of endometriosis-associated pain. Obstet Gynecol Clin 2003;30(1):133–150.

Nickel J: Interstitial cystitis: A chronic pelvic pain syndrome. Med Clin N Am 2004;88:467–481.

Stenchever MA: Comprehensive Gynecology, 4th ed. St. Louis, Mosby Inc., 2001.

105 Degenerative Disc Disease

1. PATHOPHYSIOLOGY

a. Degenerative disc disease (DDD) is most often due to age-related changes, but the condition also is affected by lifestyle, genetics, smoking, nutrition, and physical activity.

b. Circumferential tears form in the annulus fibrosus after repetitive use.

c. Several circumferential tears coalesce into radial tears, which progress into radial fissures. The disc then disrupts with tears passing throughout the disc.

d. Loss of disc height occurs with peripheral annular bulging. Proteoglycans and water escape through fissures formed from nuclear degeneration, resulting in further thinning of the disc space.

e. The innervated outer disc annulus serves as a major pain generator.

f. Radiculopathy results from nerve root compression secondary to herniated disc material, stenosis, or proteoglycan-mediated chemical inflammation released from discs.

2. IMAGING FINDINGS

a. Computed tomography (CT) scan
   i. Valuable diagnostic tool in assessing fractures and other osseous abnormalities of the spine
   ii. CT-myelography aids with presurgical planning by allowing identification of osseous structures causing neural compression.

b. Magnetic resonance imaging (MRI)
   i. Useful in identifying abnormalities of the soft tissues and neural structures
   ii. Neoplasms, osteomyelitis, and fractures can also be identified.
   iii. Detects early disc degeneration and annular tears and disc herniation
   iv. As the discs desiccate, the MRI signal decreases on T2-weighted images.

c. Plain radiography
   i. Anteroposterior (AP) and lateral lumbar spine x-rays are helpful for identifying loss of disc height as a result of disc degeneration, spondylosis/osteophyte formation, and facet arthropathy.
   ii. Oblique views are helpful to identify spondylolysis.
   iii. Flexion/extension films are necessary to identify dynamic instability and can assist in identifying appropriate surgical candidates for fusion procedures.

3. DIFFERENTIAL DIAGNOSIS

a. Spinal stenosis
b. Fractures (e.g., osteoporotic compression fractures)
c. Spondylolysis, spondylolisthesis
d. Osteomyelitis of the spine
e. Discitis
f. Cervical/lumbar myofascial pain
g. Piriformis syndrome
h. Fibromyalgia
i. Osteoarthritis
j. Osteoporosis
k. Paget disease
l. Rheumatoid arthritis

4. CLINICAL ISSUES

a. Presentation
   i. Cervical
      (1) Discogenic pain without nerve root involvement is vague, diffuse, and distributed axially.
      (2) Pain referred from disc to the upper extremity usually is nondermatomal.
      (3) Activities that increase intradiscal pressure (e.g., lifting, Valsalva maneuver) intensify symptoms.
      (4) Lying supine provides relief by decreasing intradiscal pressure.
      (5) Vibrational stress from driving also exacerbates discogenic pain.
      (6) Radicular pain is deep, dull, and achy or sharp, burning, and shooting.
      (7) Radicular pain follows a dermatomal pattern into the upper extremity.
      (8) Patients may present with distal limb numbness and proximal weakness in addition to pain.
      (9) Patient with radicular pain also displays decreased cervical range of motion.
   ii. Lumbar
      (1) Chronic back pain and stiffness
      (2) Limited range of motion
      (3) Sciatic syndrome consists of stiffness in the back and pain radiating down to the thighs, calves, and feet, associated with paresthesias, weakness, and reflex changes.
      (4) Pain is exacerbated by coughing, sneezing, or physical activity.
      (5) Pain is usually worse when sitting, and with straightening or elevating the leg.
      (6) Pain gets worse when bending, lifting, or twisting.

(7) Pain may be relieved with frequent changing of positions or with lying down supine.

b. General points

i. Cervical DDD occurs most commonly at the levels of C5-6 and C6-7. This is due to the mechanical influence on the cervical intervertebral discs by the extensive movement carried out in the cervical spine in relation to the rigid thoracic spine.

ii. Symptomatic thoracic discs are uncommon; most common level is T11-12.

iii. Calcification is more common in thoracic disc fragments and parent discs than in cervical or lumbar region.

iv. For the lumbar spine, disc degeneration occurs most often at the lower levels, 90% at L5-5 and L5-S1, given they undergo the greatest torsion and compressive loads.

v. DDD may be observed with MRI in 25% of asymptomatic individuals younger than 40 years and in 60% of those older than 40 years.

vi. Smoking and certain occupational activities also predispose patients to cervical/lumbar radiculopathy.

vii. Provocative discography is currently the only technique to correlate structural abnormalities of the intravertebral disc seen on advanced imaging studies with a patient's pain response.

viii. Electrodiagnostic studies are useful for identification of compression neuropathy, radiculopathy, or systemic motor and sensory diseases.

c. Natural history

i. Most of the acute low-back symptoms are myofascial in origin and typically resolve within 4 to 6 weeks.

ii. The benign nature of degenerative conditions of the spine should be emphasized as well as the fact that acute exacerbations tend to improve over time regardless of therapy.

5. TREATMENT

a. Nonsurgical therapy

i. Therapy directed toward management of the condition

ii. Anti-inflammatory medications

iii. Muscle relaxants

iv. Membrane-stabilizing agents (gabapentin, carbamazepine) for neuropathic pain

v. Opioid medications for severe symptom exacerbation

vi. Functionally oriented physical therapy program

vii. Trigger point injection for myofascial pain

viii. Low-dose tricyclic antidepressants for improvement of sleep

ix. Epidural steroid injection for temporary relief of radicular symptoms

x. Facet injections for temporary pain relief and establishment of facet-mediated pain; facet rhizotomies for longer symptomatic relief for patients with clearly identified facet pain

    xi. Intradiscal electrothermal therapy (IDET) to modify collagen in the posterior annulus in an attempt to seal annular fissures and to ablate nociceptive fibers

  b. Surgical therapy

    i. The surgical indications for DDD of the lumbar spine are highly debated and evolving.

    ii. Surgery is considered when intensive nonsurgical therapies have failed and the patient continues to have functionally limiting pain.

    iii. Current data are incomplete to judge the scientific validity of spinal fusion for low-back pain syndromes. However, if the intervertebral disc is clearly identified as the source of low-back pain, interbody fusion with discectomy appears to have favorable results.

6. PROGNOSIS

  a. DDD ultimately may progress to internal disc disruption.

  b. In general, DDD is a benign condition.

  c. Functional limitations can occur when neural compression and symptoms of spinal stenosis, neural claudication, and segmental instability develop.

  d. Persistent neurologic deficits from these conditions are rare and can be avoided if the conditions are diagnosed early and appropriate treatment is begun.

  e. A few patients may develop chronic pain syndromes.

  f. Low-back pain is the most common cause of the chronic pain syndrome.

SUGGESTED READINGS

Carette S, Leclaire R, Marcoux S, et al: Epidural corticosteroid injections for sciatica due to herniated nucleus pulposus. N Engl J Med 1997;336(23):1634–1640.

Carette S, Marcoux S, Truchon R, et al: A controlled trial of corticosteroid injections into the facet joints for chronic low back pain. N Engl J Med 1998;325(14):1002–1007.

Carragee EJ, Tanner CM, Khurana S, et al: The rates of false-positive lumbar discography in select patients without low back symptoms. Spine 2000;25(11):1373–1380.

Chen TY: The clinical presentation of uppermost cervical disc protrusion. Spine 2000;25(4):439–442.

Cicala RS, Thoni K, Angel JJ: Long-term results of cervical epidural steroid injections. Clin J Pain 1989;5(2):143–145.

Cohen SP, Larkin TM, Barna SA, et al: Lumbar discography: A comprehensive review of outcome studies, diagnostic accuracy, and principles. Reg Anesth Pain Med 2005;30(2):163–183.

Connor PM, Darden BV II: Cervical discography complications and clinical efficacy. Spine 1993;18(14):2035–2038.

Dreyfuss P, Halbrook B, Pauza K, et al: Efficacy and validity of radiofrequency neurotomy for chronic lumbar zygapophysial joint pain. Spine 2000;25(10):1270–1277.

Freemont AJ, Peacock TE, Goupille P, et al: Nerve ingrowth into diseased intervertebral disc in chronic back pain. Lancet 1997;350(9072):178–181.

Saal JA, Saal JS: Intradiscal electrothermal treatment for chronic discogenic low
back pain: A prospective outcome study with minimum 1-year follow-up. Spine
2000;25(20):2622–2627.

Schwarzer AC, Aprill CN, Derby R, et al: The prevalence and clinical features
of internal disc disruption in patients with chronic low back pain. Spine
1995;20(17):1878–1883.

106 Spinal Stenosis

1. PATHOPHYSIOLOGY

a. Spinal stenosis refers to the narrowing of the spinal canal anywhere along its axis with compression of the nerve roots in the central canal or in the neural foramina.

b. It may be due to acquired or degenerative processes or to congenital stenosis.

c. Congenital stenosis is due to inadequate development of the canal or foramina (congenitally short pedicle, thickened lamina and facets, or excessive scoliotic or lordotic curves).

d. The narrowed canal may lead to clinically significant stenosis if additional degenerative changes further reduce the diameter of the canal and contribute to nerve root impingement.

e. Loss of disc height from degenerative changes or loss of vertebral body height from osteoporosis or compression fracture can cause foraminal narrowing.

f. Spondylolisthesis may also lead to narrower foramen.

g. Degenerative spinal stenosis begins with progressive intervertebral disc degeneration.

h. Progressive disc degeneration causes increased axial loading of the posterior elements of the spine, including the facet joints.
   i. This leads to facet arthropathy with osteophyte formation.
   ii. Concomitantly, hypertrophy of the ligamentum flavum and protrusion of the degenerative disc material occur.

i. Facet osteophytes, ligamentum flavum hypertrophy, and disc bulging results in encroachment on the central spinal canal and the neural foramina.

j. Pain, weakness, or numbness in the extremities occurs when there is a nerve root compression.

2. IMAGING FINDINGS

a. Computed tomography (CT)
   i. Provides general information about canal diameter, spur formation, and foraminal
   ii. Shows the shape, size, and nearby structures of the spinal canal
   iii. CT myelogram demonstrates central or lateral canal stenosis in both sagittal and axial planes with good visualization of the bony anatomy.
   iv. On CT scans, spinal stenosis is well defined as the diminished diameter(s) and cross-sectional area of the spinal canal.
   v. CT of the cervical spine can be improved by using intravenous contrast agents to enhance the epidural veins, thus better defining the margins of the epidural space.

b. Magnetic resonance imaging (MRI)
   i. Useful in delineating the extent and causes of the narrowing
   ii. Most useful in evaluating soft tissues and neural structures
   iii. Reveals disc degeneration, ligamentous and facet hypertrophy, malalignment, central or lateral canal stenosis, and intrinsic cord or root abnormalities
   iv. Hourglass configuration of the thecal sac is displayed in the sagittal planes of a T2-weighted scan
   v. Not optimal for visualization of bony details
c. Plain radiography
   i. Reveals narrow anteroposterior diameter in both congenital and acquired forms of spinal stenosis
   ii. Shows degenerative changes and spondylolisthesis
   iii. Spondylosis appears as curvilinear bony outgrowths from the lateral and posterior margins of the vertebral body endplates
   iv. Useful in ruling out tumors, injuries, or abnormalities

3. DIFFERENTIAL DIAGNOSIS

a. Conus medullaris and cauda equina neoplasms
b. Degenerative spondylolisthesis
c. Discitis
d. Peripheral vascular disease
e. Sciatic claudication
f. Venous claudication after thrombosis
g. Peripheral neuropathy
h. Osteoarthritis of the hips and knees
i. Neurofibromas, ependymomas, hemangioblastomas, dermoids, epidermoids, lipomas
j. Metastatic spread of tumor
k. Epidural abscess
l. Inflammatory arachnoiditis
m. Trauma/fractures
n. Lumbar facet syndrome
o. Pathologic vertebral fracture with bony stenosis (osteoporosis)

4. CLINICAL ISSUES

a. Presentation
   i. Cervical stenosis
      (1) Subtle loss of hand dexterity and mild proximal upper extremity weakness
      (2) Pain in the cervical neck and arms
      (3) Numbness and tingling in one or both upper extremities
      (4) Sharp radicular pain into the affected arm with associated paresthesias and weakness secondary to the compressed nerve root

    ii. Lumbar stenosis
- (1) Claudication-like leg pain or weakness when walking, which is relieved by resting or sitting down (neurogenic claudication)
- (2) Pain radiating from the lower back to the buttocks, or lower legs, often causing the patient to stop walking
- (3) Numbness and tingling in one or both lower extremities
- (4) Worsening pain with extension of the lumbar spine and improvement with forward flexion of the hips, knees, or lumbar spine
- (5) The degree of axial and extremity pain varies between individuals.
- (6) Symptoms from central canal narrowing tend to be diffuse (nondermatomal) compared with foraminal narrowing, where irritation of the exiting nerve root often produces symptoms in a dermatomal distribution.
- (7) Lower extremity symptoms are almost always described as burning, numbness, tingling, or dull fatigue in the thighs and legs.

b. General points
- i. Few causes of spinal stenosis are truly congenital.
- ii. Although many conditions may be associated with spinal stenosis, most cases are caused by acquired degenerative changes of the intervertebral discs, ligaments, and facet joints surrounding the spinal canal.
- iii. For the cervical spine, stenosis most commonly occurs at C5-6 and C6-7.
- iv. For the lumbar spine, stenosis most commonly occurs at L4-5 and L5-S1.
- v. The most common nerve affected is the L5, with associated weakness of extensor hallucis longus.
- vi. Degenerative spondylolisthesis is commonly associated with spinal stenosis and tends to exacerbate the nerve root compression.
- vii. Thoracic spinal stenosis is rare and often is associated with focal disease of long-standing nature.
  - (1) It is more likely to directly affect the spinal cord because of the relatively narrow thoracic spinal canal.
  - (2) Compression of the thoracic spinal cord can result in myelopathy
- viii. Spinal stenosis of the cervical and thoracic regions may contribute to neurologic injury, such as development of a central spinal cord syndrome following spinal trauma.
- ix. Spinal stenosis of the lumbar spine is associated most commonly with axial back pain and radiculopathy.
- x. In cases of severe lumbar stenosis, innervation of the urinary bladder and the rectum may be affected (cauda equina syndrome), but most often, lumbar stenosis results in back pain

with lower extremity weakness and numbness along the distribution of nerve roots of the lumbar plexus.

  xi. Symptom severity does not always correlate with the degree of lumbar canal narrowing.

5. NATURAL HISTORY

a. Cervical stenosis
   i. The stenosis progresses in one-third of affected individuals.
   ii. Stenosis of the central cervical spine may result in myelopathy from cord compression.
   iii. There is a propensity for initial deterioration, followed by a period of stability and subsequent progression of myelopathy.
b. Lumbar stenosis
   i. Natural history of lumbar spinal stenosis is not well understood. A slow progression appears to occur in all affected individuals.
   ii. Canal stenosis in the lumbosacral region will result in pain, neurogenic claudication, or both.
   iii. Disease onset is usually insidious; early symptoms may be mild and progress to become extremely disabling.
   iv. Even with significant narrowing, a patient is very unlikely to develop an acute cauda equina syndrome in the absence of significant disc herniation.

6. TREATMENT

a. Nonsurgical therapy
   i. Minimize stress on the lumbar spine by maintaining ideal body weight
   ii. Lumbar bracing
   iii. Bed rest
   iv. Anti-inflammatory drugs
   v. Physical therapy, such as, heat, aquatherapy, and exercise, to strengthen abdominal muscles and reduce lumbar lordosis
   vi. Epidural steroid injection
   vii. Nonsurgical measures for spinal stenosis are aimed at symptomatic relief. They have few proven benefits in the long run, however.
b. Surgical therapy
   i. Surgery is recommended when significant radiculopathy, myelopathy (cervicothoracic), neurogenic claudication (lumbar), or incapacitating pain is present.
   ii. Surgical decompression techniques include laminectomy, laminotomy, laminoplasty, foraminotomy, and anterior discectomy.
   iii. The ideal technique to use depends on where the narrowing is located, what is causing the narrowing, how stable the spine is, and how great is the surgeon's expertise.

7. PROGNOSIS

a. Patients with spinal stenosis often show no improvement on long-term follow-up when managed conservatively. Their symptoms rapidly return with the resumption of activity.

b. For patients with severe pain limiting their activities, early surgery is the best way to return them to full activity and independent living.

SUGGESTED READINGS

Amundsen T, Weber H, Nordal HJ, et al: Lumbar spinal stenosis: Conservative or surgical management?: A prospective 10-year study. Spine 2000; 25(11):1424–1436.

Atlas SJ, Keller RB, Robson D, et al: Surgical and nonsurgical management of lumbar spinal stenosis: Four-year outcomes from the Maine lumbar spine study. Spine 2000;25:556.

Epstein NE: Circumferential surgery for the management of cervical ossification of the posterior longitudinal ligament. J Spinal Disord 1998;11(3):200–207.

Epstein NE, Epstein JE: Lumbar stenosis. In Youmans JR (ed): Neurological Surgery, 4th ed. Philadelphia, Saunders, 1996, pp 2396–2397.

Loeser JD, Butler SH, Chapman CR, Turk DC: Bonica's Management of Pain. Philadelphia: Lippincott Williams & Wilkins, 2001: pp 1522–1523.

Silvers HR, Lewis PJ, Asch HL: Decompressive lumbar laminectomy for spinal stenosis. J Neurosurg 1993;78:695–701.

Wallace MS, Staats PS: Pain Medicine & Management. New York, McGraw-Hill, 2005, pp 141–146.

Warfield CA, Bajawa ZH: Principles & Practice of Pain Medicine. New York, McGraw-Hill, 2004, 273–282.

107 Herniated Nucleus Pulposus

1. PATHOPHYSIOLOGY

a. Herniation of the nucleus pulposus through the annulus fibrosis
b. Pain and nerve dysfunction occurs when the herniated fragment irritates and/or compresses the nerve root.
c. Caused by aging, degenerative disc diseases, or injury to the spine

2. IMAGING FINDINGS

a. Computed tomography (CT) myelography
   i. Delineate bony structure better than magnetic resonance imaging (MRI)
   ii. May be performed to define the size and location of disc herniation
b. MRI
   i. Very sensitive in delineating disc herniations
   ii. Shows spinal canal compression by the herniated disc
c. Plain radiograph
   i. Useful adjunct to other radiographic evaluations, especially with weight-bearing flexion and extension views
   ii. May be performed to rule out other causes of back or neck pain

3. DIFFERENTIAL DIAGNOSIS

a. Myofascial pain
b. Spinal stenosis
c. Spondylosis
d. Spondylolisthesis
e. Discogenic pain
f. Facet arthropathy
g. Compression fracture
h. Epidural fibrosis

4. CLINICAL ISSUES

a. Presentation
   i. Lumbar herniation
     (1) Low-back pain
     (2) Pain radiating to the leg in a dermatomal distribution
     (3) Radicular pain that is often characterized as achy, burning, shooting, or stabbing
     (4) Maneuvers associated with an elevation of intrathecal pressure, such as coughing, sneezing, laughing, or prolonged sitting, usually aggravate this pain.

(5) Pain usually improves when the patient is in the supine position with the legs slightly elevated.

(6) Sensory loss, muscle weakness, or diminished reflexes in the distribution of the affected nerve root may be present.

(7) In severe cases, bowel, bladder or sexual disturbances may be present.

  ii. Cervical herniation

(1) Neck pain, especially in the back and sides

(2) Deep pain near or over the shoulder blades on the affected side

(3) Pain radiating to the shoulder, upper arm, forearm, and rarely the hand, fingers, or chest in a dermatomal distribution

(4) Pain exacerbated with coughing, laughing, or straining

(5) Increased pain when bending the neck or turning head to the side

(6) Spasm of the neck muscles

(7) Upper extremity muscle weakness

  iii. General points

(1) Most herniation occurs in the lumbar area of the spine

(2) Lumbar disc herniation occurs 15 times more often than cervical disc herniation, and it is one of the most common causes of lower back pain.

(3) The cervical discs are affected 8% of the time and the thoracic discs only 1% to 2% of the time

(4) In 95% of cases, either L4-L5 or L5-S1 disc is affected.

(5) Most common age for disc rupture is during the 3rd and 4th decades of life

(6) Diagnosis is generally made by CT myelography or MRI.

(7) Electromyography (EMG) findings can be helpful in patients with nerve root impingement.

b. Natural history

  i. Ninety percent to 95% of patients will recover over time (1 to 6 months) without any specific treatment.

  ii. Small percentage of people will require further treatment, including physical therapy, steroid injections, or surgery.

5. TREATMENT

a. Nonsurgical therapy

  i. Bed rest, followed by a gradual increase in activity

  ii. Medication to control pain and inflammation (steroidal and/or nonsteroidal)

  iii. Neuropathic medication for patients with radicular symptoms

  iv. Physical therapy

  v. Epidural corticosteroid injection can provide pain relief in patients with acute onset or exacerbation of sciatica

  vi. Nucleoplasty

   b. Surgical therapy
      i. Microdiscectomy
     ii. Hemilaminotomy or hemilaminectomy

6. PROGNOSIS

   a. Spontaneous resolution of symptoms from nerve root compression occurs in 90% of all cases, most within 6 to 12 weeks.
   b. Surgery has a 90% success rate in improving the symptoms of herniated disc and allowing patients to return to work.
   c. The relief of radicular pain with surgical intervention is a much more predictable result (>90%) than the relief of back pain (>50%).

SUGGESTED READINGS

Deyo RA, Phillips WR: Low back pain: A primary care challenge. Spine 1996;21: 2826–2832.

Ehni BL, Benzel EC: Lumbar discectomy. Spine Surg 1999;1:389–400.

Loeser JD, Butler SH, Chapman CR, Turk DC: Bonica's Management of Pain. Philadelphia: Lippincott Williams & Wilkins, 2001: pp 1509–1539.

Schwarzer AC, April CN, Derby R, et al: The prevalence and clinical features of internal disc disruption in patients with chronic low back pain. Spine 1995;20:1878–1883.

Wallace MS, Staats PS: Pain Medicine & Management. New York, McGraw-Hill, 2005, pp. 141–146.

Warfield CA, Bajawa ZH. Principles & Practice of Pain Medicine. New York, McGraw-Hill, 2004, 277–278.

108 Facet Hypertrophy

1. PATHOPHYSIOLOGY

a. Facet hypertrophy is a manifestation of arthrosis and spondylotic changes of the spine.

b. Any acquired, traumatic, or degenerative process that distorts the normal anatomy or function of a facet joint can disrupt the normal biomechanics of the joint and result in facet joint hypertrophy.

c. Facet joint hypertrophy, along with osteophyte formation, can encroach on the lateral recesses of the spinal canal and the neural foramina.

d. Compression of the exiting nerve roots results in a radicular pain syndrome (lateral recess syndrome).

e. Facet joint can be a source of spine pain due to trauma, inflammation, synovial impingement, and chondromalacia.

2. IMAGING FINDINGS

a. Computed tomography (CT)
   i. CT scan of the spine provides excellent anatomic imaging of the osseous structures of the spine, especially to rule out fractures or arthritic changes.
   ii. With facet joint hypertrophy, one may find arthritic changes in the facets and degenerative disk disease.
   iii. Generally, a CT scan is not necessary unless other bony pathology (e.g., a fracture) must be excluded.

b. Magnetic resonance imaging (MRI)
   i. MRI provides detailed anatomic images of the soft structures of the spine, such as the intervertebral disks, which often show degenerative changes prior to facet joint pathology.
   ii. MRI also may illustrate nerve root entrapment secondary to facet joint hypertrophy and may help visualize the neural foramen.
   iii. In general, an MRI is not necessary for nonradicular cervical/lumbar spine pain.

c. Plain radiography
   i. Plain radiographs are traditionally ordered as the initial step in the workup of spine pain.
   ii. The main purpose of plain films is to determine underlying structural pathology.
   iii. X-ray films may reveal degenerative changes, but, in general, no abnormalities are seen in persons with facet joint pathology.

d. Bone scan
   i. Bone scans can be helpful when a tumor, infection, or fracture (occult or traumatic) is suggested.
   ii. Bone scans are not usually indicated in the initial workup, and the results are normal in persons with facet joint syndrome.

3. DIFFERENTIAL DIAGNOSIS

a. Radiculopathy
b. Internal disc disruption
c. Discogenic pain
d. Myofascial pain syndrome
e. Nerve root compression
f. Spondylolysis/spondylolisthesis
g. Spinal stenosis
h. Spondylosis
i. Sacroiliac joint dysfunction
j. Piriformis syndrome

4. CLINICAL ISSUES

a. Presentation
  i. Cervical spine
    (1) Generalized posterior neck and suboccipital pain
    (2) Localized tenderness over the posterolateral aspect of the neck
    (3) Pain often exacerbated by cervical extension and axial rotation
  ii. Lumbar spine
    (1) Axial low-back pain
    (2) Pain tends to be localized to the back with radiation to the buttock and posterior thigh and, occasionally, below the knee.
    (3) Pain is often exacerbated by twisting the back, by stretching, by lateral bending, and in the presence of a torsional load.
    (4) Pain is worse in the morning, aggravated by rest and hyperextension, and relieved by repeated motion.
b. General points
  i. Facet joint derangement is commonly seen in patients with prior neck/back surgery.
  ii. Axial spine pain originating from the facet joints has a similar presentation to discogenic pain.
  iii. Pain originating from facet joints is likely to be the etiology of 15% to 40% of nonradicular low-back pain and 40% to 60% of nonradicular neck pain.
c. Natural history
  i. Facet hypertrophy is usually due to degenerative process of the spine.
  ii. This condition is often progressive, resulting in chronic, intractable spinal pain.
  iii. It often coexists with spinal disc abnormalities, further leading to chronic pain.
  iv. This subsequently results in diminished spinal motion and weakness.

5. TREATMENT

a. Nonsurgical therapy
  i. Nonsteroidal anti-inflammatory drugs
  ii. Physical therapy
  iii. Medial branch nerve block
  iv. Intra-articular facet joint injection with corticosteroids and a local anesthetic
  v. Medial branch neurotomy through radiofrequency (rhizotomy), chemical neurolysis, or cryoneurolysis

b. Surgical therapy
  i. Surgery is rarely indicated in primary and isolated facet arthropathies.
  ii. Surgical spinal fusion may be performed for discogenic pain, which may affect secondary cases of facet arthropathies.

6. PROGNOSIS

a. With an active and focused spine rehabilitation program, the prognosis for these patients to achieve pain-free activity is good.
b. However, the definitive diagnosis of facet joint syndrome is often difficult to make and challenging to confirm.

SUGGESTED READINGS

Adams MA, Hutton WC: The mechanical function of the lumbar apophyseal joints. Spine 1983;8(3):327–330.

Bogduk N: International Spinal Injection Society Guidelines for the performance of spinal injection procedures. Part I. Zygapophysial joint blocks. Clin J Pain 1997;13:285–302.

Carette S, Marcoux S, Truchon R, et al: A controlled trial of corticosteroid injections into facet joints for chronic low back pain. N Engl J Med 1991;325(14): 1002–1007.

Cavanaugh JM, Ozaktay AC, Yamashita T, et al: Mechanisms of low back pain: A neurophysiological and neuroanatomic study. Clin Orthop 1997;335:166–180.

Cho J, Park YG, Chung SS: Percutaneous radiofrequency lumbar facet rhizotomy in mechanical low back pain syndrome. Stereotact Funct Neurosurg 1997; (1-4 Pt 1):212–217.

Dreyer SJ, Dreyfuss P: Low back pain and the zygapophyseal joints. Arch Phys Med Rehabil 1996;77:290–300.

Dreyfuss P, Halbrook B, Pauza K, et al: Efficacy and validity of radiofrequency neurotomy for chronic lumbar zygapophyseal joint pain. Spine 2000;25(10): 1270–1277.

Dreyfuss P, Halbrook B, Pauza K, et al: Lumbar radiofrequency neurotomy for chronic zygapophyseal joint pain: A pilot study using dual medial branch blocks. Int Spinal Inject Soc Sci News 1999;3(2):13–31.

Fukui S, Ohseto K, Shiotani M, et al: Distribution of referred pain from the lumbar zygapophyseal joints and dorsal rami. Clin J Pain 1997;13:303–307.

Kleef M, Barendse G, Kessels A, et al: Randomised trial of radiofrequency lumbar facet denervation for chronic low back pain. Spine 1999;24:1937–1942.

Lewinnek GE, Warfield CA: Facet joint degeneration as a cause of low back pain. Clin Orthop 1986;213:216–222.

Mooney V, Robertson J: The facet syndrome. Clin Orthop 1976;115:149–156.

North RB, Han M, Zahurak M, Kidd DH: Radiofrequency lumbar facet denervation: Analysis of prognostic factors. Pain 1994;57:77–83.

Niosi CA, Oxland TR: Degenerative mechanics of the lumbar spine. Spine 2004; 46:202S–208S.

Van Wijk RM, Geurts JW, Wynne HJ, et al: Radiofrequency denervation of lumbar facet joints in the treatment of chronic low back pain: A randomized, double-blinded, sham lesion-controlled trials. Clin J Pain 2005;21(5):462.

109 Failed Back Surgery Syndrome

1. PATHOPHYSIOLOGY

  a. Axial low-back pain
  b. May be due to mechanical disruption of the facet joints, disc, or musculoskeletal components
  c. Facet joint arthritis, fusion arthritis, degenerative changes of adjacent discs
  d. Lower extremity pain
  e. May be referred pain from mechanical components, such as facet joints, discs, or sacroiliac joints
  f. Pain from nerve root irritation related to epidural scarring entangling one or more nerve roots or from the foraminal narrowing due to loss of disc or vertebral body height

2. IMAGING FINDINGS

  a. Computed tomography (CT) scan
      i. Delineates bony structure better than magnetic resonance imaging (MRI)
  b. MRI
      i. Gadolinium-enhanced MRI helps to differentiate between postsurgical scar and recurrent or retained disc fragments
      ii. Limited functions in defining bony anatomy
  c. Plain radiograph
      i. Useful adjunct to other radiographic evaluations
      ii. May be performed to rule out other causes of back pain

3. DIFFERENTIAL DIAGNOSIS

  a. Herniated disc
  b. Myofascial pain
  c. Spinal stenosis
  d. Lumbar spondylosis
  e. Osteoarthritis root compression
  f. Spondylolisthesis
  g. Facet arthropathy

4. CLINICAL ISSUES

  a. Presentation
      i. Depending on the surgical procedure and the original condition, pain associated with failed back surgery syndrome (FBSS) varies between patients in terms of distribution, character, and associated neurologic abnormalities.

    ii. Most commonly, patients present with axial low-back pain with unilateral lower extremity pain.

    iii. Pain is often diffuse, dull, and achy in quality.

b. General points

    i. FBSS is a general term that refers to persistent or recurrent chronic pain following lumbosacral spine surgery.

    ii. Fifteen percent of patients who have spinal surgery develop FBSS.

    iii. Etiology is multifactorial.

       (1) Poor patient selection

       (2) Inaccurate diagnostic evaluation

       (3) Faulty technique

       (4) Recurring or persistent herniated disc

       (5) Inadequate relief of pressure from spinal stenosis

       (6) Instability of facet joints

       (7) Nerve injury

       (8) Complications from surgery

    iv. Most common causes are recurrent disc herniation, spinal stenosis, epidural scarring, and arachnoiditis

    v. Electromyography (EMG) is useful in differentiating acute and chronic muscle denervation.

    vi. Nerve conduction studies are useful in correlating clinical symptoms with noncompressed nerve roots (from MRI).

    vii. Provocative discography is performed to determine whether mechanical loading of individual discs reproduces an individual patient's characteristic pain.

    viii. Diagnostic blocks are performed to localize a peripheral pain pathway.

c. Natural history

    i. FBSS is technically not a syndrome, and there are no typical scenarios.

    ii. Every patient is different, and a patient's continued treatment and workup need to be individualized to his or her particular condition and situation.

5. TREATMENT

a. Nonsurgical options

    i. Physical therapy

    ii. Pharmacologic management

       (1) Nonsteroidal anti-inflammatory drugs: first-line medical treatment against the pain associated with musculoskeletal disorders

       (2) Systemic opioids: Stable plasma levels of opioid analgesics improve quality of life and cause fewer side effects.

       (3) Neuropathic medication for patients with radicular symptoms (anticonvulsants and tricyclic antidepressants)

    iii. Facet joint injection

    iv. Epidural corticosteroid injection
    v. Intradiscal electrothermal annuloplasty
    vi. Spinal cord stimulation
    vii. Implantation of intrathecal pump
  b. Surgical therapy
    i. Decompression
    ii. Fusion
    iii. Dorsal root ganglionectomy

6. PROGNOSIS

  a. The rate of success of reoperation varies from 12% to 100%.
  b. Reoperation should only be considered if there is a clear anatomic reason for worsening pain and conservative measures have failed.
  c. Epidural fibrosis requiring surgical lysis is an adverse prognostic factor.
  d. Favorable prognostic indicators:
    i. Women have been reported to do better than men.
    ii. Patients with good results from prior surgeries.
    iii. Patients who have undergone a small number of operations do better after reoperation.
    iv. Patients with radicular pain have fared better than those with axial back pain.
    v. Patients who are employed immediately before surgery have been reported to have superior outcome from reoperation.

SUGGESTED READINGS

Loeser JD, Butler SH, Chapman CR, Turk DC: Bonica's management of pain. Philadelphia: Lippincott Williams & Wilkins, 2001: pp 1540–1548.

North RB, Campbell JN, James CS, et al: Failed back surgery syndrome: 5-year follow-up in 102 patients undergoing repeated operation. Neurosurgery 1991;28:685–691.

North RB, Ewend MG, Lawton MT, et al: Failed back surgery syndrome: 5-year follow-up after spinal cord stimulator implantation. Neurosurgery. 1991; 28(5):692–699.

Onesti ST: Failed back syndrome. Neurologist 2004;10(5):259–264.

Rowlingson J: Epidural steroids in treating failed back surgery syndrome. Anesth Analg 1999;88:240–242.

Sanders WP, Truumees E: Imaging of the postoperative spine. Semin Ultrasound CT and MR 2004;25(6):523–535.

Warfield CA, Bajawa ZH: Principles & Practice of Pain Medicine. New York, McGraw-Hill, 2004.

1. PATHOPHYSIOLOGY

a. Acute vascular insufficiency is largely caused by atherosclerosis and embolization, resulting in muscle necrosis and irreversible changes.

b. Claudication refers to cramping pain, resulting from an abnormal balance between blood supply and metabolic demands of activity.

c. Ischemic rest pain, which represents severe arterial insufficiency, occurs when basal resting tissue requirements outstrip blood flow.

d. Artery entrapment syndrome is the result of compression by muscle or connective tissue resulting in claudication.

e. Arterial cystic disease is due to arterial occlusion by mucoprotein cysts within the adventitial layer.

f. Thromboangiitis obliterans (Buerger disease) is a panangiitis of the neurovascular bundles of the hands and feet. It is the result of infiltration by giant cells and lymphocytes.

g. Raynaud disease is defined by episodic digital vasospasm initiated by cold or stress and may be mediated by adrenoreceptors or adrenoreceptor-immune complexes.

h. Causes for venous thrombosis include venous stasis, vessel wall injury, and hypercoagulability (Virchow triad).

i. Compartment syndrome is the result of either vasospasm, venous hypertension, or increased transmural tissue pressure that results in premature vascular closure, muscle necrosis, neurologic injury, and acute pain.

j. Arterial aneurysms are the result of septic embolization (mycotic), infectious causes (i.e., abscess, cellulitis), or traumatic injury.

2. DIFFERENTIAL DIAGNOSIS

a. Arterial insufficiency

b. Artery entrapment syndromes (i.e., popliteal)

c. Thromboangiitis obliterans (Buerger disease)

d. Raynaud disease

e. Thrombophlebitis

f. Deep venous thrombosis

g. Compartment syndrome

h. Arterial aneurysms

3. CLINICAL ISSUES

a. General points

  i. Young patients with unilateral claudication symptoms suggest artery entrapment syndromes.

  ii. Adventitial cystic disease mostly occurs in young males with rapid onset of severe claudication.

    iii. Buerger disease typically affects Eastern European males who are heavy smokers and younger than 40 years.

    iv. Raynaud disease occurs in women more than 70% of the time and is associated with connective tissue diseases and certain occupational hazards (vibration tool operators).

    v. Cellulitis of an extremity may be distinguished from thrombophlebitis by lymphangiitis, regional lymph node enlargement and tenderness, and diffuse systemic symptoms.

b. Diagnosis

    i. Ankle pressure index (API) is the ratio of the ankle-to-arm blood pressure (normal range, 1.10 to 1.2). An API of less than one suggests arterial insufficiency.

    ii. Angiographic (magnetic resonance angiography [MRA] or percutaneous angiography) evaluation correlates well with API data.

    iii. An "hourglass" appearance with angiography is consistent with adventitial cystic disease.

    iv. Pathologic findings consistent with Buerger disease include small artery occlusions, proximal tapering, and no plaques observed with angiography.

    v. Raynaud disease is diagnosed by the ice-water immersion test, where return to baseline digit temperature is prolonged in patients inflicted with this disorder.

    vi. Venous thrombosis is diagnosed by decreased flow by Doppler ultrasound, impedance plethysmography, or radioactive fibrinogen uptake testing.

    vii. Compartment syndrome can be diagnosed by measuring tissue pressures in the compartment, with normal tissue pressures between 0 and 10 mm Hg.

c. Clinical features

    i. Acute vascular insufficiency is characterized by its sudden onset, focal localization, and the "five P's," including pallor, pain, paresthesias, paralysis, and pulselessness.

    ii. Chronic arterial insufficiency typically presents with numbness, coldness, tingling, or paresis.

    iii. Claudication is always relieved by rest and is reproducible with exercise in a functional muscle group.

    iv. Ischemic rest pain is constant, nonfocal, and aggravated by limb elevation and cold.

    v. Increased collateral blood flow at the knees (i.e., geniculate arteries) suggests chronic arterial entrapment syndromes.

    vi. Venous thrombosis can produce tenderness with dorsiflexion (Homan sign), increased skin temperature, swelling, pain, discoloration, paresthesias, and weakness.

    vii. Buerger disease presents as intermittent claudication of the arch of the foot, which can progress to ischemic rest pain and gangrene.

    viii. Raynaud disease classically presents with blanching and numbness, followed by cyanosis and reactive hyperemia.

ix. Acute compartment syndromes provoke intense pain that is localized to the involved muscle group, especially with passive range of motion. Palpable pulses are diagnostically unreliable, and may be present with ongoing tissue ischemia.

x. Mycotic aneurysms typically present as warm, tender, pulsatile masses with audible systolic bruits.

d. Natural history

i. Nondiabetic patients with intermittent claudication, as opposed to ischemic rest pain, typically do not require limb amputations.

ii. Raynaud disease becomes more severe as the condition progresses, resulting in ulceration and pulp loss after digital artery occlusion.

iii. Acute venous thrombosis outflow obstruction can interfere with arterial inflow, cause limb cyanosis, and progress to venous gangrene.

4. TREATMENT

a. Management of venous thrombosis involves treatment of the underlying disease, bed rest, elevation of the extremity, and moist compresses.

b. Smoking cessation and regular exercise may improve outcome and quality of life in patients with claudication symptoms.

c. Percutaneous treatments have a higher success rate for larger vessels, whereas vascular stenting is reserved for complex or repeat lesions.

d. Arterial reconstruction and bypass surgery is reserved for diffuse small vessel disease.

e. Palliative measures for failed arterial reconstruction include lumbar sympathectomy, spinal cord stimulation (SCS), and medical management.

f. Lumbar sympathetic (L3) blocks may be beneficial in patients with a popliteal inflow index greater than 0.7, resulting in improved blood flow, rest pain, heal ulceration, and skin necrosis.

g. In anticoagulated patients, intravenous regional anesthesia technique (IVRA) may be an alternative therapy in blocking postganglionic neurons.

h. Spinal cord stimulation (T9-11) has a long-term efficacy of greater than 70%, possibly due to increased peripheral blood flow, decreased edema, and long-term pain relief.

i. Medical therapies for ischemic limb pain have been disappointing. They include vasodilators, phosphodiesterase inhibitors (Cilostazol and pentoxifylline), antithrombotics, fibrinolytics, antiplatelet drugs, and gene therapy (vascular endothelial growth factor).

j. Uncontrolled studies have shown that medical therapies (i.e., nifedipine), sympathetic blockade (i.e., stellate ganglion), IVRA, and surgical sympathectomy may provide clinical benefit in Raynaud disease.

k. In addition to smoking cessation, sympathetic blockade and SCS may have a role in treatment of complicated cases of Buerger disease.

l. Several prospective controlled studies have confirmed that long-term risk for recurrent events is decreased in patients anticoagulated for deep venous thrombosis.

SUGGESTED READINGS

Erdek MA, Staats PS: Spinal cord stimulation for angina pectoris and peripheral vascular disease. Anesthesiol Clin N Am 2003;21:797–804.

Warfield CA, Cohen SA, Stabile MJ: Pain in the extremities. In Warfield CA (ed): Principles and Practice of Pain Medicine, 2nd ed. New York, McGraw-Hill, 2004, pp 315–342.

1. PATHOPHYSIOLOGY

a. Pathophysiologic mechanisms for neuropathic limb pain may include ectopic generation, afferent sensitization, hyperexcitability, amplification of neural pacemakers, and electrical cross-communication.

b. A neuroma is a tangled mass of neuronal tissue formed after axonal injury by the process of wallerian degeneration. Electrically active neuromas are termed ectopic generators.

c. Neuropathic limb pain may also be due to altered neural modulation in the thalamus, cortex, and central nervous system (CNS).

d. Diabetic neuropathy may be due to metabolic (i.e., glycosylation, nitric oxide) or vascular derangements of nerve cell membranes.

e. HIV-associated neuropathy is attributed to direct HIV infection, immune-mediated nerve injury, coinfection (cytomegalovirus), or antiviral agents (i.e., didanosine).

f. Mononeuropathy multiplex (MM), or multifocal neuropathy, is the result of ischemic injury to peripheral nerves due to small- and medium-vessel vasculitis (i.e., rheumatoid arthritis, HIV-associated, leprosy, Lyme disease).

g. Compression neuropathy refers to external pressure injury to peripheral nerves and is categorized as neurapraxia (impairment with normal axonal structure), axonotmesis (wallerian degeneration), and neurotmesis (completely severed nerve).

2. DIFFERENTIAL DIAGNOSIS

a. Compression neuropathy
b. Diabetic neuropathy
c. HIV neuropathy
d. Neuroma
e. Guillain-Barre syndrome
f. Toxic neuropathy
g. Metabolic neuropathy
h. Paraneoplastic neuropathy
i. Autoimmune neuropathy
j. Lyme disease
k. Leprosy

3. CLINICAL ISSUES

a. General points
   i. Neuropathy refers loosely to any peripheral nerve lesion, focal or diffuse.

    ii. Polyneuropathy (PN) implies a symmetric and generalized condition, which may overlap clinically with multifocal neuropathy.

    iii. Large axonopathies, or axon degeneration, are the most common form of PN (i.e., diabetes mellitus, HIV, toxic-metabolic).

    iv. Myelinopathies, or segmental demyelination, are less common and are usually the result of an autoimmune insult on peripheral nerves (i.e., Guillain-Barre syndrome).

    v. Diabetic neuropathy
      (1) Generally presents as a chronic distal sensory deficit that is not painful.
      (2) Painful diabetic neuropathy is an acute small-fiber syndrome, which includes lumbar and thoracic radiculoplexopathy and distal sensory PN.

    vi. HIV-associated PN affects up to one-third of infected patients.

    vii. Guillain-Barre syndrome is the most common form of acute inflammatory demyelinating PN.

    viii. Median nerve syndrome is the most common compression neuropathy, predominately affecting women between 40 and 60 years, and occurring bilaterally more than 50% of the time.

  b. Diagnosis

    i. Nerve conduction studies (NCS) and electromyography will diagnose most PN, differentiating axonal from demyelinating, time course and severity, as well as motor from sensory fibers.

    ii. NCS will not diagnose rare pure small-fiber neuropathies (pain and temperature).

    iii. Quantitative sensory testing (QST) provides a noninvasive quantitative evaluation of sensory threshold and function. QST has a sensitivity of 60% in the diagnosis of pure small-fiber neuropathies.

    iv. Initial laboratory studies include complete blood count, liver function tests, erythrocyte sedimentation rate (ESR), antinuclear antibodies, rheumatoid arthritis (RA) factor, Lyme titer, thyroid-stimulating hormone, B_{12} level, and serum/urine electrophoresis.

    v. Nerve biopsy is rarely indicated in the diagnosis of PN (i.e., leprosy, sarcoidosis, amyloidosis).

    vi. Intraepidermal nerve fiber density may be a sensitive indicator for certain small-fiber neuropathies, although routine use is not clinically available.

  c. Clinical features

    i. Clinical history should include the time course, anatomic and fiber-type distribution, and pathophysiology consideration of the pain disorder.

    ii. Positive symptoms typical of PN include paresthesias, dysesthesias, hyperesthesia, allodynia, and hyperalgesia.

    iii. Symmetric pain is a prominent feature of small-fiber neuropathies, whereas variable pain is consistent with demyelinating PN.

    iv. MM presents as a rapid onset of severe pain, numbness, and neurologic deficits (i.e., ulnar, sciatic nerves) for days.

    v. Diabetic neuropathy presents with diminished pain and temperature sensation, preserved proprioception and reflexes, and possible autonomic dysfunction.

    vi. HIV neuropathy is usually a distal, symmetric, sensory polyneuropathy. Clinical features include decreased pinprick, temperature, and proprioceptive senses as well as depressed tendon reflexes.

    vii. Guillain-Barre syndrome develops over several days, resulting in limb paresthesias, distal to proximal weakness, loss of tendon reflexes, and deep aching proximal muscle pain.

    viii. Compression neuropathy presents with paresthesias, numbness, and pain in the cutaneous nerve distribution (i.e., median, ulnar). Chronic signs include muscle atrophy and decreased sensation.

  d. Natural history

    i. Diffuse axonal insult (axonotmesis) is less likely to recover compared with segmental demyelination.

    ii. Axonal regeneration occurs roughly at a pace of 1 inch per month from the site of injury.

    iii. Recovery from pure myelinopathy typically takes 6 to 8 weeks, whereas mixed PN may take several months to years to recover.

4. TREATMENT

  a. Therapeutic modalities are often successful in PN, and failed therapy is usually due to inadequate dosing schedules.

  b. Tricyclic antidepressants (i.e., amitriptyline, nortriptyline) have been shown, in randomized controlled studies, to be effective and safe in the treatment of painful PN.

  c. Tricyclic antidepressants exert their analgesic effect by inhibiting norepinephrine and serotonin reuptake in the CNS. Typical side effects include sedation, orthostasis, cardiac arrhythmias, and urinary retention.

  d. Controlled trials confirm anticonvulsants (i.e., carbamazepine, gabapentin) as efficacious in painful PN, but the risk of adverse effects equals their likelihood of clinical benefit.

  e. In a double-blind, randomized, controlled trial, tramadol (210 mg/day) was shown to improve pain scores and physical and social function in patients with diabetic neuropathy.

  f. Long-acting opioids (i.e., MS Contin, methadone) may have a role in PN when traditional therapies have failed.

  g. Although topical agents (i.e., capsaicin) and N-methyl-D-aspartate antagonists (dextromethorphan) may reduce peripheral nerve pain, clinical efficacy has been unimpressive.

SUGGESTED READINGS

Aminoff MJ: Electrophysiologic testing for the diagnosis of peripheral nerve injuries. Anesthesiology 2004;100:1298–1303.

Warfield CA, Cohen SA, Stabile MJ: Pain in the extremities. In Warfield CA (ed): Principles & Practice of Pain Medicine, 2nd ed. New York, McGraw-Hill, 2004, pp 315–342.

1. PATHOPHYSIOLOGY

a. The mechanisms underlying phantom limb pain after amputation have not been fully elucidated.

b. A series of elements are involved in generating phantom pain, including the peripheral nervous system, spinal cord, and brain.

c. Inciting events occur in the periphery, which subsequently generates a cascade of events that transmit more centrally.

d. Peripheral pain generators include spontaneous activity within neuromas or dorsal root ganglion (DRG) as well as sympathetic nervous system-mediated pain.

e. Spinal plasticity (sensitization) may result from increased N-methyl-D-aspartate (NMDA) receptor activity, loss of afferent C-fiber inhibition, and A-beta mechanoreceptor modulation of spinal column laminae (I and II).

f. Electrophysiologic studies performed on patients with phantom limb pain have shown cerebral reorganization of the primary somatosensory cortex, subcortex, and thalamus.

g. Potential genetic and psychological coping factors may contribute to the phantom limb phenomenon.

2. DIFFERENTIAL DIAGNOSIS

a. Virtually all amputees experience phantom sensations after limb amputation.

b. Phantom limb pain refers to the painful sensation to the absent limb.

c. Phantom limb sensation refers to any sensation in the absent limb, excluding pain.

d. Stump pain refers to pain localized in the stump.

e. Reasons for amputation include traumatic, peripheral vascular disease, and neoplasm.

f. Persistent limb pain may be due to infection, bone spurs, neuromas, and wrinkled scar tissue.

3. CLINICAL ISSUES

a. General points

i. The incidence of phantom limb pain ranges from 60% to 80% after amputation.

ii. Phantom limb pain appears to be independent of age, gender, or side of amputation.

iii. Phantom pain is less frequent in children and congenital amputees.

iv. Phantom limb sensation is a risk factor for phantom limb pain and stump pain.

v. Preamputation pain is a risk factor for postoperative phantom pain.

b. Clinical features

  i. Onset of pain typically occurs within the first few days after amputation, but it may be delayed for months to years.

  ii. Phantom pain is usually intermittent, rarely constant, ranging from a few times per day to weekly.

  iii. Pain is described as shooting, stabbing, squeezing, throbbing, and burning and is localized to the distal parts of the amputated limb.

  iv. Stump pain typically subsides with healing, but hyperalgesia, allodynia, and wind-up pain (repeat pricking stimuli) may persist 5% to 10% of the time.

  v. "Telescoping" refers to the phenomenon of the distal phantom limb gradually felt within the residual limb or stump.

  vi. Phantom pain may be modulated by stress control, stump massage, weather changes, rehabilitation, or use of prosthetic devices.

c. Natural history

  i. Although the incidence and intensity of phantom pain persists, both frequency and duration of pain attacks abate over time.

  ii. Median phantom pain scores were shown to decrease 1, 2, and 5 years after amputation.

4. TREATMENT

a. Clear evidence-based guidelines for the treatment of phantom limb pain are lacking.

b. Treatment can be classified as medical, nonmedical, and surgical.

c. Medical treatment is the most effective and includes tricyclic antidepressants (doxepin, amitriptyline), anticonvulsants (carbamazepine, gabapentin, lamotrigine), sodium channel blockers (lidocaine, mexiletine), calcitonin, and NMDA receptor antagonists (ketamine, memantine).

d. Opioids administered via the oral or intrathecal route may provide some benefit with limited risk of dependence.

e. Anesthetic blocks have been claimed to be effective in phantom pain, but none of them have a proven efficacy in well-controlled trials.

f. Nonmedical treatment

  i. Transcutaneous electrical nerve stimulation

  ii. Vibration therapy

  iii. Acupuncture

  iv. Biofeedback

  v. Electroconvulsive therapy

g. Proximal surgical extension of the amputation is almost never indicated, unless there is local pathology (neuroma, infections, scar tissue).
h. Neurosurgical options
    i. Dorsal root entry zone rhizotomy
    ii. Cordotomy
    iii. Thalamotomy
    iv. Sympathectomy
    v. Most surgical options have been abandoned because of lack of efficacy.
i. Preemptive analgesia is hypothesized to abate preamputation pain and subsequent phantom limb pain. To date, the clinical evidence is indeterminate regarding preemptive strategies (epidurals, nerve sheath catheters) in reducing phantom pain.

5. PROGNOSIS

a. Prospective studies have shown that amputees experience phantom limb pain approximately 70%, 65%, and 60% after 1 week, 6 months, and 2 years, respectively.
b. Survey studies of longstanding phantom limb pain revealed that pain disappeared in 16%, decreased markedly in 37%, and remained similar in 44%, with roughly 3% of patients with worse pain.
c. It is thought that as the incidence and intensity of phantom pain persists, both frequency and duration of pain attacks abate over time.

SUGGESTED READINGS

Halbert J, Crotty M, Cameron ID: Evidence for the optimal management of acute and chronic phantom pain: A systemic review. Clin J Pain 2002;18:84–92.
Nikolajsen L, Jensen TS: Phantom limb pain. Br J Anaesth 2001;87(1):107–116.

1. PATHOPHYSIOLOGY

   a. Osteoarthritis (OA) is the result of joint space narrowing, joint space sclerosis, and periarticular osteophyte formation.
   b. Trochanteric bursitis is caused by overuse of the gluteus medius tendon and tensor fascia over the femur. The result is bursal wall thickening, fibrosis, and loss of lubrication.
   c. Meralgia paresthetica is an entrapment syndrome of the lateral femoral cutaneous nerve resulting in neurologic deficits.
   d. Osteonecrosis is likely the result of vascular insufficiency, with subsequent periosteum, bone marrow, and joint destruction.
   e. Chronic steroid use and excess alcohol ingestion are risk factors for osteonecrosis.

2. DIFFERENTIAL DIAGNOSIS

   a. Hip and femur fracture
   b. OA
   c. Osteonecrosis
   d. Trochanteric bursitis
   e. Iliopsoas and ischiogluteal bursitis
   f. Sacroiliitis
   g. Neoplasm
   h. Meralgia paresthetica
   i. Lumbar nerve root syndrome
   j. Facet arthropathy
   k. Aortoiliac insufficiency (Leriche syndrome)

3. CLINICAL FEATURES

   a. General points
      i. Greater than 14% of patients older than 60 years report significant hip pain.
      ii. The most common causes for hip pain include trochanteric bursitis, OA, and femur fractures.
      iii. The hip joint is a relatively immobile ball-and-socket joint due to its articulation of the femur with the acetabulum and pelvic girdle.
      iv. Pain referred from the hip to the lower back, and vice versa, is common.
      v. Pain with weight bearing and improvement with rest is suggestive of OA.
      vi. In high-risk patients (i.e., chronic steroids), pain worsening with weight bearing and with rest should raise suspicion of osteonecrosis.

vii. The medial femoral circumflex artery is the major blood supply to the neck of the femur, and occult fractures can result in osteonecrosis.

viii. Occult hip fracture is suggested with anterolateral hip tenderness, severe pain with weight bearing, and intolerance to passive hip rotation.

ix. Lumbar nerve root syndrome, facet arthropathy, and sacroiliitis should be suspected when hip pain is associated with lower back pain or neurologic findings (i.e., paresthesias, hypesthesias, deep tendon reflexes).

x. Constant nocturnal pain suggests infectious, inflammatory, or neoplastic disease.

b. Diagnosis

i. Radiography should be performed on patients with acute or moderate chronic hip pain to exclude fractures.

ii. Weight-bearing plain films revealing joint space narrowing, sclerosis, and osteophyte formation are consistent with OA.

iii. Radioimmunoassay (RA) with gadolinium enhancement may be necessary to evaluate occult fractures, osteonecrosis, infection, or neoplasm.

iv. Ultrasonography is reserved for diagnostic needle-guided joint aspiration.

c. Clinical findings

i. OA presents primarily with morning stiffness and groin pain and becomes worse with internal rotation and flexion.

ii. Meralgia paresthetica classically presents with upper lateral thigh pain, hypesthesia, paresthesias, and normal tendon reflexes.

iii. Lateral hip pain with point tenderness is consistent with trochanteric bursitis.

iv. Severe hip pain with passive range of motion suggests the need for immediate evaluation for osteonecrosis, occult fracture, synovitis, or neoplastic disease.

v. Aortoiliac insufficiency may present with thigh claudication, aching pain in the buttock, weakness of the hip, and muscle atrophy. Diminished pulses and bruits over the iliac and femoral arteries may be present.

vi. The Patrick test assesses the hip and sacroiliac joint. A positive test occurs when, after flexion, abduction, and external rotation of the affected leg so that the ankle of that leg is on top of the opposite knee, the patient experiences pain in the absence of pain with passive hip joint motion.

vii. A positive straight-leg raise test elicits radicular pain in the affected leg at 60 degrees or less of leg elevation. It has a sensitivity of 80% and specificity of 40%.

d. Natural history

i. OA commonly presents in patients older than 40 years.

ii. With advanced OA, pain is noted to occur with less activity, at rest, and at nighttime.

    iii. Early diagnosis of osteonecrosis may prevent joint destruction and hip replacement.

4. TREATMENT

a. Empiric treatment for mild hip pain, stiffness, and normal range of motion includes minimizing weight-bearing activity and direct pressure, sleeping with pillow between legs, passive stretching exercises, and nonsteroidal anti-inflammatory drugs (7–10 days).

b. Local anesthetic blocks are useful in differentiating pain from the hip, lateral femoral cutaneous nerve, lumbar nerve root, lumbar facet joint, and sacroiliac joint.

c. Arthrocentesis is recommended when hip pain is acute and severe or there is evidence of infection (i.e., septic arthritis).

SUGGESTED READINGS

Anderson BC: Evaluation of the adult with hip pain. Available at: http://patients.uptodate.com/topic.asp?file=ad_orth/8074&title=Hip+pain.

Steinberg GG, Seybold EA: Hip and pelvis. In Orthopaedics in Primary Care, 3rd ed. New York, Elsevier, 1999.

1. CENTRAL PAIN SYNDROMES

a. Neuropathic pain caused by lesion or dysfunction in the central nervous system (CNS)

b. Key features of central pain:

   i. Result from damage to somatosensory pathways; damage may be slight (no detectable sensory loss) to massive

   ii. Idiosyncratic

   iii. Occurs in distribution of sensory damage, if present

   iv. Onset may be delayed

   v. May be reversible

   vi. Three common components:

      (1) Steady/constant and neuralgic

      (2) Spontaneous

      (3) Evoked (allodynia and hypesthesia)

   vii. Somatosensory local anesthetic blockade and sympathetic blocks may help temporarily if evoked element is present.

   viii. Steady pain is better relieved by intravenous sodium thiopental (STP) rather than opiate infusion.

   ix. Steady pain that is not relieved by proximal transection may respond to chronic stimulation that induces paresthesia in painful area.

   x. Evoked and neuralgic components may be relieved by proximal neural interruption.

2. CENTRAL PAIN–SPINAL CORD

a. General points

   i. Incidence of central pain in spinal cord damage: 6% to 94%

   ii. Usually results from trauma

   iii. Etiology and degree or completeness of lesion usually does not correlate with presence, severity, or quality of pain.

   iv. Onset possibly delayed (up to years) after inciting insult

      (1) Longer delay in onset of pain, the more likely syrinx is present

      (2) Decompression of syrinx seldom improves pain

b. Main components of pain

   i. Steady (burning, dysesthetic, or aching, 96%)

   ii. Shooting (2%)

   iii. Evoked (4% allodynia)

   iv. Visceral

   v. Musculoskeletal

c. Clinical correlation of pain

   i. Evoked pain requires some preserved sensation, often in a radicular distribution at upper level with complete lesion, or more diffuse in lower complete lesions.

ii. Facial cord pain always associated with syrinx
iii. Visceral-like pain may be difficult to differentiate from intra-abdominal pathology.
iv. Musculoskeletal-like pain suggests nociceptive pain.
v. Neuralgic pain correlates strongly with conus-cauda lesions.
vi. In general, variable patterns of sensory loss

d. Pathophysiology
  i. Animal studies correlate poorly with clinical observation.
    (1) Conflicting observation in human patients showed:
      (a) Often delayed onset of pain
      (b) Not alleviated by cord transection proximal to lesion
      (c) Not alleviated by lesions (rostral to causative lesion) made in same structures responsible for pain
  ii. Single-photon emission computed tomography and positron emission tomography scans suggest diminished thalamic perfusion contralateral to the cord pain and normalization of perfusion after treatments that successfully abolish pain.
  iii. Both points suggest pain is generated centrally at the cortical level.

3. TREATMENT

a. Medical treatment
  i. Tricyclic antidepressant: amitriptyline
  ii. Nonsteroidal anti-inflammatory drugs
  iii. Clonidine
  iv. Clonazepam
  v. 5-Hydroxytryptophane
  vi. Desipramine
  vii. Intrathecal baclofen, morphine
  viii. Ketamine
  ix. Alfentanil
  x. Drugs found to be ineffective: trazodone, valproate, mexiletine
  xi. No controlled studies to look at anticonvulsant and opioids
  xii. Therapy often fails, complete relief of pain unlikely, often recurs over time

b. Interventional treatment
  i. Local anesthetic block
    (1) Difficult to localize and unpredictable depths of penetration to target fibers
    (2) Not very useful
  ii. Percutaneous radiofrequency rhizotomy
    (1) Usually only in quadriplegic
    (2) Severe allodynia/ hyperpathia
    (3) Singe root
    (4) Identify with local anesthetic diagnostic block and rule out sensory compromise

    iii. Cordectomy: rostral to injury site

        (1) Efficacy is limited, secondary to proposed pattern generating mechanism at the cortical level (as mentioned above)

        (2) Useful for lancinating and evoked element

        (3) With lesions at or above T10, only 25% received pain relief after cordectomy

        (4) With lesions below T10, ALL patients enjoyed some relief

        (5) Abolishes any hope of eventual recovery of cord function (stringent patient selection needed)

    iv. Cordotomy

        (1) Good for neuralgic and evoked components

        (2) Disappointing for steady component

        (3) Small risk of ipsilateral arm paresis

    v. Dorsal root entry zone procedure

        (1) Radicular root pain

        (2) Less useful for diffuse, steady, burning, phantom body pain

    vi. Dorsal column stimulation

        (1) Most useful strategy for diffuse steady pain

        (2) Seldom successful

          (a) Injury or surgical scarring limit access to dorsal column.

          (b) Nerve fibers die back to the dorsal column after major cord transactions, so it is very difficult to produce paresthesia in that distribution by stimulating the dorsal column.

        (3) Most useful in conus-cauda lesions, in which case damaged roots may contribute to pain

    vii. Destructive brain operations

        (1) Limited role

        (2) Not effective for steady pain

          (a) Mesencephalic tractotomy

          (b) Thalamotomy

    viii. Deep brain stimulation

        (1) Alternative to dorsal column stimulation (when technically impossible)

        (2) Sensory thalamus: encouraging results in 56% of patients with neuropathic pain, not helpful for nociceptive pain

        (3) Periventricular-periaqueductal gray: successful in 59% with nociceptive pain, 23% with neuropathic pain

4. CENTRAL PAIN—BRAIN

  a. Background

    i. Etiology: brain injury that interferes with sensory pathways between foramen magnum to cerebral cortex

        (1) Independent of etiology or severity of injury

        (2) Ninety-one percent of a series resulted from vascular lesion

    ii. One percent to 4% of strokes resulted in pain/allodynia

    iii. No correlation of extent of sensory/motor compromise and pain

    iv. Mechanism remains obscure and treatment disappointing

  b. Clinical features

    i. In small study of 73 cases:

      (1) Steady: 98%

        (a) Burning: 64.4%

        (b) Dysesthetic: 31.6%

        (c) Aching: 38.6%

      (2) Neuralgic or intermittent: 16.4%

      (3) Evoked: 65% had allodynia, hyperpathia, or both

    ii. No correlation between pain and lesion size, location, or degree/quality of sensory loss

    iii. Injury site can occur anywhere that affects sensory pathways, despite older indications of thalamus injury

    iv. Interestingly, craniotomy and certain neurosurgical operations rarely cause central pain.

      (1) Spinoreticulothalamic tract, limbic system, hypothalamus, dorsomedian, center median, intralaminar and reticular nuclei of thalamus, kinesthetic pathway, and basal ganglia

    v. Onset

      (1) Immediate: 29%

      (2) Delayed up to 1 month: 18%

      (3) One month to 1 year: 26%

      (4) Occasionally delayed for years

    vi. Reversibility

      (1) Stroke in same area as instigating lesion

      (2) Removal of tumor

      (3) Resection of cortex: not consistently reversible by surgery

    vii. Occasional associated symptoms

      (1) Dystonia: on same side of pain, usually with thalamus stroke

      (2) Action tremor

  c. Pathophysiology

    i. Central disinhibition resulting from damage to some portion of the spinothalamic tract suggested by recent observation

    ii. In patients with similar anatomic lesions and sensory loss, some develop central pain while others do not.

    iii. Pain severity and characteristics independent of severity or completeness of stroke

      (1) Central pain observed after hemispherectomy, indiscernible from those of minor stroke and intact thalamus and cortex

      (2) It is assumed that the mechanisms are the same regardless of stroke severity

    iv. Signaled by somatosensory cortical mechanism that is somato-topographically organized
       (1) Can be ipsilateral or contralateral depending on location of stroke
    v. Disconnect between sensory receptors, likely nociceptors, from the cortex
       (1) Disconnect can be large, resulting in sensory loss, or so slight, that patient has no clinically detectable sensory loss
       (2) Disconnect leading to disinhibition of somatotopographically organized somatosensory pathways (nociceptive pathways)
          (a) For example, contralateral pathways eliminated by stroke, leaving ipsilateral fibers intact
          (b) It is known in primates that there are ipsilateral projections of spinothalamic tract
    vi. Tasker proposed "steady stroke pain is the result of hyperactivity in brainstem nuclei that mediate the polysynaptic nonsomatotopic portion of the pain pathway induced by disinhibition of those structures by the stroke, with resultant signaling of pain in the paucisynaptic somoto-topographically organized system on the side of the brain contralateral to the pain in small strokes and ipsilateral in massive ones."

  d. Medical treatment
    i. Neither surgical nor medical treatment shown to be promising, as with central cord pain
    ii. Amitriptyline and carbamazepine
       (1) Most frequently used
       (2) Statistically significant results in placebo-controlled study
    iii. Distal local anesthetic blockade provides only temporary relief
    iv. Intravenous lidocaine
    v. Oral mexiletine
    vi. Antidepressant
    vii. Naloxone
    viii. Intrathecal baclofen

  e. Surgical treatment
    i. Peripheral and cord procedures: In general, treatment should be aimed at the brain.
       (1) Chronic trigeminal stimulation is the only modality that seems promising for brain central pain in the face
       (2) Cordotomy: not very useful, few case reports
       (3) Trigeminal dorsal root entry zone: disappointing
       (4) Dorsal column stimulation: disappointing
    ii. Mesencephalic tractotomy
       (1) Previous data showed low success rate
       (2) More recent studies may show better response
    iii. Medial thalamotomy
       (1) Low success rate
       (2) High rate of recurrence

iv. Deep brain stimulation
   (1) Most frequently used surgical procedure
   (2) Stimulate periventricular gray, periaqueductal gray, and thalamus or medial lemniscus to produce paresthesia in area of pain
   (3) Thalamic lead placement often too painful in stroke pain with allodynia and hyperpathia
   (4) Zero to 80% incidence of significant pain relief, usually in less than 50% of cases
v. Motor cortex stimulation
   (1) Very little information currently available
   (2) Appears promising
   (3) Difficult to accurately localize electrode in patients with massive cortical destruction

SUGGESTED READING

Bendok B, Levy M: Bain stimulation for persistent pain management. In Gildenberg PL, Tasker R (eds): Textbook of Stereotactic and Functional Neurosurgery. New York, McGraw-Hill, 1998, pp 1539–1546.

Boivie J, Leijon G: Clinical findings in patients with central post-stroke pain. In Casey KL (ed): Pain and Central Nervous System Disease. New York, Raven Press, 1991, pp 65–75.

Casey KL: Pain and central nervous system disease: A summary and overview. In Casey KL (ed): Pain and Central Nervous system Disease: The Central Pain Syndromes. New York, Raven Press, 1991, pp 1–11.

Cesaro P, Defer G, Moretti JL, Dagos JD: Central pain and thalamic activation. Pain 1990;(suppl 5):S433.

Jefferson A: Cordectomy for intractable pain. In Lipton S, Miles J (eds): Persistent Pain. Vol 4. New York, Grune & Stratton, 1981, pp 112–115.

Marshall J: Sensory disturbances in cortical wounds with special reference to pain. J Neurol Neurosurg Psychiatry 1951;14:187–204.

Pagni CA, Canavero S: Functional thalamic depression in a case of reversible central pain due to a spinal intramedullary cyst. J Neurosurg 1995;83:163–165.

Tasker R: Central pain states. In Warfield CA, Bajwa ZH (eds): Principals and Practice of Pain Medicine, 2nd ed. New York, McGraw-Hill, 2004, pp 394–404.

Yezierski RP: Pain following spinal cord injury: The clinical problem and experimental studies. Pain 1996;68:185–194.

115 Brachial Plexopathy

1. ANATOMY OF BRACHIAL PLEXUS

a. Anterior rami of C5-T1 nerve roots (variable inclusion of C4 and T2)
   i. Contributions from both anterior and posterior rootlets (motor and sensory, respectively)
   ii. Anterior rami located just distal to neural foramina and continue to form trunks of brachial plexus
   iii. Posterior rami innervate paraspinal muscles (not brachial plexus)
b. Roots: located in neural foramina
c. Trunks: between scalene muscles
d. Divisions: posterior to clavicle
e. Cord: inferior to clavicle
f. Superficial in supraclavicular fossa where it lies in close proximity to lung apex

2. SYMPTOMS AND FINDINGS

a. General
   i. Usually vague and nonspecific symptoms (delay diagnosis)
   ii. Purely or mostly motor symptoms
      (1) Due to stretch injuries (neurapraxia) or avulsions
         (a) Young/trauma patients
         (b) Neonates after breech deliveries with shoulder dystocia
         (c) Motor vehicle accident (MVA), especially motorcycle accidents
      (2) Complete flaccid paralysis: avulsions of brachial plexus
      (3) Avulsion, usually permanent loss of function
      (4) Neurapraxia injuries: 80% to 90% patients recover some function
   iii. Mixed motor and sensory
      (1) Tumor invasion of brachial plexus and often extension into spinal column and neural foramina
      (2) Older patients
   iv. Predominantly sensory
      (1) Postradiation for cancer (especially breast or lung)
b. Specific findings
   i. C5
      (1) Loss of shoulder abduction, deltoids, biceps
      (2) Sensory deficit: radial arm
      (3) Loss of biceps reflex
   ii. C6
      (1) Loss of wrist extension

        (2) Sensory deficit of lateral forearm

        (3) Loss of brachioradialis reflex

   iii. C7

        (1) Loss of wrist flexion, finger extension

        (2) Sensory loss of middle finger

        (3) Loss of triceps reflex

   iv. C8

        (1) Loss of finger flexion

        (2) Sensory loss of medial forearm

   v. T1

        (1) Loss of finger abduction

        (2) Sensory loss of medial aspect of arm

c. Symptoms by anatomy

   i. Superior plexus lesions (C5-C6)

        (1) Deltoid, biceps, brachioradialis, brachialis

        (2) Inability to abduct and externally rotate shoulder

        (3) Inability to flex elbow

        (4) Inability to pronate forearm

        (5) Arm hangs loose, internally rotated (porter's tip position)

        (6) Sensory loss: deltoid and radial side of forearm

   ii. Middle plexus lesion (C7)

        (1) Unusual

        (2) Sensory loss over back of forearm, radial aspect of dorsum of hand

   iii. Inferior plexus lesions (C8, T1)

        (1) Paralysis of small hand muscles and finger flexors

        (2) Preserved finger and wrist extensors

        (3) Hyperextension at metacarpophalangeal joints and flexion at interphalangeal joints

        (4) May result from upward pulling on shoulder

   iv. Long-term complications of plexus lesions

        (1) Skin blisters

        (2) Ulceration and secondary infection joint contractures

        (3) Complex regional pain syndrome

        (4) Osteoporosis

3. ETIOLOGY

a. Trauma

   i. Birth injuries (stretch injuries)

        (1) Breech delivery

        (2) Shoulder dystocia

   ii. MVAs

   iii. Football injuries

   iv. Backpack injuries

   v. Laborers carrying heavy loads

        (1) Upper plexus injury

        (2) Superficial position of plexus in supraclavicular fossa susceptible to exogenous compression and traction

        (3) Rucksack paralysis in soldier

b. Neoplasm: most common cause in adults

    i. Primary

        (1) Nerve and nerve sheath tumors arise from brachial plexus

    ii. Secondary (most common in adults)

        (1) Pancoast tumor (grave prognosis, often irresectable)

        (2) Lymphoma

        (3) Leukemia

        (4) Multiple myeloma

        (5) Lipoma

    iii. Metastases

        (1) Breast carcinoma most common

        (2) Metastases vs. radiation therapy

            (a) Postradiation time less than 3 months or more than 5 years favors metastases

            (b) Intense pain, lower plexus lesions, Horner syndrome favors metastases

    iv. Radiation therapy

        (1) Especially for breast and lung

        (2) Usually sensory

        (3) Skin changes

        (4) Lymphedema of extremity

        (5) Induration over supraclavicular fossa

        (6) Upper plexus lesion

        (7) Paresthesia after tapping supraclavicular fossa

    v. Iatrogenic

        (1) Positioning injury during general anesthesia

            (a) Shoulder braces/maxillary roll placed too medially, compressing the plexus before it descends behind clavicle

            (b) Arm abducted more than 90 degrees

                (i) Head of humerus descends into axilla, compressing plexus as it enters the axilla

            (c) Trendelenburg position, resulting in excessive depression of shoulder girdle stretching upper roots of plexus

        (2) Axillary artery injury (cardiac catheterization, transarterial axillary nerve block)

    vi. Vascular

        (1) Embolism: rare cause

        (2) Generalized vasculopathies: rare cause

        (3) Hematoma after anticoagulation or artery cannulation

    vii. Anatomic

        (1) Thoracic outlet syndrome

            (a) Young to middle-aged women

            (b) Unilateral and intermittent

        (c) Anterior and posterior shoulder region, radiating down lateral arm to hand

        (d) Paresthesia, particularly C8-T1 ulnar distribution

        (e) Elevating arm or increased arm activity can initiate/aggravate symptoms

  viii. Cryptogenic

    (1) Neuralgic amyotrophy

        (a) May be precipitated by infection

        (b) Third and fourth decades

        (c) Acute onset of shoulder pain

        (d) Worst at night and with movement

        (e) Usually right side (25% bilateral)

        (f) Motor more than sensory (infrequent)

    (2) Familial brachial plexopathy

        (a) Recurrent episodes over years, separated by intervals of full recovery

        (b) May have first attack in first decade, but third and fourth decades most common

        (c) Minor dysmorphic features (hypertelorism, epicanthic folds, cleft palate)

        (d) Nerve involvement outside brachial plexus

        (e) Pain is initial manifestation: sharp and burning in shoulder, exacerbated by movement

        (f) Weakness follows: motor symptoms more than sensory

        (g) Upper trunk affected most often, though not exclusively

    (3) Serum sickness

        (a) Typhoid or parathyroid vaccinations

        (b) Sudden onset of pain in shoulder or upper arm

        (c) Followed by weakness over shoulder muscles

        (d) Paralysis and atrophy possible

        (e) Decreased reflex

        (f) Vasomotor changes

        (g) Uncommon: sensory findings and radial nerve involvement

        (h) Pathogenesis

          (i) Immune complex causing vasculitis and nerve edema, which cause impingement while exiting foramina

          (ii) May result in ischemia and nerve necrosis (lancinating pain)

4. TREATMENT

  a. Physical rehabilitation: cornerstone of all brachial plexus injury

    i. Stretch injuries (infants): significant impact

    ii. Avulsion: limited impact

  b. Control phantom pain

  c. Avulsion injuries

    i. Lesions at root entry zone (pseudomeningoceles)
       (1) Grave prognosis
       (2) Usually not amenable to surgery
    ii. Supraganglionic nerve avulsions
       (1) No current treatment
       (2) Early microanastomoses of nerve roots and nerve roots to spinal cord appear promising with some nerve regeneration
         (a) Regeneration leads to muscle function in one-third of patients, most have improved pain
    iii. Juxtaforaminal and more distal avulsion
       (1) Microsurgical grafting and anastomoses using phrenic, spinal accessory, intercostals, and medial pectoral nerves
    iv. Avoid prolonged immobilization of affected shoulder
       (1) Avoid frozen extremity
    v. Accurate anatomic identification of injury site
       (1) History and physical findings
       (2) Magnetic resonance imaging

SUGGESTED READINGS

Bertelli JA, Dorsi MJ, Storm PB, Moriarity JL: Surgical repair of brachial plexus injury: A multinational survey of experienced peripheral nerve surgeons. J Neurosurg 2004;101:365–376.

Cohen SA, Michael JS, Warfield CA: Pain in the extremities. In Warfield CA, Bajwa ZH (eds): Principles and Practice of Pain Medicine, 2nd ed. New York, McGraw-Hill, 2004, pp 315–327.

Geiger LR, Mancall EL, Penn AS, Tucker SH: Familial neuralgic amyotrophy. Brain 1974;97:87.

Guha A, Graham B, Kline DG, Hudson AR: Brachial plexus injuries. In Wilkins RH, Rengachary SS (eds): Neurosurgery, 2nd ed. New York, McGraw-Hill, 1996, pp 3121–3134.

1. PATHOPHYSIOLOGY

a. Complex regional pain syndrome (CRPS) is a neurologic disorder affecting both the central and peripheral nervous systems.

b. The sympathetic nervous system has a likely role in neuropathic and inflammatory pain states, although there is little agreement as to whether it plays a primary role in CRPS causation.

c. Peripheral (A delta, C, A-beta) and central (WDR neurons) nociceptor stimulation may result in central plasticity or ongoing nociceptor activity.

d. Increased density of α_1-adrenoceptors in hyperalgesic skin may be responsible for excitation and sensitization of nociceptor afferents.

e. Potential genetic factors, such as increased HLA antigen expression, may be associated with poor clinical outcomes.

2. DIAGNOSTIC TESTING

a. CRPS is suggested if regional pain and sensory changes after trauma exceed the magnitude or duration of the typical healing period.

b. There is no definitive test for CRPS, but additional studies may confirm clinical suspicion.

c. Diagnostic tests include sensory (quantitative sensory test), motor (electromyography [EMG], nerve conduction), autonomic (quantitative sudomotor axon-reflex test, thermography, Doppler flow), and trophic (bone scintigraphy).

d. Regional anesthetic blocks (sympathetic or intravenous) help determine the sympathetic-maintained pain (SMP) component of CRPS.

e. Phentolamine infusion test also determines the involvement of SMP.

3. DIFFERENTIAL DIAGNOSIS

a. Neuropathic syndromes (i.e., small fiber, diabetic, entrapment)
b. Thoracic outlet syndrome
c. Discogenic disease
d. Deep venous thrombosis
e. Cellulitis
f. Lymphedema
g. Erythromelalgia
h. Fibromyalgia
i. Peripheral vascular disorders

4. CLINICAL ISSUES

a. General points
   i. Women predominate (2.5:1) with a mean age between 36 and 42 years.
   ii. CRPS is usually linked to a history of trauma, immobilization, or procedures (i.e. surgery, venopuncture, or injection).
   iii. There is no correlation between severity of insult to the ensuing painful syndrome.
   iv. Upper extremity involvement tends to be more frequent than lower extremity (55:45).
   v. Incidence of CRPS is not fully known, ranging from 7% to 37% for extremity fractures.
   vi. Psychological factors, such as stress and inadequate coping mechanisms, are potential risk factors.
      (1) No psychiatric disorder is known to predispose an individual to CRPS.

b. Diagnosis
   i. The International Association for the Study of Pain (IASP) established the differential criteria for CRPS I and II.
   ii. The diagnosis of CRPS I (reflex sympathetic dystrophy) includes sensory changes (allodynia, hyperalgesia, hypoalgesia), edema, temperature abnormalities, and sweating.
   iii. The distinction between CRPS I and II (causalgia) is the evidence of a definable nerve injury.
   iv. The signs and symptoms for both conditions are clinically indistinguishable.

c. Clinical features
   i. Pain out of proportion to clinical signs is the cardinal feature of CRPS.
   ii. Clinical triad consists of sensory, autonomic, and motor signs and symptoms.
   iii. Pain is described as burning (81%), aching, and shooting in nature.
   iv. Most prevalent signs include allodynia (74%), decreased range of motion (70%) and weakness, color and temperature changes, and edema.
   v. Pain is typically exacerbated by temperature changes and emotional factors.
   vi. Typical skin changes include hyperkeratosis, glossy skin, and ulcer formation.
   vii. Atrophy of musculoskeletal system (i.e., osteopenia) from disuse or contracture generally occurs later in the disease (several months).

d. Natural history
   i. CRPS may progress through distinct, sequential stages with an early, intermediate (dystrophic), and late (atrophic) stage.
   ii. Later atrophic changes are presumably irreversible in nature.

    iii. However, certain subsets of patients with CRPS exhibit early fulminate features, independent of the duration of the disease course.

    iv. Optimal clinical improvement may result from early institution of therapeutic interventions.

5. TREATMENT

a. Because the mechanisms of CRPS are not fully elucidated, treatment focuses on functional restoration.

b. Most patients improve with pain management, rehabilitation, and psychological therapy.

c. The functional restoration pathway allows for the physician to apply the necessary interventional modality to promote continued clinical improvement.

d. Psychological therapy includes relaxation techniques, biofeedback, stress management, and cognitive behavioral therapy.

e. Full psychological evaluation is recommended in patients with CRPS after 2 months, including psychometric testing.

f. Medical therapies with proven benefit include:
    i. Antidepressants (amitriptyline)
    ii. Antiepileptics (gabapentin)
    iii. Bisphosphonates (alendronate)
    iv. Topical dimethylsulfoxide
    v. Topical clonidine
    vi. Oral corticosteroids
    vii. Intravenous bretylium, lidocaine, or phentolamine
    viii. Intranasal calcitonin.

g. Systemic α_1 blockers (phenoxybenzamine, prazosin) may improve peripheral blood flow and reduce SMP.

h. Regional anesthetic blocks (sympathetic or intravenous) provide pain relief and facilitate the functional restoration pathway.

i. Neuromodulation therapy, including spinal cord and thalamic stimulation, as well as intrathecal therapy, are reserved for treatment standstill.

j. Palliative therapies include surgical or radiofrequency ablation of sympathetic ganglia and limb amputation secondary to severe tissue breakdown.

k. Functional rehabilitation and physiotherapy focuses on:
    i. Desensitization of the affected region
    ii. Mobilization and isometric strengthening
    iii. Stress loading and increased range of motion
    iv. Postural normalization
    v. Aerobic conditioning
    vi. Vocational and ergonomic reconditioning.

6. PROGNOSIS

a. Up to 60% of children will respond well to physical therapeutic measures and pharmacologic therapy.

b. A 5-year follow-up study showed that 26% of patients had to change their job while 72% continued to work full time.

c. Severe cases of CRPS may lead to marked limitation of function, disability, and possible amputation.

d. Although most experts agree that prognosis is poor with late-stage symptoms, the precise prognostic implications regarding sensory, autonomic, and motor disturbances in CRPS are unknown.

SUGGESTED READINGS

Raja SN, Grabow TS: Complex regional pain syndrome I (reflex sympathetic dystrophy). Anesthesiology 2002;96:1254–1260.

Stanton-Hicks M: Complex regional pain syndrome. Anesthesiol Clin N Am 2003;21:733–744.

Warfield CA, Stanton-Hicks M: Complex regional pain syndrome. In Warfield CA, Bajwa ZH (eds): Principles & Practice of Pain Medicine, 2nd ed. New York, McGraw-Hill, 2004, pp 405–416.

117 Neuroma

1. PATHOPHYSIOLOGY

    a. Axonal injury and usually complete separation from cell body

        i. Wallerian degeneration

    b. Nerve regeneration via axonal sprouting toward separated end

        i. Poor realignment or obstacles lead to axonal growing in a disorganized fashion forming a bulbous mass of tangled neuronal tissue

    c. Neuroma may become the nerve's sensory terminal with abnormal activity

        i. Abnormal persistent pain: continue firing/propagating information even after noxious stimulus removed

    d. Neuroma may function as impulse generator that has spontaneous pacemaker activity

        i. Spontaneously depolarize and fire in absence of stimuli

2. ECTOPIC GENERATION

    a. Neuroma responsible for chronic ongoing neuropathic pain and paresthesia by altering normal property of the axon

        i. Depolarized by various types of stimulation (noxious and nonnoxious)

        ii. Fire continuously despite removal of stimulus

        iii. Depolarize in absence of stimulus (intrinsic pulse generator activity)

    b. Ectopic generator stimulated by various stimuli

        i. Ischemia

        ii. Mechanical

        iii. Neuroactive substances (histamine, prostaglandins, catecholamines)

3. ETIOLOGY

    a. Any nerve injury/transaction/trauma can result in neuroma formation and development of chronic neuropathic pain.

        i. Examples:

            (1) Morton neuroma: neurofibroma or neuritis (not always true neuroma) caused by compression of interdigital nerves by adjacent metatarsal heads (usually 3rd and 4th toes)

                (a) Burning pain radiates from neuroma into toes

                (b) Reproduce symptoms by exerting pressure between implicated toes

                (c) Triggered or worsened with walking; eventually becomes continuous pain

(d) Treatment
    (i) Interdigital injection of local anesthetic agent and corticosteroids
    (ii) Correction of foot abnormalities that caused compression
    (iii) If pain is persistent and intractable, consider surgery
(2) Amputation with stump neuroma
(3) Nerve transaction during surgery
(4) Tumor (acoustic neuroma, facial nerve neuroma)
(5) Diagnostic nerve biopsy
(6) More often with cryoneurolysis and electrocauterization than scissor cut or tight ligation

4. DIAGNOSIS

a. Palpable directly over site of nerve injury
b. Unusually tender, especially to pressure over site
c. High-resolution computed tomography or magnetic resonance with gadolinium

5. TREATMENT

a. Medical management of neuropathic pain
b. Most surgical results disappointing in the long run
c. Surgical intervention targeted to prevent re-formation of neuroma after excision
d. Some interventions may even enhance neuropathic pain.
e. Many nerve regeneration enhancement techniques in which neuroma and subsequent pain development have not been studied.
f. Surgical excision of neuroma
    i. Often complicated by recurrence and multiple subsequent interventions
    ii. Resected nerves usually need to be replaced by graft
g. Mechanically prevent nerve fiber proliferation
    i. Cover nerve stump with cap to prevent neuroma development and regeneration.
        (1) Autologous cap (muscle, vein, fascia, bone canal, fatty tissue, etc.)
        (2) Epineurial flap technique and epineural grafting (rarely used)
        (3) Synthetic (silicone, collagen, etc.)
    ii. Implantation of transected nerve into muscles or bone
        (1) Only postamputation neuroma responded well
        (2) Nevertheless, suggests that scar formation should be minimized in peripheral nerve surgery
    iii. Nerve stump ligation

      iv. Stump electrocoagulation or freezing may decrease neuroma size
- h. All of these methods assume reduction in quality of life by preventing any restoration of nerve function.
- i. Pharmacologically hinder nerve fiber growth
    - i. Alcohol
    - ii. Steroids
    - iii. Formalin
    - iv. Pepsin
    - v. Nitrogen mustard
    - vi. Hydrochloric acid
    - vii. Phenol injection
    - viii. Selective dorsal root ganglion destruction
    - ix. Repeat procaine injection into neuroma
- j. Resection of damaged nerve and insertion of sural graft with microsurgical technique followed inevitably by recurrence of pain
    - i. Suggest peripheral nerve injury had induced changes in central nervous system not reversed by treating injured nerve

SUGGESTED READINGS

Battista AD, Cravioto H, Budsilovich GN: Painful neuroma: Changes produced in peripheral nerve after fascicle ligation. Neurosurgery 1981;9:589–600.

Devor M, Rappaport Z: Pain and the pathophysiology of damaged nerve. In Fields H (ed): Pain Syndromes in Neurology. London, Butterworth & Co., 1990, pp 42–83.

Lewin-Kowalik J, Marcol W, Kotulska K, et al: Prevention and management of painful neuroma. Neurol Med Chir (Tokyo) 2006;46:62–68.

Noordenbos W, Wall PD: Implications of the failure of nerve resection and graft to cure chronic pain produced by nerve lesions. J Neurol Neurosurg Psychiatry 1981;44:1068–1073.

Raynor E, Kleiner-Fisman G: Polyneuropathy. In Warfield C, Bajwa Z (eds): Principles & Practice of Pain Medicine, 2nd ed. New York, McGraw-Hill, 2004, pp 387–388.

118 Postherpetic Neuralgia

1. BACKGROUND

a. Herpes zoster is a viral infection that is usually associated with acute pain.
b. When pain persists for at least 3 to 6 months after the zoster rash resolution, the diagnosis of postherpetic neuralgia (PHN) is made.

2. HERPES ZOSTER

a. Epidemiology
   i. After primary chicken pox infection, the varicella-zoster virus (VZV) is dormant in the sensory ganglia of the nervous system.
   ii. Herpes zoster is reactivation of the virus and its spread from dorsal root or cranial nerve ganglion to the corresponding dermatome.
   iii. Incidence of 500,000 in the United States annually.
   iv. Twenty percent to 30% of population will have reactivation during their lifetime.
   v. Fifty percent lifetime occurrence of those who live to 85 years
   vi. Incidence increases with age.
   vii. Incidence increases with suppression of cell-mediated immunity (AIDS, organ transplant, chemotherapy).
b. Natural history
   i. Usually prodromal pain precedes unilateral rash by a few days
   ii. Thoracic dermatome most common, representing 50% to 70% of all cases
   iii. Acute pain usually resolves as rash resolves (2 to 4 weeks)
   iv. Subacute herpetic neuralgia can persist (1 to 4 months)
   v. PHN (>4 to 6 months)

3. POSTHERPETIC NEURALGIA

a. Epidemiology
   i. PHN is defined as a debilitating neuropathic pain state that persists for at least 3 months (6 months according to some sources) after resolution of the zoster rash.
   ii. Nine percent to 34% of adult patients with herpes zoster are reported to develop PHN (depending on definition and time criteria used).
   iii. Incidence of 0.8 to 14 per 1000 persons per year.
   iv. Age is the most important risk factor.
      (1) Most common in older patients, though can be seen at all ages

      (2) Eighty-five percent of patients with PHN older than 40 years

      (3) Seventy percent of patients older than 50 years

      (4) More than 50% of patients older than 60 years with zoster will develop PHN.

      (5) More than 70% of patients older than 80 years with zoster will develop PHN.

    v. Other well-established risk factors for developing PHN in those with acute zoster outbreaks:

      (1) Older age

      (2) More intense acute pain

      (3) More severe rash

      (4) Prodrome of dermatomal pain before the rash appears

b. Pathophysiology

   i. Hypothesis that normal age-related decrease in T cell-mediated immunity is responsible for increase incidence of VZV reactivation

      (1) Patients with HIV, certain malignancy, chemotherapy, long-term use of corticosteroids, and other immunosuppressive states are at increased risk

c. Prevention

   i. Antiviral agents

      (1) Antiviral agents reduce duration of acute zoster pain.

      (2) May reduce severity of PHN if given within 72 hours of zoster rash outbreak.

      (3) No clear evidence exists that antivirals reduce incidence of PHN, although some studies suggest the possibility. Given the excellent safety profile of antivirals, aggressive early treatment during acute outbreak may be valuable.

   ii. Vaccines

      (1) Trials of vaccines to boost T cell-mediated immunity demonstrated efficacy, safety, and immunogenicity.

d. Natural history

   i. PHN usually resolves within 12 months; 10% to 20% persist.

   ii. Can be discontinuous, with pain-free intervals of varying duration

   iii. Can develop in patients without acute zoster pain or without rash (zoster sine herpete)

      (1) Diagnosis: VZV DNA in cerebrospinal fluid (CSF)

e. Clinical manifestations

   i. Thoracic dermatomes and ophthalmic distribution of trigeminal nerve are most common regions involved.

      (1) Ophthalmic involvement may develop into keratitis; when severe enough, can result in vision loss. Early ophthalmology consult is warranted.

   ii. Pain often described as severe, excruciating, debilitating, and incapacitating

   iii. Constant aching, burning, jabbing, shooting, or lancinating

    iv. Characterized most commonly by cutaneous allodynia and hyperalgesia to mechanical stimulation

      (1) Allodynia: pain elicited by non-noxious stimuli such as clothing or air movement

      (2) Hyperalgesia: exaggerated pain response to a mildly noxious stimulus

      (3) Allodynia reported in 70% to 90% of patients with PHN

      (4) Paresthesia may also occur: abnormal sensations ("pins and needles" or numbness)

      (5) Dysesthesias sometimes present: unpleasant abnormal sensations

f. Pharmacologic treatments

  i. Topical preparations

    (1) Good starting point, especially for those system treatment results in side effects that are undesirable or contraindicated

    (2) Peripheral drive responsible for pain in subgroup of patients secondary to ectopic discharges within the cutaneous nociceptive afferents (irritable nociceptor hypothesis)

    (a) Local anesthetics

    (b) Transdermal lidocaine (lignocaine), 5% Lidoderm patch

      (i) Specific indication for PHN

      (ii) First-line therapy

      (iii) Especially effective for allodynia

      (iv) Topical patch (5%) to affected area

      (v) Up to 3 patches can be worn simultaneously for 12 hours each day

    (c) Eutectic mixture of local anesthetics (EMLA): 2.5% lidocaine and 2.5% prilocaine

      (i) Evidence of significant pain relief for up to 10 hours

    (d) Lidocaine gel (5%)

      (i) Some evidence for effectiveness in PHN

    (e) Aspirin/nonsteroidal anti-inflammatory drugs (NSAIDs)

      (i) During active and early postherpetic phase, pain associated with tissue trauma, inflammation, and increased tissue prostaglandins

      (ii) NSAIDs inhibit cyclooxygenase, thus decrease prostaglandin synthesis

    (f) Topical aspirin

      (i) Shown to be better than placebo in reducing PHN

    (g) Other topical NSAIDs (diclofenac, indomethacin, benzydamine) no better than placebo

    (h) Capsaicin: approved by Food and Drug Administration (FDA) for topical treatment of PHN

    (i) Selective neurotoxin specific for small C-fiber afferents (particularly those activated by noxious heat)

    (j) Adverse events: Burning and hyperalgesia leads to noncompliance and discontinuation of treatment in more than 30% of patients.

        (i) EMLA cream may reduce capsaicin-induced discomfort.

 ii. Antidepressants

    (1) Tricyclic antidepressants (TCAs): comprehensively studied for PHN

        (a) Block reuptake of norepinephrine and serotonin (5-HT), thus may relieve pain by increasing neurotransmitters of the descending inhibitory pathways for pain perception

        (b) Amitriptyline: trials suggest 48% to 67% patients with excellent response

        (c) Nortriptyline: (metabolite of amitriptyline) selective inhibitor of norepinephrine reuptake

        (d) Start at low doses (10-25 mg) administered at bedtime.

        (e) Increase dose every 5 to 7 days based on patient's response.

        (f) Adverse effects: (anticholinergic effects) sedation, confusion, urinary retention, dry month, postural hypotension, arrhythmia

        (g) Limits usefulness in elderly patients

        (h) Anticholinergic ophthalmic drops for glaucoma should not be used concurrently

        (i) Nortriptyline is TCA least likely to cause postural hypotension.

    (2) Serotonin-norepinephrine reuptake inhibitor (SNRI)

        (a) Duloxetine: indicated for management of neuropathic pain associated with diabetic peripheral neuropathy (DPN)

        (b) SNRIs increase activity of norepinephrine and 5-HT in CNS

        (c) Decrease in pain as early as week 1

        (d) Generally well tolerated. Side effects include nausea, constipation, decreased appetite, somnolence, headache, dizziness, dry mouth.

        (e) Dose of 30 to 120 mg daily. No evidence of 120 mg/day offering any therapeutic advantage over 60 mg/day, but clearly less well tolerated.

        (f) Contraindicated in those with liver dysfunction, heavy alcohol consumption, narrow-angle glaucoma, concurrent use of monoamine oxidase inhibitor (MAOI) and thioridazine

iii. Antiepileptic
  (1) Gabapentin: FDA approved and randomized controlled trial (RCT) shown to be efficacious for PHN and DPN
    (a) Large multicenter RCT showed doses of 1800 to 2400 mg/day (maximum dose, 3600 mg/day) resulted in statistically significant 34% reduction in PHN pain.
    (b) Bind $\alpha_2\delta$ subunits of voltage-activated calcium channels, decrease Ca^{2+} influx into nerve terminals, and reduce release of neurotransmitters (glutamate and norepinephrine)
    (c) Adverse effects: dizziness and somnolence
  (2) Pregabalin: FDA approved for PHN and DPN
    (a) Neuronal calcium channel modulator: bind $\alpha_2\delta$ subunits of voltage-activated calcium channels, decrease Ca^{2+} influx into nerve terminals, and reduce release of NT (glutamate and norepinephrine)
    (b) Three double-blinded, placebo-controlled, multicenter studies showed significant decrease in pain scores and improved sleep.
    (c) PHN: 150 to 300 mg/day (divided twice or three times daily)
  (3) Carbamazepine
    (a) Shown to reduce neuralgic lancinating pain
    (b) Ineffective for continuous pain
    (c) Marginal efficacy for PHN
    (d) Monitoring requirements
iv. Opioids
  (1) Second-line therapy if TCA and membrane stabilizer fails to produce desire response
  (2) Can be used safely and effectively in chronic noncancer pain, but there are concerns for tolerance, physical dependence, and addiction
  (3) RCT double-blinded placebo-controlled crossover trial showed opioids are as effective as TCAs in treatment of PHN. More patients preferred treatment with opioids (50%) than TCAs (30%) [$P = 0.02$].
    (a) Controlled-release morphine
    (b) Methadone
    (c) Controlled-release oxycodone
v. N-Methyl-D-aspartate antagonists
  (1) Weak clinical evidence for ketamine and dextromethorphan efficacy as adjuvant agents in selected patients with PHN
  (2) Limited use secondary to intolerable side effects, especially with ketamine
    (a) Ketamine
    (b) Dextromethorphan
    (c) Methadone

g. Invasive treatments
    i. Considered if conventional medical therapy has failed
    ii. Sympathetic blocks
        (1) If anatomically amendable
        (2) May provide temporary relief but typically no long-lasting benefits
    iii. Intercostal nerve block/neurolysis
        (1) Thoracic dermatomes
        (2) Diagnostic/therapeutic
    iv. Intrathecal steroids
        (1) Intrathecal methylprednisolone
        (2) Limited clinical trials in the United States
        (3) Suggest good pain relief up to 2 years into follow-up
        (4) Concerns about safety (i.e., adhesive arachnoiditis) greatly limits use in the United States
    v. Spinal cord stimulation
        (1) May provide significant long-term pain control and improvements in daily function
        (2) High rate of spontaneous resolution of PHN makes patient selection for spinal cord stimulation crucial
    vi. Intrathecal pump
        (1) Safe long-term pain control with intrathecal medication (opioids, local anesthetics, clonidine, etc.)
        (2) Though no RCTs have documented benefit in PHN, this approach may offer significant pain relief for patients who have not responded to other options.
        (3) Cost effective for selected chronic pain syndromes in the long run

SUGGESTED READINGS

Dworkin RH, Schmader KE: Herpes zoster and postherpetic neuralgia. In Benzon HT, Raja SN (eds): Essentials of Pain Medicine and Regional Anesthesia. Philadelphia, Elsevier, 2005, pp 386–391.

Gidal B, Billington R: New and emerging treatment options for neuropathic pain. Am J Manag Care 2006;12:S269–S278.

Pappagollo M, Hadley EJ: Pharmacological management of postherpetic neuralgia. CNS Drugs 2003;17(11):771–780.

Raja SN, Haythornthwaite JA, Pappagallo M, et al: A placebo-controlled trial comparing the analgesic and cognitive effects of opioids and tricyclic antidepressants in postherpetic neuralgia. Neurology 2002;59(7):1015–1021.

Watson CPN: Postherpetic neuralgia: Clinical features and treatment. In Fields HL (ed): Pain Syndromes in Neurology. London, Butterworth and Co., Ltd., 1990, pp 223–238.

Wood MJ, Kay R, Dworkin RH, et al: Oral acyclovir therapy accelerates pain resolution in patients with herpes zoster: A meta-analysis of placebo-controlled trials. Clin Infect Dis 1996;22(2):341–347.

1. GENERAL

a. Entrapment neuropathies occur where nerves normally would be somewhat confined, and neuropathy ensues due to increased pressure causing insult to peripheral nerves.

b. Degree of compressive damage to peripheral nerves
   i. Neurapraxia: functional impairment without axonal structural loss
      (1) Can recover in days by removal of compressive stimulus
   ii. Axonotmesis: wallerian degeneration follows axonal loss
      (1) Regeneration can take months to years
   iii. Neurotmesis: severance of entire nerve and supporting connective tissue
      (1) Poor spontaneous regeneration

c. Ulnar nerve entrapment
   i. Elbow: most common site of ulnar entrapment in the condylar groove and cubital tunnel
      (1) Improper arm positioning during general anesthesia
      (2) Deformity from injuries to elbow
      (3) Prolonged flexion tightening of aponeurosis
   ii. Symptoms
      (1) Pain at elbow radiating proximally or distally
      (2) Paresthesia along medial portion of palm and 4th and 5th digits
      (3) Muscle wasting in hypothenar eminence
      (4) Weakness of interossei
      (5) Weakness of flexor carpi ulnaris and flexor digitorum profundus (proximal entrapment)
      (6) Claw-hand deformity in severe cases

d. Radial nerve entrapment
   i. Between upper arm and elbow, nerve courses laterally around spiral groove and passes superficially along humerus
      (1) Humeral shaft fractures with callus formation
      (2) Compression in radial tunnel by superficial and deep heads of supinator
         (a) Radial tunnel syndrome: deep ache of extensor supinator muscles in dorsal forearm
         (b) Unable to extend thumbs and fingers at metacarpophalangeal (MCP) joint
         (c) Pain and paresthesias on dorsum of thumb and index finger

e. Medial nerve entrapment
   i. Carpal tunnel: most common compressive neuropathy in the upper extremity
      (1) Most common in women between 40 and 60 years

        (2) Any condition that may decrease the capacity of the carpal tunnel

           (a) Fractures, ganglions, xanthomas, synovial disorders, obesity, pregnancy, hypothyroidism, acromegaly, myeloma, amyloidosis, Raynaud disease, chronic renal failure, diabetes

        (3) Symptoms

           (a) Paresthesias and pain during sleep

           (b) Symptoms localize over palmar aspects of finger and hands (but may include wrist and forearm pain)

           (c) Clumsiness and hand weakness

           (d) Aggravated by repeated wrist and finger flexion

        (4) Signs

           (a) Palmar aspect of thumb to ring finger: decreased sensation

           (b) Thenar muscles atrophy

           (c) Tinel sign: distal paresthesia by percussion of median nerve proximal to flexor retinaculum or distally at base of palm

           (d) Phalen test: tourniquet to 60 mm Hg or acute flexion of wrist elicits paresthesia

    ii. Proximal to carpal tunnel

        (1) Pronator syndrome: median nerve entrapment between two heads of pronator teres

           (a) Tennis players/excessive forearm pronation

           (b) Localized forearm pain and numbness in median nerve distribution in the hand

           (c) Weakness of flexor digitorum and flexor pollicis longus (cannot oppose thumb and 2nd digit forcefully)

           (d) Weakness to pronation

f. Suprascapular nerve entrapment

    i. Pure motor nerve arising from upper brachial plexus

    ii. Course under trapezius through a notch on upper scapula border

    iii. Damage to scapula may injure nerve

        (1) Supraspinatus and infraspinatus weakness without sensory deficit

        (2) Pain after shoulder abduction

        (3) Tenderness on palpation of suprascapular notch

g. Femoral nerve entrapment

    i. Entrapment beneath inguinal ligament secondary to scar or prolonged lithotomy most common

    ii. Compression in iliacus compartment from hematomas secondary to trauma or anticoagulant

h. Lateral femoral cutaneous nerve entrapment

    i. Also known as meralgia paresthetica, Roth or Bernhardt disease

    ii. Entrapment most common as it exits the pelvis into the thigh

    iii. Belts, girdles, tight pants, pelvic surgery

    iv. Direct trauma to anterior-superior iliac spine

    v. Presents as burning pain and dysesthesias along anterolateral thigh, exaggerated by walking or standing.

    vi. Diagnostic block of the lateral femoral cutaneous

i. Sciatic nerve entrapment

    i. Common sites of entrapment/compression

      (1) Exiting sciatic notch under piriformis

      (2) Between greater trochanter and ischial tuberosity, compression by gluteus maximus and hamstrings

    ii. Hip fracture dislocation and hip arthroplasty

    iii. Muscle fibrosis from deep injections into buttock

    iv. Piriformis syndrome: spasm or scarring of piriformis muscle

      (1) Presentation similar to sciatica: burning buttock pain radiating down posterior leg

      (2) Foot drop, impaired hip extension, lateral leg/foot sensory compromise

    v. Common peroneal nerve entrapment

      (1) Lies superficially at fibular neck before dividing into superficial and deep peroneal nerves

      (2) Susceptible to compression at fibular neck (just distal to fibular head)

        (a) General anesthesia or coma

        (b) Prolonged squatting

        (c) Crossing legs

        (d) Mass compression: ganglions or cyst in knee joint

      (3) Symptoms: foot drop and anterolateral lower leg and dorsum of foot sensory deficit

    vi. Anterior tibial entrapment

      (1) Anterior tibial/compartment syndrome

        (a) Compression of deep peroneal nerve most commonly caused by muscle swelling in anterior compartment of leg

        (b) Common etiology

          (i) Trauma

          (ii) Reperfusion after arterial occlusion

          (iii) Excessive exercise

      (2) Distal tibial nerve syndrome

        (a) Becomes superficial at medial ankle as it passes under flexor retinaculum into foot

        (b) Sensory and motor to sole of foot

        (c) Symptoms

          (i) Diffuse foot pain and parenthesis in sole

          (ii) Compression or palpation over medial Achilles tendon may elicit symptoms (tarsal tunnel syndrome)

    (3) Sural nerve
        (a) Prolonged pressure over posterior lateral thigh
        (b) Paresthesias and pain over lateral aspect of ankle and foot

SUGGESTED READINGS

Cohen SA, Stabile MJ, Warfield CA: Pain in the extremities. In Warfield CA, Bajwa ZH (eds): Principles & Practice of Pain Medicine, 2nd ed. New York, McGraw-Hill, 2004, pp 319–325.

Stewart JK, Aguayo AJ: Compression and entrapment neuropathies. In Dyck PJ, Thomas PK, Lambert EH, Bunge R (eds): Peripheral Neuropathy, 2nd ed. Philadelphia, WB Saunders, 1984, p 1435.

1. CHEMOTHERAPY-INDUCED PERIPHERAL NEUROPATHY

a. Background
   i. Common limiting factor in therapy with chemotherapeutic drugs
   ii. Severe limitation on quality of life as chemotherapeutic agents become more successful in cancer treatment
b. Clinical course
   i. Variable time of onset, from immediately during administration of drugs to delayed onset
   ii. Usually incomplete recovery, requiring long period of regeneration
   iii. May be irreversible
   iv. Currently no reliable prophylactic or therapeutic treatment option
c. Etiology
   i. Vinca alkaloids
      (1) Vincristine
      (2) Cisplatinum
   ii. Paclitaxel
   iii. Taxol
   iv. Suramin
   v. Cytarabine
   vi. Etoposide, methotrexate, and Ara-C
      (1) Capable of inducing polyneuropathy but rarely used, or usually used at low enough doses that will not cause neuropathies
d. Pathophysiology
   i. Mechanism poorly understood
   ii. Some studies suggest impaired cellular Ca^{2+} regulation contributing to chemically induced neuropathy.
   iii. Some drugs have direct effects on nerve excitability by altering ion conductance of axon and/or Schwann cells.
   iv. Cisplatin has high affinity for peripheral nervous system and has been shown to accumulate in dorsal root ganglion, inducing shrinking of the nuclear and cytoplasmic compartments, disturbing cellular metabolism and axoplasmatic transport.
e. Factors determining degree of damage
   i. Type of drug used
   ii. Duration of administration
   iii. Rate of infusion
   iv. Cumulative dose applied (can occur even after single dose)
   v. Sensory, motor, and autonomic deficits

    vi. Preexisting nerve damage from:
- (1) Diabetic neuropathy
- (2) Alcohol neuropathy
- (3) Inherited neuropathy
- (4) Paraneoplastic syndrome

    vii. Combination of Taxol and cisplatin can lead to rapidly progressing neuropathy exceeding symptoms known from either agent alone.

   viii. Rate of infusion

f. Symptom characteristics
    i. Depressed deep tendon reflex (DTR): most common manifestation
    ii. Painful dysesthesias in hands and feet (glove and stocking distribution)
    iii. Sensory, motor, and autonomic deficits: depends on chemotherapeutic agent
    iv. Agent-specific symptoms
- (1) Vincristine: primarily sensory neuropathy
  - (a) Early: paresthesia and pain of hands and feet
  - (b) Distally accentuated hyperesthesia
  - (c) DTR vanishes early
  - (d) Advance stages: muscle cramps and weakness of distal muscles
  - (e) Autonomic dysfunction in more than one-third of patients: orthostatic hypotension, constipation, ileus, bladder and erectile dysfunction
  - (f) Usually reversible after months or years, but sometimes irreversible
  - (g) Cases of onset of neuropathy or symptom progression even after cessation of therapy ("coasting")
- (2) Platinum compounds (cisplatin, carboplatin, oxaliplatin)
  - (a) All platinum compounds produce hypesthesia of distal extremities, reversible in 80% of patients, and completely resolved after 6 to 8 months in 40% of all patients
  - (b) Cisplatin
    - (i) Onset of sensory deficit about 1 month after initiation of therapy
    - (ii) Decreased vibratory perception, loss of DTR, uncomfortable paresthesia starting in lower extremities
    - (iii) Affect mostly small and thinly myelinated axon (pain and temperature perception): paresthesia range from light tingling to extensive pain
    - (iv) Advanced: pronounced ataxia and gait difficulty
    - (v) Muscle cramps
    - (vi) Lhermitte sign or electric sensation in shoulder girdle: due to demyelination of dorsal roots and columns

(vii) Electroneurography detects pure sensory neuropathy late in course

(viii) Motor nerves usually spared (normal electromyography [EMG])

(ix) Characteristic phenomenon of "coasting"

(c) Oxaliplatin (relatively new compound for colorectal cancer)

(i) Induce sensory symptoms 30 to 60 minutes after infusion

(ii) Paresthesia and dysesthesia aggravated by cold

(iii) Dose: more than 540 mg/m^2 nearly always produces neuropathy

(iv) Symptoms completely disappear in days to a few weeks and reappear with each drug application

(3) Taxol (docetaxel and paclitaxel)

(a) May produce neuropathy after single dose of Taxol, especially if used with cisplatin

(b) More that 50% of patients develop paresthesia/dysesthesia with Taxol greater than 250 mg/m^2, which appears 24 to 72 hours after administration.

(c) Symmetrical hypesthesia and hyperalgesia of upper and lower extremities

(d) Affects all sensory modalities preferring thick myelinated fibers that conduct vibration and proprioception

(e) Autonomic neuropathy

(f) Muscle weakness and disabling motor neuropathy reported

(g) Nerve conduction velocity (NCV) studies and EMG reveal damage to motor nerves even in asymptomatic cases.

(h) Muscle pain starts in 1 to 2 days and resolves in 4 to 7 days.

(i) Synergistic effect of Taxol and cisplatin

(i) Pain and paresthesia in fingers and toes

(ii) Paralysis

(iii) Cranial nerve involvement

(iv) Autonomic dysfunction

g. Diagnosis

i. Clinical examination and history

ii. No reliable test or technical tool to detect and evaluate early stages

iii. NCV studies and EMG insensitive for early stages and unreliable even after prominent neuropathy ensues

h. Treatment

i. No effective drugs for prophylaxis or therapy of this neuropathy

ii. First-line treatments for symptom management

(1) Carbamazepine: 600 to 1200 mg

(2) Particularly effective for early hyperpathic symptoms under oxaliplatin therapy

  (3) Gabapentin
  (4) Tricyclic antidepressants
 iii. Prophylactic measures
  (1) Neurotropic factors (animal models, not clinically applicable yet)
   (a) Insulin-like and nerve growth factors reduce or prevented cisplatin, vincristine, and Taxol-induced neuropathy
   (b) Glia-derived neurotrophic factor: analgesic effect in neuropathic pain states
  (2) Neuroprotective compounds (promising, but need further studies)
   (a) Amifostine
    (i) Given 30 minutes before start of therapy has slight significance
   (b) Glutathione
    (i) 30 minutes before start of therapy significantly reduces chemically induced neuropathy

2. RADIATION MYELOPATHY, PLEXOPATHY, AND NEUROPATHY

 a. Radiation myelopathy
  i. Etiology
   (1) Subacute radiation myelopathy
    (a) Myelopathy most often found in cervical cord after head-and-neck cancer radiotherapy
    (b) Hodgkin disease radiotherapy
     (i) Mechanism unknown but related to transient demyelination
   (2) Chronic myelopathy
    (a) Late complication of spinal cord irradiation
    (b) Early delayed type (occurs 6 to 8 months after radiation)
     (i) Related to demyelination and necrosis of white matter
    (c) Late delayed type (1 to 4 years after radiation)
     (i) Vascular damage
  ii. Symptoms
   (1) Subacute myelopathy in cervical cord
    (a) Shock-like pain in neck precipitated by neck flexion (Lhermitte sign)
    (b) May radiate down spine into extremities
   (2) Chronic myelopathy
    (a) Pain precedes neurologic deficit
    (b) Pain localized to dermatomes at or below level of damage
    (c) Partial transverse myelopathy symptoms eventually develop

        (d) Some patients develop Brown-Séquard syndrome
           (i) Unilateral weakness
           (ii) Pyramidal tract signs
           (iii) Contralateral sensory deficits

  iii. Treatment
      (1) No specific therapy proven to be successful
      (2) Corticosteroids often used to reduce edema

b. Radiation plexopathy
  i. Etiology
    (1) Chest wall and axillary radiotherapy
       (a) Brachial plexopathy
          (i) Fourteen percent of 128 patients with breast cancer developed radiation-induced brachial plexopathy (RIBP)
          (ii) Increased likelihood of RIBP when combined with cytotoxic chemotherapy
       (b) Malignant peripheral nerve tumors
       (c) Nerve entrapment in lymphedematous shoulder
       (d) Ischemia
    (2) Lower extremity pain reported to occur 2 to 3 months after sacral plexus irradiation

  ii. Symptoms of RIBP
    (1) Shoulder and arm pain
       (a) Forty-seven percent of patients with RIBP had pain
    (2) Initial symptoms
       (a) Paresthesia
       (b) Numbness
       (c) Heaviness
       (d) Weakness
       (e) Swelling
       (f) Pain is presenting symptom in 18%, but becomes major symptom in 35%
    (3) Progressive sensory and motor loss

  iii. Differential diagnosis of RIBP
    (1) Radiation-induced brachial plexopathy
    (2) Metastatic brachial plexopathy (MBP)
    (3) Cervical radiculopathy
    (4) Osteoarthritis of shoulder
    (5) Shoulder bursitis
    (6) Myofascial pain
    (7) Iatrogenic plexus injury during surgery or central line placement
    (8) Chemotherapeutic neurotoxicity
    (9) Plexus tumors after radiation
       (a) MBP
          (i) Rapidly progressive ipsilateral shoulder/arm pain
          (ii) Selective lower plexus initially

        (iii) Horner syndrome more common in MBP than RIBP and associated with epidural tumor spread (35% patients with MBP)

   (b) RIBP
      (i) Upper plexus involvement initially
      (ii) Magnetic resonance imaging (MRI) best modality to differentiate MBP from RIBP
      (iii) Computed tomography with intravenous contrast

  (c) EMG shows fibrillation and myokymia in RIBP, but not in pure MBP
       (i) MBP can have some radiation fibrosis, so EMG cannot rule out MBP
       (ii) MRI and biopsy should be utilized to rule out recurrence of tumor and radiation-induced tumor

iv. Clinical course of RIBP
  (1) Early-onset RIBP
    (a) Three to 14 months onset
    (b) Occurs in 1.4% to 20% of irradiated breast cancer patients
    (c) Usually self-limiting
  (2) Late-onset RIBP
    (a) One to 20 years after treatment, about 5% after total dose of 60 Gy
    (b) Higher incidence when large fraction dose (3 Gy)
    (c) Less commonly associated with pain
    (d) Mostly involves upper plexus

v. Confounding factors
  (1) Radiation plus cytotoxic chemotherapy increase likelihood of RIBP
  (2) Dose of radiation
  (3) Treatment technique

vi. Pathophysiology
  (1) Progressive fibrous constriction of nerve bundles
  (2) Thickening of endoneurium
  (3) Loss of myelin
  (4) Obliteration of small blood vessels

vii. Treatments
  (1) Lack of promising therapy
  (2) Rehabilitation therapy
  (3) Spinal cord stimulation
  (4) Dorsal root entry zone rhizotomy
  (5) Neurolysis of dorsal root ganglion

SUGGESTED READINGS

Hough SW, Kanner RM: Cancer pain syndromes. In Warfield CA, Bajwa ZH (eds): Principles & Practice of Pain Medicine, 2nd ed. New York, McGraw-Hill, 2004, pp 458–459.

Kori SH: Diagnosis and management of brachial plexus lesions in cancer patients. Oncology 1995;8:756.

Martin LA, Hagen NA: Neuropathic pain in cancer patients: Mechanisms, syndromes, and clinical controversies. J Pain Sympt Manage 1997;14(2):99–117.

Quasthoff S, Hartung HP: Chemotherapy-induced peripheral neuropathy. J Neurol 2002;249:9–17.

Siau C, Bennett GJ: Dysregulation of cellular calcium homeostasis in chemotherapy-evoked painful peripheral neuropathy. Anesth Analg 2006;102:1485–1490.

121 Fibromyalgia

1. CLINICAL FEATURES

a. Diffuse, widespread musculoskeletal pain and stiffness with multiple tender points located in specific areas
b. Affects approximately 5 million people in the United States
c. Females between 20 and 60 years account for 75% of patients.
d. Unknown etiology
e. Sleep disturbance is present in 90% of patients; stage 4 of the sleep cycle is usually affected.
f. Pain occurs in muscles, tendons, and joints all over the body.
g. Pain is in 11 of 18 tender points, with bilateral involvement, above and below the waist.
   i. Anterior tender points
      (1) C5-C7 intertransverse space
      (2) 2nd rib, costochondral junction
      (3) Lateral epicondyle
      (4) Knee: medial fat pad
   ii. Posterior tender points
      (1) Occipital area
      (2) Midpoint of upper trapezius
      (3) Supraspinatus muscle
      (4) Gluteal muscles
      (5) Greater trochanter

2. POSSIBLE ETIOLOGIES

a. Stress
b. Disordered sleep
c. Chemical or hormonal imbalance
d. Lower pain threshold
e. Metabolic
f. Central nervous system (CNS) injury
g. Infection
h. Endocrine disorder

3. ASSOCIATED SYMPTOMS

a. Sleep disturbance
b. Memory difficulties
c. Irritable bowel
d. Raynaud phenomena
e. Weakness
f. Subjective extremity swelling
g. Depression

h. Daytime fatigue
i. Dizziness
j. Headache
k. Morning stiffness
l. Dysmenorrhea

4. AGGRAVATING FACTORS

a. Change in weather
b. Cold environments
c. Premenstrual and menopausal states
d. Hormonal imbalance
e. Overexertion
f. Depression

5. PROGNOSIS

a. Chronic in nature and may last a lifetime with waxing and waning possible
b. It is not disfiguring and does not progress to other rheumatologic or medical diseases.
c. If there is a focal trigger, the symptoms cease when the focal issue is resolved.

6. TREATMENT

a. The most highly recommended modalities include lifestyle changes, medication, relaxation techniques, exercise techniques.
b. Medications include Flexeril, tramadol, Tylenol, tricyclic antidepressants, selective serotonin reuptake inhibitors, and serotonin-norepinephrine reuptake inhibitors.
c. Relaxation techniques include massage, yoga, self-hypnosis, Tai Chi, and biofeedback.
d. Additional rehabilitation modalities include heat, ice, manual therapy, transcutaneous electrical nerve stimulation, and aquatics.

SUGGESTED READINGS

Goldenberg DL: Fibromyalgia syndrome. A decade later. Arch Intern Med 1999;159:777–795.

Leventhal LJ: Management of Fibromyalgia. Ann Intern Med 1999;131:850–858.

Stralanyl D, Copeland ME: Fibromyalgia and Chronic Myofascial Pain Syndrome. Oakland, CA, New Harbinger, 1996.

1. DEFINITION

a. Sites in muscle fascia or tendon that, when palpated, produce a local or referred pain pattern in a reproducible manner that is non-myotomal, sclerotomal, dermatomal.
b. Trigger points are often found in taut bonds of muscle as well as ligaments, tendons, joint capsule, skin, and periosteum.

2. EPIDEMIOLOGY

a. Affects women more than men
b. Seen in children and young adults, most common in the 30- to 50-year age range.
c. Muscle groups most commonly affected: trapezius, levator scapulae, axial postural muscles

3. ETIOLOGY

a. May occur in any skeletal muscle
b. Stress and tension: most frequent cause, also nonrestorative sleep, prolonged spasm, fatigue, and chill
c. Occurs most frequently in axial muscles
d. May develop in areas of pain due to nerve root compression, peripheral nerve entrapment, and after a laminectomy

4. CLASSIFICATION OF TRIGGER POINTS

a. Primary: independently develop
b. Secondary: may develop in antagonistic or neighboring protective muscles secondary to stress or spasm
c. Always painful, tender, and symptomatic either at rest or in motion.
d. Referred pain elicited more frequently by needling
e. "Jump response": Patient suddenly jumps or moves when trigger point palpated.
f. Referred pain patterns are specific and reproducible for primary trigger points (TRFs).

5. LATENT

a. Asymptomatic, no treatment, often found coincidentally; tender on palpation
b. May predispose to active TRFs
c. Can cause muscle shortening and weakness

6. TREATMENT

a. Stretch and spray
   i. Vapocoolant spray: Temporary anesthesia allows stretching of the muscles.
   ii. Cooling: relieves muscle spasm

7. TRIGGER POINT INJECTION AND PAIN RELIEF

a. Mechanical disruption (dry needling)
   i. Disrupts muscle elements or nerve endings
   ii. Release of intracellular potassium and nerve fiber depolarization
b. Fluid injection (saline, steroid, local anesthetic)
   i. Dilutes nerve: sensitizing substances
   ii. Local anesthetic interrupts feedback mechanism
   iii. Fecal necrosis: by some local anesthetics
   iv. No advantage over dry needling

8. HISTOLOGY OF TRIGGER POINTS

a. Biopsy findings: nonspecific and inconsistent
   i. Waxy degeneration of muscle fiber.
   ii. Moth-eaten fibers, ragged red fibers
   iii. Swollen mitochondria, decreased glycogen stores, irregularity of sarcomeres
b. Botulinum toxin type A injection
   i. Results of three randomized, controlled trials mixed but promising: 30% pain reduction for 5 to 6 weeks, no difference compared with saline for refractory unilateral cervicothoracic paraspinal muscle pain, no statistical difference at 30 days compared with steroid injection

SUGGESTED READINGS

Rachlin ES, Rachlin IS: Myofascial Pain and Fibromyalgia: Trigger Point Management. St. Louis, Mosby, Inc., 2002.

Simons DG, Travell JG, Simons LS, Cummings BD: Myofascial Pain and Dysfunction: The Trigger Point Manual. Philadelphia, Lippincott Williams & Wilkins, 1999.

123 HIV/AIDS

1. PATHOPHYSIOLOGY

a. HIV mainly infects the host's CD4 lymphocytes.
  i. HIV causes the destruction of CD4 cells through multiple mechanisms, including apoptosis.
  ii. With the loss of CD4 cells, the infected person becomes susceptible to opportunistic infections.
b. Pain secondary to many causes
  i. Viral infection itself
  ii. Antiviral, antineoplastic, or antibacterial medications
  iii. Secondary infections
  iv. Interventional procedures

2. EPIDEMIOLOGY

a. Patients with AIDS are living nearly normal lives secondary to reduced viral burdens.
b. Up to 90% of HIV-positive patients live with pain.
c. Pain in HIV-positive patients is at least as prevalent as pain in patients with cancer.

3. DIFFERENTIAL DIAGNOSIS

a. Cutaneous causes
  i. Kaposi sarcoma
  ii. Oral cavity pain from cytomegalovirus (CMV) or Herpes
b. Visceral causes
  i. Tumor: Kaposi' sarcoma or lymphoma
  ii. Gastritis or ulcerative gastritis
  iii. Pancreatitis from antiretroviral medications, especially didanosine (DDI) and pentamidine
  iv. Infection from mycobacterium avium intracellulare (MAI), CMV, fungi, and parasites causing diarrhea
  v. Biliary tract disorders caused by *Cryptosporidium* or CMV
c. Deep somatic causes
  i. Reactive arthritis, Reiter syndrome, psoriatic arthritis
  ii. Nonspecific polyarthralgia (acute phase)
  iii. Painful myopathy, diffuse inflammatory myopathy
  iv. Inflammatory myopathy or toxic painful neuropathy as a medication side effect, especially secondary to zidovudine-induced electrolyte disturbances
  v. HIV neuropathic pain
  vi. Postherpetic neuralgia
  vii. Diabetic neuropathy due to its high prevalence

    d. Headache
       i. HIV-related: meningitis, encephalitis, or neoplasm
       ii. HIV-unrelated: tension or migraine
       iii. Iatrogenic: zidovudine therapy

3. DIAGNOSIS

    a. Cutaneous and visceral causes
       i. Diagnosis made by medical consultation using typical radiographic, laboratory, and tissue findings
    b. Deep somatic causes
       i. Nonspecific polyarthralgias usually occur in the acute phase of HIV infection, which can lead to a painful articular syndrome that usually affects large joints.
       ii. Psoriatic arthritis is often severe and accompanied by erosive changes and crippling deformity.
       iii. Painful myopathy in the early to intermediate stages of HIV is characterized by proximal muscle weakness and is often a side effect of antiretroviral therapy.
       iv. Neuropathic pain is often described as burning, electric, stabbing, brief, or shooting pain that can begin after healing has stopped or despite the absence of tissue injury.
       v. Allodynia is not uncommon with neuropathic pain.
    c. Headache
       i. Need to check immune status in addition to central nervous system signs and symptoms.
       ii. Consider radiographic evidence of mass but still need tissue diagnosis prior to treatment of underlying cause.
       iii. Cerebrospinal fluid studies, including cultures and polymerase chain reaction, can help differentiate primary cause.

4. TREATMENT

    a. Treat underlying cause
    b. No specific validated guidelines: look to World Health Organization (WHO) cancer guidelines
    c. Nonsteroidal anti-inflammatory drugs (NSAIDs) or Tylenol, weak opiates, strong opiates
       i. NSAIDs or Tylenol
          (1) Tylenol: risk of dose-dependent hepatotoxicity
          (2) NSAIDs: gastrointestinal and renal side effects
       ii. Weak opioids
          (1) Mild to moderate pain
          (2) Can combine with NSAIDs or Tylenol for synergistic effect
       iii. Strong opiates
          (1) Severe pain
          (2) Sustained release formulations for constant pain

(3) With advanced AIDS, PO medications may not be tolerated; consider terlipressin (TP) administration.
  iv. Adjuvant medications
    (1) Neuropathic pain, depression: antidepressants and anticonvulsants
    (2) Diarrhea-decreased bowel motility from opioid and tricyclic antidepressants
  v. Antidepressants
    (1) Can have helpful side effects
    (2) Carbamazepine can cause bone marrow depression
    (3) Lidoderm patch is sometimes effective for postherpetic neuralgia
  vi. Behavioral therapy
    (1) Hypnosis, visualization, biofeedback, cognitive-behavioral therapy

SUGGESTED READINGS

Carr DB, Goudas LC: Evaluating and managing pain for patients with HIV/AIDS: An overview. In Nedeljkovic SS (ed): Pain Management, Anesthesia and HIV/AIDS. Philadelphia, Butterworth-Heineman, 2001, pp 119–141.

Paranjape RS: Immunopathogenesis of HIV infection. Indian J Med Res 2005; 121(4):240–255.

124 Osteoarthritis

1. PATHOPHYSIOLOGY

a. Heterogeneous group of disorders with a characteristic pathology
   i. Articular cartilage damage in load-bearing areas
   ii. New bone formation at the joint margin called osteophytosis
   iii. Subchondral bone changes
   iv. Synovitis
   v. Joint capsule thickening
b. Occurs most commonly in synovial joints
   i. Hands, hips, knees, and spine
c. Pathogenesis of pain
   i. Articular cartilage has no nerve endings.
   ii. Cartilage matrix is rich in collagen and proteoglycans, which, in osteoarthritis, gradually breakdown from proteolytic degradation.
   iii. Increased synthesis of similar but slightly altered matrix by chondrocytes leads to cartilage surface fibrillation, cleft formation, and loss of cartilage volume.
   iv. Ossification of cartilage outgrowths leads to osteophytes.
   v. Loss of cartilage leads to bone pain.
   vi. Cytokines released from cartilage, synovium, and bone affect chondrocyte function, which increases progression to osteoarthritis.

2. EPIDEMIOLOGY

a. Ten percent to 15% of population in the United Kingdom is suffering from osteoarthritis at any one time.
b. Risk factors
   i. Increasing age, family history, previous joint injuries, and obesity

3. DIAGNOSIS

a. Increased age
   i. Unusual before age 40 years
b. Pain
   i. Joint pain in relation to use and relieved by rest
c. Stiffness
   i. Related to inactivity
d. Reduced movement
   i. Pain on movement and joint mobility is restricted
e. Swelling
   i. Palpable firm swelling at the joint margins
f. Crepitus
   i. Joint cracking with movement

g. Differential diagnosis
   i. Referred pain, periarticular conditions, and somatization

4. RADIOGRAPHIC FINDINGS

a. Osteophytes, bone shape change, subchondral bone cysts, and loss of cartilage

5. TREATMENT

a. Information
   i. Disease education, weight loss, exercise, lifestyle alterations
b. Self-help
   i. Simple analgesics and topical agents
c. Simple nonsurgical interventions
   i. Nonsteroidal anti-inflammatory drugs, physiotherapy or occupational therapy, orthoses
d. Advanced nonsurgical interventions
   i. Joint injections
e. Surgery
   i. Partial or total joint replacement, osteotomy, or resurfacing

SUGGESTED READING

Dieppe, PA, Lohmander LS: Pathogenesis and management of pain in osteoarthritis. Lancet 2005;365:965–973.

125 Sickle Cell Disease

1. EPIDEMIOLOGY

  a. Acute pain crises account for approximately 95% of all hospital admissions for patients with sickle cell disease.

  b. On average, each admission last 7 days.

  c. Males are more likely than females to present to the hospital secondary to their higher hemoglobin and increased blood viscosity.

  d. Sickle cell crisis can be precipitated by:

    i. Infection

    ii. Fever

    iii. Temperature extremes

    iv. Dehydration

    v. Sleep difficulties

  e. Increasing number of painful crises is correlated with an increased mortality.

2. TREATMENT

  a. In-patient treatment

    i. Parenteral opioids either around the clock or patient-controlled analgesia (PCA)

    ii. Intravenous hydration

    iii. Oxygen

    iv. Blood transfusion

    v. Antibiotics as needed

    vi. Heating pads/massage

  b. Out-patient treatment

    i. Daily oral penicillin in younger children if not allergic

    ii. Over-the-counter pain medication

    iii. Prescribed analgesics

    iv. Avoiding temperature extremes

    v. Drinking at least 150 mL/kg per day

    vi. Adequate rest

    vii. Stress avoidance

    viii. Regular physician visits

SUGGESTED READINGS

Ballas SK, Lusardi M: Hospital readmission for acute sickle cell painful episodes: Frequency, etiology, and prognostic significance. Am J Hematol 2005;79: 17–25.

Chen E, Cole SW, Kato PM: A review of empirically supported psychosocial interventions for pain and adherence outcomes in sickle cell disease. J Pediatr Psychol 2004;29(3):197–207.

126 Multiple Sclerosis

1. PATHOPHYSIOLOGY

a. Multiple sclerosis (MS)
   i. Central nervous system (CNS) disease of heterogeneous symptoms related to inflammation and demyelination
b. Spasticity in MS
   i. Demyelination in the descending corticospinal, vestibulospinal, and reticulospinal pathways
c. Pain in MS
   i. Linked to deafferentation of central pathways
   ii. Injury of spinothalamic pathway causes disinhibition of other pain pathways.
   iii. CNS lesions can cause hyperexcitability.
   iv. Spinal cord injury can cause increased neuronal activity at that site and thalamus.
   v. Central pain associated with posterior column involvement

2. EPIDEMIOLOGY

a. Pain in MS was first described by Charcot in 1872.
b. Spasticity affects 40% to 75% of patients with MS.
c. Reports of pain prevalence vary from 30% to 80%.
   i. Forty percent of patients with MS report that pain has an important affect on activities of daily living.
   ii. Pain can worsen with increasing age or disease progression.
   iii. Chronic pain affects 60% to 90% of patients with pain.
   iv. Acute pain affects 16% to 40% of patients with pain.

3. DIAGNOSIS

a. Spasticity
   i. Can be quantified by the Ashworth scale, a subjective measure
   ii. Test quadriceps hypertonicity and pendulum test for an objective measure
   iii. Treating spasticity can unmask pain
b. Acute pain
   i. Stereotypical paroxysmal attacks characterized by intense pain
   ii. Often originates with trigeminal nerve
c. Chronic pain
   i. Usually low-back pain and extremities
   ii. Characteristically described as burning, paresthesias, and deep muscular aching

4. TREATMENT

a. Spasticity
   i. Nonpharmacologic treatment: full range of motion and aerobic exercise, relaxation methods such as yoga or biofeedback
   ii. Pharmacologic treatment: baclofen, which stimulates gamma-aminobutyric acid (GABA) receptors, tizanidine, a centrally acting α_2-adrenergic receptor agonist
   iii. Supplemental medication: benzodiazepines or dantrolene
   iv. Interventional treatment: intrathecal baclofen pump for those who cannot tolerate the side effects of baclofen, botulism toxin, phenol injections, and surgical neurectomy and rhizotomy
b. Acute pain
   i. Trigeminal neuralgia typically responds to such anticonvulsants as carbamazepine (first-line treatment).
   ii. As the disease progresses, may need adjuvant therapy with other anticonvulsants
   iii. Other adjuvant medications: baclofen, misoprostol, and topiramate
   iv. Interventional treatment: percutaneous glycerol rhizotomy or radiofrequency ablation
c. Chronic pain
   i. Pharmacologic treatment for low-back pain in MS includes anticonvulsants, which remain the first-line treatment.
   ii. Nonsteroidal anti-inflammatory drugs, opioids, and nerve blocks can be used in patients who do not respond to anticonvulsants.
   iii. Patients suffering from complex regional pain syndrome may respond to tricyclic antidepressants.

SUGGESTED READINGS

Beiske AG, Pedersen ED, Czujko B, Myhr KM: Pain and sensory complaints in multiple sclerosis. Eur J Neurol 2004;11:479–482.

Crayton H, Heyman RA, Rossman HS: A multimodal approach to managing the symptoms of multiple sclerosis. Neurology 2004;63:S12–S18.

Svendsen KB, Jensen TS, Hansen HJ, Bach FW: Sensory function and quality of life in patients with multiple sclerosis pain. Pain 2005;114:473–481.

127 Parkinson Disease

1. PATHOPHYSIOLOGY

a. Presence of neuronal loss and Lewy bodies in the substantia nigra
   i. Need neuronal loss in excess of 60% to show symptoms
   ii. Onset is usually 4 to 5 years before symptoms start

2. EPIDEMIOLOGY

a. Prevalence is estimated between 87 and 330/100,000 in United States.
b. Up to half of patients with Parkinson disease suffer from pain.

3. DIAGNOSIS

a. Pain from complications of Parkinson disease
   i. Patients usually older than 60 years
   ii. Associated gait disorder can lead to trauma
   iii. Possibly associated with rheumatic illness
b. Limb rigidity
   i. Most common cause of pain
   ii. Lower limb rigidity can be misdiagnosed as radiculopathy with radiation of pain into the lower leg.
   iii. No weakness associated with Parkinson disease
   iv. Axial and upper extremity rigidity can also be present.
   v. Rigidity of face, chin, or jaw can be a presenting feature.
c. Dystonia
   i. Painful agonist or antagonist pulling of foot musculature
   ii. Usually occurs as an "off" phenomenon
   iii. Can occur as medication efficacy changes
   iv. Less commonly, posturing can take place in the face, arm, jaw, neck, or leg
d. Sleep disorders
   i. Restless leg syndrome can cause severe insomnia.
   ii. Unpleasant and painful sensation in the legs during inactivity and transition from wakefulness to sleep
   iii. Rigidity can make rolling over in bed difficult.
   iv. Rapid eye movement behavior disorder is common in patients with Parkinson disease, which can cause them to injure their partner.
e. Gastrointestinal pain
   i. Constipation is common secondary to intestinal slowing and medication.
   ii. Esophageal symptoms (dysphagia, acid regurgitation, pyrosis, and noncardiac chest pain) are common.

      iii. Medication can lead to abdominal cramping, bloating, and nausea

      iv. Bromocriptine mesylate can cause retroperitoneal fibrosis.

  f. Neck pain and headache

      i. Usually secondary to orthostatic hypotension

      ii. Seen in both Parkinson disease and syndrome

  g. Primary pain disorders

      i. Diffuse sensation of tension, discomfort, or paresthesias.

      ii. More common in younger patients.

      iii. Up to 25% of patients describe a burning in their mouth.

      iv. Chronic, severe oral or genital pains are primary disturbances.

4. TREATMENT

  a. Pain from complications

      i. Treat underlying cause

  b. Limb rigidity

      i. Anti-Parkinson therapy reduces rigidity and pain.

      ii. Physical therapy and massage are important adjuvant treatments.

  c. Dystonia

      i. Increase dose of current anti-Parkinson medication.

      ii. Start diary of symptoms.

      iii. "Off" dystonias may respond to botulism toxin type A.

  d. Primary pain disorders

      i. Burning in the mouth can be treated with gabapentin.

      ii. Primary pain secondary to Parkinson disease may respond to levodopa therapy.

SUGGESTED READING

Wright AF: Neurogenetics II: Complex disorders. J Neurol Neurosurg Psychiatry 2005;76:623–631.

128 Diabetic Peripheral Neuropathy

1. PATHOPHYSIOLOGY

a. Genetic predisposition
   i. ApoE4, ARZ2 alleles, angiotensin-converting enzyme (ACE) inhibitor polymorphism, and Toll recC polymorphism
b. Inflammation
   i. Oxidative/nitrative stress, protein kinase C (PKC), selectin, vascular cell adhesion molecules (VCAMs), IL6, TNF α, NF kB, reactive oxygen species (ROS), and nitrotyrosine
c. Combination of genetics, inflammation, and glucotoxicity leads to endothelial injury with functional changes.

2. EPIDEMIOLOGY

a. Prevalence is 45% after 25 years
   i. About 7 million patients with diabetic neuropathy
   ii. Most common neuropathy in developed countries
   iii. More hospitalizations than for all other diabetic complications combined
   iv. Responsible for 50% to 75% of all nontraumatic amputations
b. Morbidity
   i. Foot ulceration leading to gangrene and limb loss
   ii. Risk for amputation: increases 1.7-fold
   iii. Risk of amputation (if concomitant deformity): increases 12-fold
c. Progresses at 1 meter squared of body area per year after diagnosis

3. DIAGNOSIS

a. Diagnosis of exclusion
   i. "Presence of symptoms or signs of peripheral nerve disease in people with diabetes after exclusion of other causes"
b. Need a minimum of two abnormalities
   i. Symptoms, signs, nerve conduction abnormalities, qualitative sensory tests, or qualitative autonomic tests
c. Focal neuropathies
   i. Primarily in older population
   ii. Vascular obstruction after which adjacent neuronal fascicles take over
   iii. Carpal tunnel syndrome is three times more likely in a person with diabetes
d. Diffuse neuropathies
   i. Primarily in older patients
   ii. Starts in thighs and buttocks and is followed by weakness
   iii. Begins in a unilateral distribution and progresses to a bilateral distribution

e. Distal symmetric polyneuropathies
   i. Most common diabetic neuropathy
   ii. Either sensory or motor
   iii. Involves both small and large fibers
   iv. Pain and hyperalgesia in the lower limbs followed by loss of thermal sensitivity and decreased light touch
   v. Reflexes and strength remain intact
f. Acute painful neuropathy
   i. Time course less than 6 months
   ii. Associated with the onset of diabetes and can be worsened by insulin or sulfonylureas
   iii. Symptoms are often worse at night and manifest in the feet more than the hands.
   iv. Can be associated with profound weight loss
g. Chronic painful neuropathy
   i. Occurs later in the course of diabetes
   ii. Pain lasts longer than 6 months
   iii. Extremely resistant to all forms of treatment and can result in tolerance to opioid and analgesics, ultimately leading to addiction
h. Differential diagnosis
   i. Claudication
   ii. Morton neuroma
   iii. Charcot neuropathy
   iv. Fascitis
   v. Osteoarthritis
   vi. Radiculopathy

4. TREATMENT

a. Hyperglycemic control
   i. Fifty percent reduction in clinical or electrophysiologic evidence of diabetic neuropathy in patients treated with intensive insulin therapy
   ii. In United Kingdom Prospective Diabetes Study, control of blood sugar was associated with an improvement in vibration perception.
b. α-Lipoic acid
   i. Thiol-replenishing and redox-modulating agent
   ii. Effective in ameliorating both the somatic and autonomic neuropathies
   iii. Currently undergoing clinical trials in the United States
c. Capsaicin
   i. Number needed to treat (NNT) to reduce pain by 50% is 5.9
   ii. One to three teaspoons to a jar of cold cream and apply locally
   iii. Likely depletes substance P

   d. Clonidine
     i. Treats sympathetic-mediated C-fiber pain
     ii. Applied topically but can be difficult to titrate
   e. Insulin infusion
     i. Treats A delta-fiber pain
     ii. Used in the setting of normoglycemia for 48 hours
   f. Nerve blocks
     i. Lidocaine by slow infusion can give relief up to 21 days
     ii. Follow nerve block with oral mexiletine
     iii. Mexiletine NNT is 10
   g. Tramadol
     i. Centrally acting weak opioid analgesic with a NNT 3.4
     ii. Shown to be better than placebo in a randomized controlled trial
     iii. Side effects are common and similar to other opioids
   h. Dextromethorphan
     i. Target is spinal N-methyl-D-aspartate (NMDA) glutaminergic receptors with NNT 1.9
     ii. Sugar-free solution can be prepared
   i. Antidepressants
     i. Tricyclic antidepressants NNT is 1.4 for an optimal dose
     ii. Selective serotonin reuptake inhibitor NNT is 6.7
     iii. Both classes accentuate the central neurotransmitters that activate endogenous pain-inhibitory systems.
   j. Carbamazepine
     i. NNT is 3.3
     ii. Double-blinded, placebo-controlled studies have demonstrated efficacy
     iii. Especially useful for lightning or shooting pain
   k. Gabapentin
     i. NNT is 3.7
     ii. Monotherapy appears efficacious in doses from 1800 to 3600 mg/day
   l. Lamotrigine
     i. Antiepileptic with antinociceptive properties
     ii. Single randomized, placebo-controlled trial has shown efficacy of this agent
   m. Transcutaneous nerve stimulation
     i. May be beneficial with low side-effect profile
     ii. Need to change electrode position to identify sensitive areas

5. MANAGEMENT

   a. Small-fiber neuropathies
     i. Careful foot care with daily inspection
     ii. Monofilament for self-testing
     iii. Well-fitting shoes
     iv. Emollient creams for drying and cracking

  b. Large-fiber neuropathies
      i. Gait and strength training
      ii. Pain management

SUGGESTED READING

Vinik AI, Mehrabyan A: Diabetic neuropathies. Med Clin N Am 2004;88: 947–990.

1. CHARACTERISTICS OF CANCER PAIN

a. Periodic exacerbations (waxes and wanes)
b. Acute
c. Chronic
d. Acute on chronic
e. Baseline (continuous) pain: treat with sustained-release medications
f. Breakthrough pain: "breaks through" sustained-release medications; treat with immediate-release, short-acting medications
g. Incident pain: associated with activity; treat with immediate-release, short-acting medications

2. TREATMENT MODALITIES FOR CANCER PAIN

a. Noninvasive
   i. Analgesics (opioid and nonopioid)
   ii. Adjunctive medications (anticonvulsants, antidepressants, muscle relaxants, benzodiazepines, neuroleptics)
   iii. Corticosteroids
   iv. Bisphosphonates (for bony pain: inhibit osteoclast activity and reduce bone resorption)
   v. Strontium 89 (incorporated into bone, preferentially into metastatic lesions)
   vi. Physical modalities (heat, ice, stretch, massage, touch therapy)
   vii. Psychological interventions (relaxation, imagery, reframing, hypnosis)
b. Invasive
   i. Anesthetic techniques
   ii. Surgery
   iii. Radiotherapy

3. ASSESSMENT OF CANCER PAIN

a. Acute vs. chronic (or acute on chronic)
b. Disease-related
c. Treatment-related
d. Preexisting painful condition
e. Evaluation: pain intensity, psychosocial assessment, physical and neurologic examination, diagnostic interventions if indicated

4. METASTATIC CANCER PAIN

a. Most common sites of metastases (depending on primary cell type): bone, brain, lung, liver, all of which can cause pain
b. Bone: richly innervated periosteum, pathologic fractures (long bone, vertebral compression, and ribs are most common)
c. Brain: increased intracranial pressure, meningeal irritation, rare central pain syndromes
d. Lung: pleural infiltration, pleural effusion (parenchymal infiltration not painful but causes dyspnea and cough)
e. Liver: capsular stretch, ductal distention, infarction

5. VISCERO-OBSTRUCTIVE PAIN

a. Gut: Any gastrointestinal (GI) cancer can cause complete or partial obstruction at any level of the gut with resultant distention and pain as well as nausea and vomiting.
b. Veno-occlusive disease (VOD): in hematopoietic cell transplantation
c. Pelvis: gynecologic and urologic malignancies

6. NEUROPATHIC PAIN

a. Primarily plexopathies and peripheral nerve injuries, rare central pain syndromes
b. Due to tumor invasion
c. Due to surgical nerve injury (e.g., post-thoracotomy and postmastectomy syndromes)
d. Due to chemotherapy, especially vinca alkaloids
e. Due to radiation injury

7. TUMOR INVASION

a. Local invasion or from metastatic disease
    i. Somatic pain
    ii. Visceral pain
    iii. Neuropathic pain

8. SPECIFIC THERAPY

a. Medications: control pain in 93% to 95% of cases; provide maximum flexibility but may cause intolerable and unrelenting side effects
b. Anesthetic techniques
    i. Peripheral nerve blockade or lysis (e.g., intercostal nerves)
    ii. Sympathectomy: for sympathetically mediated neuropathic pain

   iii. Cranial nerve blockade or lysis: for head and neck cancers
   iv. Plexus blockade or lysis
       (1) Stellate ganglion: for facial or upper extremity pain
       (2) Celiac plexus: upper and midabdominal pain (liver, pancreas, spleen, small bowel, colon)
       (3) Superior hypogastric plexus: for lower abdominal and pelvic pain (sigmoid colon, rectum, pelvic tumors)
       (4) Ganglion impar: for perineal pain

End-of-Life Issues and Treatment of Symptoms Other Than Pain

1. THE DYING PROCESS

a. The trajectory toward death differs from slowly progressive illness with waxing and waning cycles to sudden catastrophic illness or injury (**Table 130-1**).

b. Biologic and psychological markers near death: cognitive dysfunction, restlessness, air hunger, pain, delirium

2. SOURCES OF SOMATIC DISTRESS

a. Pain (**Table 130-2**)

b. Nausea/vomiting: anatomy, biochemistry, management (**Table 130-3**)

   i. Causes of nausea and vomiting

      (1) Disease: visceral lesions, brain lesions

      (2) Iatrogenic: medications (chemotherapy), other bodily invasions

---

TABLE 130–1 Signs that Death is Imminent

Hypersomnolence
Disorientation
Irregular breathing
Excessive secretions
Visual and auditory hallucinations
Decreased clarity of sight
Decreased urine production
Mottled skin
Cool extremities
Truncal warmth

TABLE 130–2 Sources of Somatic Distress in Patients with Cancer

Most feared symptom
Interferes with activity
Denies enjoyment in daily living
Prevents nurturing social exchanges
Frequent cause of psychiatric symptoms

Most misunderstood symptom
Disease-specific symptoms
Symptoms caused by treatment ("toxicity")
Coexisting conditions

TABLE 130–3 Biochemistry of Antiemetics

Dopamine Blockers	Histamine (H1) Blockers

Metoclopramide (Reglan)
• CNS effect
• Gastric effect
 	
Butyrophenones
• Droperidol
• Haloperidol
 	
Phenothiazines
• Prochlorperazine (Compazine)
• Promethazine (Phenergan)
 	
Side effects of dopamine blockers
  ◦ EPS
  ◦ Sedation
  ◦ Dysphoria
  ◦ Confusion
	Diphenhydramine (Benadryl)
	Hydroxyzine (Atarax, Vistaril)
	Dimenhydrinate (Dramamine)
	Side effects of antihistamines
	  ◦ Sedation
	  ◦ Confusion
	  ◦ Dry mouth/dry skin
	  ◦ Urinary retention
	  ◦ Blurred vision

Acetylcholine blockers
Scopolamine
• Transdermal
• Intravenous
 	
Belladonna
Dimenhydrinate (Dramamine)
Side effects of anticholinergics
  ◦ Dry mouth
  ◦ Confusion
  ◦ Sedation
	Serotonin blockers
	Ondansetron (Zofran)
	Granisetron (Kytril)
	Side effect
	  ◦ Headache

Substance P antagonists
Aprepitant (Emend)
Side effects
  ◦ Fatigue
  ◦ Diarrhea
  ◦ Constipation	

Nonspecific antiemetics
Benzodiazepines
Side effects of benzodiazepines
  ◦ Sedation
  ◦ Confusion
  ◦ Amnesia
  ◦ Suppression of REM sleep
 	
Cannabinoids
Corticosteroids
Sympathomimetics
Nonpharmacologic methods
	Nonpharmacologic antiemesis
	Relaxation
	Imagery
	Reframing
	Biofeedback
	Acupuncture
	
	Rarely work alone
	Excellent adjunctive therapy

     ii. Anatomy of nausea and vomiting
       (1) Central and peripheral (brain and gut)
       (2) Brainstem (area postrema)
         (a) Chemoreceptor trigger zone (CTZ), nucleus tractus solitarius
         (b) Highly vascular, ineffective blood-brain barrier
     iii. Biochemistry of nausea and vomiting
       (1) Dopamine receptors
       (2) Acetylcholine receptors
       (3) Histamine receptors
       (4) Serotonin receptors
       (5) Opioid receptors
       (6) Substance P receptors
       (7) γ-Aminobutyric acid (GABA) receptors

c. Dyspnea and cough
     i. Dyspnea is a sensation of breathlessness: increases ventilation, decreases activity
     ii. Dyspnea is not the same as respiratory distress
     iii. Characteristics: copious secretions, cough, chest pain, fatigue, air hunger, hemoptysis
     iv. Causes of dyspnea and cough
       (1) Primary pulmonary disease
       (2) Cardiac failure
       (3) Head and neck cancers
       (4) Neuromuscular pathology
       (5) Renal insufficiency
       (6) Mediastinal pathology
       (7) Intra-abdominal pathology
     v. Treatment of dyspnea and cough
       (1) Treat physiology
         (a) Pulmonary
         (b) Cardiac/renal
         (c) Intra-abdominal
         (d) Neuromuscular
         (e) Secretions
       (2) Treat psychological distress: respiratory sedatives
       (3) Hemoptysis: terrifying, a palliative care emergency

d. Cachexia
     i. Energy depletion
     ii. Malnutrition
     iii. Biochemical changes
     iv. Impaired socialization
     v. Refractory to treatment
     vi. Treatment of cachexia
       (1) Appetite stimulants: megestrol acetate, corticosteroids, cannabinoids
       (2) Suppression of metabolism (reversal of catabolism)

    e. Sedation and low energy: due to disease or medications
       i. Treatment of sedation and low energy
         (1) Discontinue offending drug
         (2) Substitute for offending drug (especially opioids, due to incomplete cross-tolerance)
         (3) Add a stimulant
            (a) Methylphenidate (~1/3 mg/kg/day in divided doses)
            (b) Dextroamphetamine (tachyphylaxis usually appears)
            (c) Modafinil (mechanism unknown)
    f. Delirium/confusion: drug side effects, paraneoplastic syndromes, sepsis, malnutrition
       i. Delirium: an acute disruption of attention and cognition
       ii. Confusion: delirium is often called "acute confusional state"
       iii. Agitation: one manifestation of delirium, namely, hyperactive delirium (restless, screaming)
       iv. Hypoactive delirium: quiet, inactive, stuporous
       v. Treatment of cognitive dysfunction and agitation
         (1) Rule out depression
         (2) Rule out medication side effects (e.g., alcohol, benzodiazepines, analgesics, antihistamines)
         (3) Rule out metabolic and hormonal imbalances
         (4) Restore normal circadian rhythms
         (5) Use antipsychotics where appropriate (e.g., "sundowning," hallucinations)
         (6) Use benzodiazepines with extreme caution
         (7) Barbiturates (especially useful for terminal agitation)
    g. Itch (pruritus): common opioid side effect
       i. Treatment of itch (pruritus)
         (1) Antihistamines
         (2) Doxepin
         (3) Mu-receptor antagonists, including mixed agonist-antagonist medications (naloxone, nalbuphine)
         (4) Attentive skin care
    h. Disturbed bladder and bowel function: due to medications, obstruction, spinal cord compromise
       i. Treatment: of constipation
         (1) Stool softeners (docusate sodium) plus gentle laxative (senna)
            (a) Lactulose often beneficial
            (b) Maintain personal dignity as much as possible
       ii. Treatment: of urinary retention
         (1) Rule out spinal cord compromise
         (2) Evaluate for infection
         (3) If due to opioids, try switching drugs (do NOT use naloxone)
         (4) If cause not reversible, catheterize

3. PSYCHOLOGICAL DISTRESS

a. Needs
   i. Dynamic
   ii. Specific fears: abandonment, dependence, pain, secretions, odor
   iii. Preferences: information/choices, comfort, control, dignity
b. "Healthy" death
   i. Presence of significant others
   ii. Physical expressions of caring
   iii. Desire for the truth
   iv. Control in decision making
   v. Discussion of practical issues
   vi. Opportunity to review the past
   vii. Personal appearance
c. Family issues
   i. Possible "burnout"
   ii. Important time in family history
   iii. Families may want desperately to help
   iv. Hospice and home health care
d. Chronic stress (including pain): Suffering escalates with unrelieved stress.
e. Psychological symptoms: Unrelieved pain can produce psychiatric symptoms that will disappear when pain control is achieved (**Table 130-4**).
f. Changes in cognitive function
   i. Disorientation
   ii. Hallucinations
   iii. Sleep disturbance
   iv. Agitation
g. Depression: Unrecognized and untreated depression will cause (reversible) cognitive dysfunction.
h. Terminal agitation: a source of psychological distress to patients and caregivers. Very high percentage of people (~50%) are agitated 24 to 48 hours prior to death.

TABLE 130–4 Psychological Symptoms Associated with Chronic Disease and Dying

Normal
Anxiety
Sadness
Abnormal
Depression
Panic disorder
Dementia

     i. Butyrophenones (haloperidol)
     ii. Benzodiazepines (including subcutaneous midazolam infusions)
     iii. Barbiturates: secobarbital, pentobarbital (start 1 to 2 mg/kg every 1 to 2 hours, titrate to effect)
     iv. Propofol
     v. Ketamine: low dose (0.5 to 1.0 mg/kg every 8 to 12 hours)
  i. Palliative methods of last resort
     i. Voluntary cessation of eating and drinking
     ii. Physician-assisted suicide
     iii. Voluntary active euthanasia
     iv. Terminal sedation
     v. Doctrine of double effect: Intervening on the patient's behalf may incur risks, including the possibility of hastening death.

1. BACKGROUND

a. Pain in children
  i. Frequently not recognized
    (1) Inability of children to accurately describe location and severity of pain
    (2) Health care workers lack knowledge of pain assessment in children
    (3) Mistaken belief that young children cannot experience pain because of immature peripheral and central nervous system
  ii. Ineffectively managed
    (1) Mistaken belief that even if young children feel pain, it is of no consequence because they will have no memory of the pain
      (a) Lack of knowledge about pathophysiology of pediatric pain
    (2) Mistaken belief that pain is an inevitable, expected consequence of illness, trauma, and surgery
    (3) Mistaken belief that pain is less harmful than risks of analgesic therapy in children
      (a) Lack of knowledge of analgesic pharmacology in children
      (b) Lack of knowledge of treatment options
        (i) Inability to appreciate the large variability in pain experienced by different patients with similar types of pain
        (ii) Health care provider and parental fear of side effects of analgesic therapy (sedation, respiratory depression, ileus, addiction, etc.)
        (iii) Inflexible prescribing with inappropriately low and infrequent dosing of analgesics on an as needed (PRN) basis
        (iv) Lack of approved labeling of potent analgesics for children: Pharmaceutical companies have been unwilling to fund pediatric studies because of small market size.
b. Facts
  i. Children, even extremely premature newborns, experience pain.
  ii. Children may suffer long-term consequences if the pain is not adequately treated, even if they have no memory of the pain.
  iii. Effective tools are available to assess pain in children of every developmental stage and age.
  iv. A large variety of analgesic therapies can be provided safely to children.

2. DEVELOPMENT OF NOCICEPTION

a. 7th week of gestation
   i. Cutaneous sensation begins in perioral region.
      (1) 15th gestational week: Cutaneous sensation spreads to extremities.
      (2) 20th gestational week: Sensory perception is present in all cutaneous and mucosal surfaces.
b. 8th week of gestation
   i. Cerebral cortex begins to develop.
      (1) Contains 10 billion neurons by the 20th week of gestation
c. 10th week of gestation
   i. Substance P appears in fetal nerve tissue.
d. 22nd week of gestation
   i. Endogenous opioids appear.
   ii. Synapses begin to form between peripheral neurons and dorsal horn neurons.
   iii. Myelination of nerve tracts in the spinal cord and brainstem begins.
      (1) Myelination of peripheral neurons is not complete until after birth.
         (a) C-fibers remain unmyelinated and A-δ fibers are thinly myelinated in adults.
   iv. Fetal electroencephalogram (EEG) patterns appear intermittent and unsynchronized.
      (1) By the 27th week of gestation, fetal EEG signals are synchronized in both hemispheres.
e. 30th week of gestation
   i. Cortical evoked potentials can be elicited and measured.
f. Beginning of third trimester
   i. All elements necessary to transmit and process noxious stimulation are present.
g. Neonates may experience more pain in response to a given noxious stimulus.
   i. Descending inhibitory pathway only component of nociceptive system lacking at birth
      (1) Develops during first 6 months of life
      (2) Neonate incapable of attenuating nociceptive signals
   ii. Dorsal horn neurons have wider receptive fields and lower excitatory thresholds.
   iii. Excitatory thresholds of dorsal horn neurons are further lowered by repetitive noxious stimulation (i.e., heel lancing).

3. RESPONSE TO NOCICEPTIVE STIMULATION

a. The experience of pain includes the perception of a noxious event via a functioning nociceptive system and a response to that

stimulation, including motor, autonomic, metabolic, behavioral, and emotional responses
  i. Neonatal stress and behavioral responses to surgery, diagnostic procedures, and therapeutic procedures well documented
    (1) Associated with increased morbidity and, in some instances, increased mortality
    (2) These responses and associated negative outcomes can be reduced by using regional anesthesia, opioids, or general anesthesia prior to painful procedures in neonates.
  b. Mounting evidence for a complex, integrated cortical response to nociceptive stimulation in neonates
    i. Neonates subjected to circumcision, repeated heel lancing, phlebotomy, and surgery
      (1) Demonstrate abnormalities in short-term behavior
        (a) Increased crying
        (b) Disrupted sleep
        (c) Feeding abnormalities
    ii. Noxious events in early infancy may affect future responses to painful events.
      (1) Future noxious events may be associated with enhanced or blunted behavioral and/or physiologic responses.
        (a) Male infants circumcised at birth without analgesia have exaggerated pain behaviors in response to vaccination between 4 and 6 months of age when compared with infants who were not circumcised or who were circumcised with topical anesthesia (EMLA).
  c. Because the stress response and short- and long-term behavioral changes can be reduced by the judicious use of analgesics, pain should be anticipated and treated appropriately in all pediatric patients, including extremely premature neonates.

4. PAIN ASSESSMENT IN CHILDREN

  a. Joint Commission on Accreditation of Healthcare Organizations (JCAHO) mandates all patients have basic right to pain assessment and management.
    i. Pain is 5th vital sign
  b. Proper and accurate pain assessment in children is essential for its successful management.
    i. Pediatric pain assessment is sometimes approximate.
      (1) Indicating that pain is either absent or possibly, probably, or definitely present
  c. Challenges of pain assessment in children
    i. Developmental stage influences perception and expression of pediatric pain.
      (1) Need to know a variety of pain assessment tools appropriate for each developmental stage

    ii. Preverbal children

   iii. Children with cognitive and/or neurologic impairment

   iv. Children may deny pain for a variety of reasons, including:

      (1) Belief that pain is a form of punishment for being bad

        (a) Admitting one is in pain is an admission of guilt

      (2) Fear that they may be separated from parents

      (3) Fear of an even more painful treatment (an injection)

      (4) Being taught not to trust or talk to strangers

        (a) Will not talk to doctors or nurses

      (5) Belief that doctors and nurses will intuitively know that they are in pain

  d. Pain assessment tools exist for children of all developmental stages.

    i. The ideal tool is practical and easy to use.

      (1) Unfortunately, many pediatric pain assessment tools are cumbersome and difficult to apply.

        (a) Especially in preverbal children and children who are cognitively impaired

    ii. Pain assessment is most accurate when the child can describe the location, nature, and severity of pain.

      (1) With appropriate words and tools, most children older than 3 years can reliably communicate their pain.

   iii. Behavioral clues (i.e., crying, restlessness, withdrawal, splinting, grimacing, increased tone) and physiologic signs (i.e., hypertension, tachycardia, sweating) are relied on in children who are younger than 3 years or are cognitively impaired.

TABLE 131–1 CRIES, Neonatal Postoperative Pain Assessment Tool

Indicator	Scoring		
	0	**1**	**2**
Crying	No	High pitched/ consolable	Inconsolable
Requires O_2 for saturation >95%	No	<30%	>30%
Increased vital signs	HR and BP = or < pre-op	HR or BP increased <20%	HR or BP increased >20%
Expression	None	Grimace	Grimace/grunt
Sleepless	No	Wakes at frequent intervals	Constantly awake

(1) Many of these signs are also associated with conditions other than pain.
    (a) Parental separation, hunger, wet diaper, fear, anxiety, hypovolemia, hypoxemia, etc.
    (b) Misinterpretation common
    (c) Parents are often helpful in differentiating pain from other conditions that may be causing distress.

iv. Useful tools
    (1) Neonate/infant pain scale: CRIES (**Table 131-1**)
    (2) Preverbal/nonverbal infant/toddler: FLACC (**Table 131-2**)
    (3) 3 to 7 year old: Wong Baker Faces Scale (**Fig. 131-1**)
    (4) 8 years and older: visual analog scale (VAS) pain score or numeric pain score

TABLE 131–2 FLACC, Behavioral Pain Assessment Scale12

Categories	Scoring		
	0	**1**	**2**
Face	No particular expression or smile	Occasional grimace or frown; withdrawn, disinterested	Frequent to constant frown, clenched jaw, quivering chin
Legs	Normal position or relaxed	Uneasy, restless, tense	Kicking or legs drawn up
Activity	Lying quietly, normal position, moves easily	Squirming, shifting back and forth, tense	Arched, rigid, or jerking
Cry	No cry (awake or asleep)	Moans or whimpers, occasional complaint	Crying steadily, screams or sobs; frequent complaints
Consolability	Content, relaxed	Reassured by occasional touching, hugging or being talked to; distractible	Difficult to console or comfort

Each of the five categories is scored from 0 to 2, resulting in a total score between 0 and 10.

WONG-BAKER FACES PAIN RATING SCALE

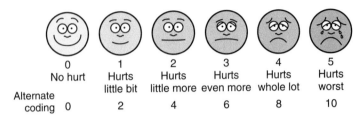

	0 No hurt	1 Hurts little bit	2 Hurts little more	3 Hurts even more	4 Hurts whole lot	5 Hurts worst
Alternate coding	0	2	4	6	8	10

Brief word instructions: Point to each face using the words to describe the pain intensity. Ask the child to choose face that best describes own pain and record the appropriate number.

Original instructions: Explain to the person that each face is for a person who feels happy because he has no pain (hurt) or sad because he has some or a lot of pain. Face 0 is very happy because he doesn't hurt at all. **Face 1** hurts just a little bit. **Face 2** hurts a little more. **Face 3** hurts even more. **Face 4** hurts a whole lot. **Face 5** hurts as much as you can imagine, although you don't have to be crying to feel this bad. Ask the person to choose the face that best describes how he is feeling.

Rating scale is recommended for persons age 3 years and older.

Figure 131–1 Wong-Baker faces pain rating scale 14. From Hockenberry MJ, Wilson D, Winkelstein ML: Wong's Essentials of Pediatric Nursing, 7th ed. St. Louis: Mosby, 2005, p 1259. Used with permission. Copyright Mosby.

SUGGESTED READINGS

Anand KJS, Hansen DD, Hickey PR: Hormonal–metabolic stress responses in neonates undergoing cardiac surgery. Anesthesiology 1990;73:661–670.

Anand KJS, Hickey PR: Halothane–morphine compared with high-dose sufentanil for anesthesia and postoperative analgesia in neonatal cardiac surgery. N Engl J Med 1992;326: 1–9.

Anand KJS, Hickey PR: Pain and its effects in the human neonate and fetus. N Engl J Med 1987;317:1321–1329.

Anand KJS, Maze M: Fetuses, fentanyl, and the stress response: Signals from the beginnings of pain? Anesthesiology 2001;95:823–825.

Anand KJS, Sippell WG, Aynsley-Green A: Randomised trial of fentanyl anaesthesia in preterm babies undergoing surgery: Effects on the stress response. Lancet 1987;8524:62–66.

Beyer JE, McGrath PJ, Berde CB: Discordance between self-report and behavioral pain measures in children aged 3–7 years after surgery. J Pain Sympt Manag 1990;5:350–356.

Breau LM, Finley GA, McGrath PJ, Camfield CS: Validation of the non-communicating children's pain checklist: Postoperative version. Anesthesiology 2002;96:528–35.

Kain ZN, Cicchetti DV, McClain BC: Measurement of pain in children: State of the art considerations. Anesthesiology 2002;96:523–526.

Krechel SW, Bildner J: CRIES: A new neonatal postoperative pain measurement score. Initial testing of validity and reliability. Paediatr Anaesth 1995;5:53–61.

Lidow MS: Long-term effects of neonatal pain on nociceptive systems. Pain 2002;99:377–383.

Merkel S, Voepel-Lewis T, Malviya S: Pain assessment in infants and young children: The FLACC Scale: A behavioral tool to measure pain in young children. AJN 2002;102:55–58.

Sturla Franck L, Miaskowski C: Measurement of neonatal responses to painful stimuli: A research review. J Pain Sympt Manag 1997;14(6):343–378.

Tyler DC, Tu A, Douthit J, Chapman CR: Toward validation of pain measurement tools for children: A pilot study. Pain 1993;52:301–309.

Whaley L, Wong D: Nursing Care of Infants and Children, 5th ed. St. Louis, Mosby, 2001, p 1301.

1. BACKGROUND

a. Most analgesics are lipophilic, requiring transformation into water-soluble substances.

b. There are significant pharmacokinetic differences in children that influence the dosage and intervals of analgesic administration.

c. There is a lack of formal pediatric drug studies, but there is significant experience using analgesic medications in children based on pediatric pharmacologic and physiologic principles.

d. Significant developmental changes in:
   i. Composition of body compartments
   ii. Plasma protein-binding capacity
   iii. Hepatic enzyme systems
   iv. Renal function

2. DEVELOPMENTAL PHARMACOLOGY

a. Body composition in neonates
   i. Larger body water content in neonates and infants results in larger volume of distribution for water-soluble drugs.
   ii. Increased volume of distribution for water-soluble drugs in neonates results in an increased duration of action and the need to increase the dosing interval for some drugs.
   iii. Smaller fat and muscle stores in neonates results in higher plasma concentrations of drugs because there is less uptake of drug in these sites.
   iv. Greater proportion of cardiac output goes to the neonatal brain, resulting in more rapid delivery of drug to active sites.
   v. Possible immature blood-brain barrier at birth facilitates entry of drugs into brain tissue.

b. Reduced protein binding in neonates
   i. Decreased quantities of albumin and α_1-acid glycoprotein
   ii. Qualitatively different albumin that binds proteins less effectively
   iii. Opioids and local anesthetics are heavily bound to α_1-acid glycoprotein. Therefore, neonates may have increased unbound concentrations of these drugs and more potential for toxicity.
   iv. Inflammatory bowel disease, malignancy, infection, and trauma increase α_1-acid glycoprotein levels, thus decreasing the unbound free fraction of protein-bound drugs.

c. Metabolism
   i. Hepatic enzyme systems responsible for phase I reactions (oxidation, reduction, hydroxylation, hydrolysis) and phase II

reactions (conjugation processes) are immature in the neonate, resulting in reduced clearance of drugs.

ii. The hepatic enzymes develop rapidly and approach adult levels in first few months of life.

iii. The cytochrome P-450 system is a crucial phase I enzyme family and is involved in the metabolism of analgesics, such as nonsteroidal anti-inflammatory drugs (NSAIDs) and opioids.

iv. Relatively large liver size in children 2 to 6 years of age relative to body weight

   (1) Metabolic capacity of liver in 2- to 6-year-old children exceeds that of adult, then decreases to adult levels by puberty.

   (2) This increased metabolic capacity in the 2- to 6-year age group necessitates increased dose of drug, with shorter intervals and higher infusion rates.

v. Increased intra-abdominal pressure (e.g., gastroschisis, omphalocele) decreases hepatic perfusion causing decreased hepatic metabolism of drugs.

d. Renal function

i. Neonates have decreased renal blood flow, glomerular filtration rate (GFR), and tubular secretory function, resulting in decreased renal secretion of drugs in neonates, especially premature neonates.

   (1) Decreased GFR in neonates results in parent drug or active metabolite accumulation; e.g., morphine metabolized to morphine-6-glucuronide (110 times more potent than morphine), which accumulates with decreased GFR.

   (2) Renal function reaches adult levels by age 1 year.

3. NSAIDS

a. NSAIDS are used for mild to moderate pain, alone or in combination with opioids (**Table 132-1**).

b. NSAIDS inhibit cyclooxygenase (COX), which is the enzyme responsible for metabolizing arachidonic acid.

i. Arachidonic acid is released from traumatized cell membranes, sensitizing peripheral nerve endings, and vasodilating vessels causing pain, erythema, and inflammation.

ii. COX-1 isoenzymes are called the constitutive form.

   (1) They are present throughout the body.

   (2) The prostaglandins and thromboxanes they produce are essential for gastric mucosa protection, renal blood flow regulation, and platelet aggregation.

iii. Potential complications of COX-1 inhibition include gastric ulceration, bleeding, altered renal function, and bronchoconstriction.

TABLE 132–1 Example Dosing of NSAIDS

Drug	Dose	Interval	Maximum Daily Dose
Aspirin	PO: 10–15 mg/kg	4–6 hr	90 mg/kg/day
Acetaminophen	PO: 10–15 mg/kg	PO: 4–6 hr	Children: lesser of 100 mg/kg/day or 4 g Infants: 75 mg/kg/day
	Rectal single dose: 35–45 mg/kg	Rectal: 6 hr	
	Rectal repeated doses: 20 mg/kg	Rectal premature newborns: 12 hr	
			Newborns: (>32 wks PCA): 60 mg/kg/day (28–32 PCA): 40 mg/kg/day
Ibuprofen	6–10 mg/kg	4–6 hr	Lesser of 40 mg/kg/day or 2.4 g
Naproxen	PO: 5–10 mg/kg	12 hr	20 mg/kg/day
Ketorolac	IV: 0.5 mg/kg	6 hr	Lesser of 2 mg/kg/day or 120 mg Maximum 20 doses or 5 days

 iv. COX-2 isoenzymes are the inducible form.
  (1) They are present only in traumatized cells or inflamed tissue.
  (2) Potential advantage of using COX-2 inhibitors is a decrease in the above-mentioned side effects of COX-1 inhibitors.
 v. Rofecoxib is a COX-2 inhibitor studied in children, but the future of COX-2-selective drugs is uncertain because of current controversy of increased cardiovascular morbidity in adults.
 c. Ibuprofen and naproxen are the most common peripheral COX inhibitors used in children.
 d. Ketorolac is the only parenteral NSAID available in the United States.
  i. It should not be used for longer than 5 days.
 e. Acetylsalicylic acid (aspirin) is used rarely in children because of its association with Reye syndrome. The main indication in children is for selected rheumatologic conditions.

   f. Acetaminophen is the most commonly used NSAID. It is a central COX inhibitor rather than a peripheral COX inhibitor, so it does not have the bleeding complications of peripheral COX inhibitors.

      i. Acetaminophen is used as an analgesic and antipyretic.

      ii. May be given orally or rectally. Higher rectal doses are required initially to obtain adequate blood levels.

      iii. Careful dosing is essential because overdose can lead to hepatic necrosis and fulminant hepatic failure.

4. OPIOIDS

   a. Opioids are used for moderate to severe pain (**Table 132-2**).

   b. Opioids bind to pre- and postsynaptic cell membranes in the central nervous system, resulting in neuronal inhibition.

   c. Morphine is the standard with which all opioids are compared.

      i. Morphine can be administered IV, PO, PR, IM, SQ, or by inhalation.

      ii. Morphine can be scheduled by interval dosing, continuous infusion, or with a patient-controlled analgesia system (**Table 132-3**).

   d. Hydromorphone is a common second-choice opioid analgesic because it may cause less nausea and pruritus than morphine.

   e. Fentanyl is 100 times more potent than morphine and has a short duration of action.

      i. In addition to IV, fentanyl is also available as a candy matrix for procedural sedation and analgesia.

      ii. Fentanyl patches are used for chronic opioid therapy, but these patches are not intended for opioid-naïve children.

   f. Methadone has a long elimination half-life and duration of action.

      i. Used for more chronic opioid therapy.

      ii. Has N-methyl-D-aspartate (NMDA) antagonist activity, so the conversion from morphine to methadone is 1:0.1 rather than 1:1.

   g. Meperidine is no longer recommended for long-term opioid therapy because of metabolite accumulation and the potential for seizures.

   h. Codeine is a common oral opioid, frequently combined with acetaminophen.

      i. It is a weak opioid, one-tenth as potent as morphine.

      ii. Four percent to 10% of population lacks the enzyme CYP2D6, which converts codeine to morphine (via O-demethylation) resulting in lack of analgesia from codeine.

      iii. This, combined with the high incidence of nausea, has led to a decrease in the use of codeine as a first-line oral opioid.

   i. Oxycodone and hydrocodone are oral opioids often combined with acetaminophen in tablet or liquid form.

      i. Liquid oxycodone may be difficult to obtain at local pharmacies. Must be absolutely clear on concentration of liquid oxycodone being used (1 mg/mL vs. 20 mg/mL).

TABLE 132–2 Example Dosing of Opioids

Opioid	Route/Age Group	Dose/Interval
Morphine	Oral: infants and children	10–25 µg/kg every 2–4 hr
	IV bolus:	25–50 µg/kg every 3–4 hr
	Preterm neonate	50–100 µg/kg every 3 hr
	Fullterm neonate	
	Infants and children	
	IV infusion:	2–5 µg/kg/hr
	Preterm neonate	5–10 µg/kg/hr
	Fullterm neonate	15–30 µg/kg/hr 3 mg/kg
	Infants and children	every 3–4 hr
Hydromorphone	Oral: infants and children	40–80 µg/kg every 4 hr
	IV bolus: infants and children	10–20 µg/kg every 3–4 hr
	IV infusion: infants and children	3–5 µg/kg/hr
Fentanyl	IV bolus	0.5–1 µg/kg every 1–2 hr
	IV infusion	0.5 µg/kg/hr
	Nasal	1–2 µg/kg
	Oral transmucosal	10–15 µg/kg (oralet)
	Transdermal	12.5, 25, 50, 75, 100 µg/hr patches
Meperidine	IV bolus: infants and children	0.8–1 mg/kg every 3–4 hr
Methadone	Oral or IV bolus: infants and children	0.1–0.2 mg/kg every 12–36 hr
Nalbuphine	IV bolus:	10–25 µg/kg every 2–4 hr
	Preterm neonate	25–50 µg/kg every 2–4 hr
	Fullterm neonate	50–100 µg/kg every 2–4hr
	Infants and children	
	IV infusion:	5–10 µg/kg/hr
	Preterm neonate	10–15 µg/kg/hr
	Fullterm neonate	20 µg/kg/hr
	Infants and children	
Codeine	Oral	0.5–1 mg/kg every 4 hr
Oxycodone	Oral	0.1–0.15 mg/kg every 4 hr

TABLE 132–3 Example PCA Dosing Guidelines

Drug	Demand Dose (µg/kg)	Lockout Interval (min)	Basal Infusion (µg/kg/hr)	1 hr Limit (µg/kg)	PRN IV Rescue Dose (mcg/kg)
Morphine	20	8–10	0–20	100	50
Hydromorphone	4	8–10	0-4	20	10

    j. Nalbuphine is an opioid agonist-antagonist useful in providing analgesia with fewer respiratory and gastrointestinal (GI) depressant effects of the pure mu-agonist opioids.
       i. It is also an effective antipruritic.
      ii. Nalbuphine does have an analgesic ceiling-effect, unlike the mu-agonist opioids.
     iii. Use caution when using nalbuphine with opioid-dependent children because it may cause withdrawal.
    k. Tramadol is an atypical opioid 10 to 15 times less potent than morphine.
       i. Fewer opioid-related side effects
      ii. Also available in combination with acetaminophen
     iii. To be avoided in patients with seizures or head trauma

5. LOCAL ANESTHETICS

    a. Local anesthetics reversibly block impulse conduction along nerve fibers by interfering with sodium channels.
    b. Local anesthetics may be administered in the intrathecal or epidural space, around peripheral nerves, or applied topically in creams or ophthalmic drops (**Table 132-4**).

TABLE 132–4 Local Anesthetic Maximum Doses

Local Anesthetic	Spinal (mg/kg)	Epidural (mg/kg)	Peripheral (mg/kg)
Lidocaine	NR	5–7*	5–7*
Bupivacaine	0.5	2.5	2.5
Ropivacaine	NR	2.5–3	2.5–3
Tetracaine	1	NR	NR

NR: not recommended
*Higher dose only with epinephrine 1:200,000.

TABLE 132–5 Local Anesthetic Epidural Infusion Maximum Doses

Age	Bupivacaine or Ropivacaine Concentration (mg/mL)	Rate (mg/kg/hr)
Neonate	0.5–1	0.15–0.25
Infant	0.5–1.25	0.15–0.3
Child	0.5–1.25	0.2–0.4

   c. Must observe dosage guidelines for local anesthetics to avoid toxicity

   d. Bupivacaine is the most commonly used local anesthetic for epidural or peripheral nerve blocks in children, although the newer agent, ropivacaine, is being used more frequently (**Table 132-5**).

      i. Because of the high protein binding of bupivacaine, the dosage of this drug must be reduced in neonates and infants.

      ii. Ropivacaine is a newer amide local anesthetic with a similar profile as bupivacaine but potentially less risk for cardiovascular toxicity.

   e. Topical anesthetics provide analgesia for painful procedures (IV placement, LP, laceration suturing, etc.).

      i. EMLA cream (eutectic mixture of local anesthetics)

         (1) Combination of lidocaine and prilocaine

         (2) Intended for intact skin

         (3) Onset time is about 60 minutes

      ii. LMX4 (liposomal 4% cream)

         (1) Newer topical agent with an onset time of about 30 minutes

      iii. LET (lidocaine, epinephrine, tetracaine)

         (1) Topical gel for open wounds such as lacerations

         (2) Onset time is 20 to 30 minutes

      iv. Lidocaine iontophoresis; onset time 20 minutes

      v. Lidocaine powder by pressurized helium: onset time 1 to 3 minutes

6. OTHER ANALGESICS

   a. Ketamine

      i. A phencyclidine derivative and a dissociative anesthetic

      ii. Potent analgesic in subanesthetic doses (0.25 to 0.5 mg/kg IV)

      iii. Used for short, painful procedures

      iv. Tendency to cause dysphoria and increased secretions

         (1) Consider using an anticholinergic to decrease secretions

    (2) Consider using a benzodiazepine to prevent dysphoric effects
- v. Increasing literature on the use of ketamine perioperatively as an adjunct to opioid analgesia
- vi. Ketamine not recommended in children with decreased intracranial compliance

b. Clonidine
  - i. An α_2-adrenergic agonist useful as an analgesic and anxiolytic
  - ii. Also used to control opioid and benzodiazepine withdrawal symptoms
  - iii. May be given orally, as transdermal patches, or as an adjunct to epidural and peripheral nerve block local anesthetics
  - iv. Dexmedetomidine is a centrally acting α_2 agonist
    - (1) Used primarily as a sedative in intensive care unit settings; it does appear to have opioid-sparing properties

7. ANTISPASMODICS

a. Muscle spasticity is a significant cause of pain in children with significant neurologic impairment (e.g., cerebral palsy).
b. Diazepam is a common agent used alone or as an adjunct to systemic or regional analgesics (0.1 to 0.3 mg/kg orally or rectally every 6 hours).
c. Baclofen is a GABA agonist given orally or administered intrathecally via implantable pumps.
d. Botulinum toxin injected intramuscularly provides up to 3 months of spasm relief.

SUGGESTED READINGS

Andersson BJ, Holford NH, Wollard GA: Perioperative pharmacodynamics of acetaminophen analgesia in children. Anesthesiology 1999;90(2): 411–421.

Berde CB, Sethna NF: Analgesics for the treatment of pain in children. N Engl J Med 2002;347:1094–1103.

Berde CB, Solodiuk J: Multidisciplinary programs for management of acute and chronic pain in children. In Schechter NL, Berde CB, Yaster M (eds): Pain in Infants, Children, and Adolescents, 2nd ed. Baltimore, Lippincott Williams & Wilkins, 2001, pp 471–486.

Birmingham PK, Tobin MJ, Henthorn TK: Twenty-four hour pharmacokinetics of rectal acetaminophen in children: An old drug with new recommendations. Anesthesiology 1997;87:244–252.

Blanco JG, Harrison PL, Evans WE, Relling MV: Human cytochrome P450 maximal activities in pediatric versus adult liver. Drug Metab Dispos 2000; 28:379–382.

Bouwmeester NJ, Anderson BJ, Tibboel D, Holford NH: Developmental pharmacokinetics of morphine and its metabolites in neonates, infants, and young children. Br J Anaesth 2004;92(2):208–217.

Collins JJ, Dunkel IJ, Gupta SK: Transdermal Fentanyl in children with cancer pain: Feasibility, tolerability, and pharmacokinetic correlates. J Pediatr 1999;134: 319–323.

Finkel JC, Rose JB, Schmitz ML: An evaluation of the efficacy and tolerability of oral tramadol hydrochloride tablets for the treatment of post-surgical pain in children. Anesth Analg 2002;94:1469–1473.

Galinken JL, Fazi LM, Cuy RM, et al: Use of intranasal fentanyl in children undergoing myringotomy and tube placement during halothane and sevoflurane anesthesia Anesthesiology 2000;93(6):1378–1383.

Hall JE, Uhrich TD, Barney JA, et al: Sedative, amnestic, and analgesic properties of small-dose dexmedetomidine infusions. Anesth Analg 2000;90:699–705.

Himmelscher S, Durieux ME: Ketamine for perioperative pain management. Anesthesiology 2005;102(1):211–220.

Kart T, Christup LL, Rasmussen M: Recommended use of morphine in neonates, infants, and children based on a literature review: Part 1 pharmacokinetics. Paediatr Anaesth 1997;7:5–11.

Kart T, Christup LL, Rasmussen M: Recommended use of morphine in neonates, infants, and children based on a literature review: Part 2 Clinical use. Paediatr Anaesth 1997;7:93–101.

Maunuksela EL, Olkhola KT: Nonsteroidal anti-inflammatory drugs in pediatric pain management. In Schechter NL, Berde CB, Yaster M (eds): Pain in Infants, Children, and Adolescents, 2nd ed. Baltimore, Lippincott Williams & Wilkins, 2003, pp 171–180.

Murat I, Gall O, Tourniaire B: Procedural pain in children: Evidence-based best practice and guidelines. Reg Anesth Pain Med 2003;28(6):561–672.

Nishina K, Mikawa K, Shiga M, Ohara H: Clonidine in paediatric anaesthesia. Paediatr Anaesth 1999;9:187–202.

Quigley C, Wiffen P: A systematic review of hydromorphone in acute and chronic pain. J Pain Sympt Manage 2003;25(2):169–178.

Ripamonti C, Groff L, Brunelli C, et al: Switching from morphine to oral methadone in treating cancer pain: What is the equianalgesic dose ratio? J Clin Oncol 1998;16:3216–3221.

Rose JB: Pediatric analgesic pharmacology. In Litman RS (ed), Hines RL (series ed): Pediatric Anesthesiology: The Requisites in Anesthesiology. St. Louis, Mosby, 2004, pp 196–205.

Rose JB: Local anesthetics and adjuvant analgesics. In Litman RS (ed), Hines RL (series ed): Pediatric Anesthesia: The Requisites in Anesthesiology. St. Louis, MO, Mosby, 2004, pp 206–211.

Schechter NL, Weisman SJ, Rosenblum M, et al: The use of oral transmucosal fentanyl citrate for painful procedures in children Pediatrics 1995;95:335–339.

Sheenan PN, Rose JB, Fazi LM, et al: Rofecoxib administration to paediatric patients undergoing adenotonsillectomy. Paediatr Anaesth 2004;14(7):579–583.

Singleton MA, Rosen JI, Fisher DM: Plasma concentrations of fentanyl in infants, children, and adolescents. Can J Anaesth 1987;34:152–155.

Williams DG, Hatch DJ, Howard RF: Codeine phosphate in paediatric medicine. Br J Anaesth 2001;86:413–421.

Yaster M: Clinical pharmacology. In Schechter NL, Berde CB, Yaster M (eds): Pain in Infants, Children, and Adolescents, 2nd ed. Baltimore, Lippincott Williams & Wilkins, 2001, pp 71–84.

Yaster M, Kost-Beyerly S, Maxwell LG: Opioid agonists and antagonists. In Schechter NL, Berde CB, Yaster M (eds) Pain in Infants, Children, and Adolescents, 2nd ed. Baltimore, Lippincott Williams & Wilkins, 2003, pp 181–224.

Yaster M, Tobin JR, Kost-Beyerly S: Local anesthetics. In Schechter NL, Berde CB, Yaster M (eds): Pain in Infants, Children, and Adolescents, 2nd ed. Baltimore, Lippincott Williams & Wilkins, 2001, pp 241–264.

Zempky WT, Cravero JP: Relief of pain and anxiety in pediatric patients in emergency medical systems. AAP Committee on Pediatric Emergency Medicine and Section on Anesthesiology and Pain Medicine. Pediatrics 2004; 114:1348–1356.

133 Epidemiology of Geriatric Pain

1. ELDERLY POPULATION IS AMONG THE FASTEST GROWING SEGMENT OF THE WORLD'S POPULATION

a. In 1998, US census shows more than 35 million people are at least 65 years old.
b. In the United States, they comprise 13% of the population.
c. Thirty percent of all prescription drugs are consumed by the elderly.
d. Fifty percent of over-the-counter medications are consumed by the elderly.

2. INCIDENCE OF CHRONIC PAIN

a. Twenty-five percent to 50% of community-dwelling elderly
b. Forty-five percent to 80% of nursing home residents
c. Prevalence is higher in those younger than 60 years old compared with those older than 60 years old.
   i. The latter group tends to be more stoic and underreport their symptoms.

3. MUSCULOSKELETAL PAIN

a. The most common complaint in patients taking analgesics
b. Arthritis: 43%
c. Other bone-and-joint pain: 31%
d. Low-back pain: 16%

4. PAIN NEGATIVELY IMPACTS ACTIVITIES OF DAILY LIVING AND AFFECTS QUALITY OF LIFE

a. Decreases degree of independence.
b. Interferes with ability to read, watch television, use the telephone.
c. Impairs cognition.
d. Chronic pain is associated with depression.
e. May impair mobility.

1. GENERAL

a. Involves the progressive decline in function of multiple organ systems, resulting in decreased reserve to compensate for the stress of surgery, anesthesia, and pain

b. Systems most relevant in the role of pain management in elderly
   i. Central nervous system
      (1) Decline in function begins as early as 50 years of age.
      (2) Mechanism is unclear, but hereditary, comorbidities, and physical and mental daily activities play important roles.
      (3) Frontal and temporal lobes are the first affected anatomic regions in the central nervous system (CNS).
      (4) Decrease in number of neurons, loss of dendritic synapses, cell receptors, intracellular enzymes
      (5) Decrease in sympathetic and parasympathetic ganglia function results in blunted cardiovascular reflexes.
      (6) Decline in serotonin system can lead to depression.
      (7) Decline in dopamine neurotransmitter often manifests as senile gait, posture, and tremor.
   ii. Hepatic system
      (1) Liver mass decreases 1% per year; therefore, clearance of drugs is prolonged.
         (a) Decrease in first pass through the liver and hepatic extraction of certain drugs
         (b) An estimated 33% decrease in hepatic perfusion with aging
      (2) Liver function tests (LFTs), conjugation, microsomal hydroxylation, and oxidation remain relatively unchanged.
      (3) Demethylation and protein synthesis decrease.
      (4) Liver regeneration decreases but the capacity to regenerate remains.
   iii. Renal system
      (1) Renal function decreases 1% per year after age 40 years.
      (2) Kidney size decreases 20% to 30%.
      (3) Glomeruli number is halved by age 70 years.
      (4) Renal blood flow drops 10% per decade after age 20 years.
      (5) Glomerular filtration rate drops 10 mL/min per decade.
      (6) Concentration ability drops 5% per decade after age 50 years.

1. POSTOPERATIVE PAIN

a. Management continues to be inadequate.
b. Elderly are more vulnerable to adverse effects of nonsteroidal anti-inflammatory drugs (NSAIDs) and opioids.
   i. Need to reduce drug dose by 25% to 50%.
c. Preemptive analgesia can be very effective.
d. Regional for postoperative pain
   i. Benefits
      (1) Maintenance of consciousness throughout surgery, therefore decreasing postoperative confusion
      (2) Provision of postoperative analgesia
      (3) Decrease in surgical stress response
      (4) Decrease in intraoperative blood loss with either spinal or epidural
      (5) Decrease in postoperative thromboembolic complications
      (6) Avoid manipulation of airway in patients with respiratory complications
      (7) Functioning epidural allows for quicker return of pulmonary status

2. ACUTE PAIN

a. Pain from a specific, brief pathologic insult (tissue damage or infectious process)
b. May be somatic or visceral
c. In the elderly, likely to be referred from site of origin in an atypical manner manifesting as behavioral symptoms.
   i. Confusion, restlessness, aggression, anorexia, fatigue
d. Likely to be less intense when reported compared with the young.
e. Prevalence decreases with age.
f. Therapy often involves NSAIDs, opioids, or treatment of the underlying disease process contributing to the pain (intra-abdominal infections, duodenal ulcers).

3. CHRONIC PAIN

a. Pain persisting beyond the usual course of an acute disease or after a reasonable time for healing to occur
b. Considerable overlap in patients with pain syndromes and cancer pain
c. Psychological mechanisms or environmental factors often playing a role
d. Often requires medications to be given on a regular schedule

e. Fifty percent compliance with therapy
    i. Inversely related to the number of medications taken
    ii. Other factors are cost, insurance coverage, physician-patient communication.
f. Neuropathic
    i. Lancinating, stabbing, burning with allodynia, hyperalgesia
    ii. Affected nerves are activated by inflammatory mechanism.
    iii. Nerve terminals proliferate in response to injury, increasing chemical and mechanical sensitivity to prostaglandins, cytokines, and catecholamines.
g. Nociceptive
    i. Aching, sharp, burning in quality
    ii. Can also be visceral that is poorly localized and crampy
h. Therapy
    i. Tricyclic antidepressants
        (1) Increase endogenous descending inhibitory pathways involving serotonin and norepinephrine
        (2) Side effects related to anticholinergic, antihistamine, and adrenergic activity (constipation, dry mouth, urinary retention, and electrocardiogram changes)
    ii. Anticonvulsants
        (1) Inhibit ectopic neuronal activity by blocking sodium channels
        (2) Carbamazepine and phenytoin can cause sedation, confusion, gastrointestinal disturbances, increased liver function tests, and depress the bone marrow.
        (3) Gabapentin and clonazepam activate inhibitory GABAergic mechanisms in dorsal horn.
            (a) Side effects are mild: sedation, nausea

1. USE SHOULD BE TAILORED TO EACH ELDERLY INDIVIDUAL

a. Elderly often have altered pharmacodynamic, pharmacokinetic, and coexisting diseases.
b. Likelihood of adverse reaction and toxicity in elderly is greater.
c. Use lowest effective dose when starting a medication and titrate slowly.

2. ACETAMINOPHEN

a. Effective and safe analgesic
b. Does not produce gastric and bleeding complications
c. Can cause dyspepsia and increase risk of end-stage renal disease
d. If dose exceeds 4 g/day can result in hepatic damage

3. CYCLOOXYGENASE 2 (COX2)

a. Decrease enzyme responsible for producing pain and inflammation
b. Decrease risk of gastrointestinal (GI) ulceration, bleeding, perforation
c. Side effects include fluid retention and edema, anemia, renal papillary necrosis, and mild elevation in liver function tests (LFTs).
d. Avoid in aspirin-sensitive patients and use with caution in patients with preexisting asthma due to cross-reactivity between aspirin and nonsteroidal anti-inflammatory drugs (NSAIDs).

4. NSAIDS

a. Most frequently used method of pain control
b. Most commonly prescribed medication in the elderly for chronic pain
c. Ten percent of chronic users have GI side effects.
d. Twenty percent of those develop ulcers and intestinal perforation.
e. Side effects include renal and hepatic failure, platelet dysfunction, bleeding complications.
f. The drug should be selected based on the needs of the patient, administered with food, lowest effective initial dose used, side effects monitored frequently, and given with antiulcer drugs (Misoprostol).
g. Mechanism of action
   i. Decrease prostaglandin synthesis at site of inflammation by reversible inhibition of COX

       (1) COX 1: found in blood vessel, stomach, kidney
       (2) COX 2: inducible form found at sites of inflammation
    ii. Decrease neutrophil migration to injured tissue
   iii. Wide range of side effects secondary to nonselective inhibition of COX 1 and COX 2
       (1) GI bleed, renal injury, fluid retention, platelet inhibition, constipation, central nervous system effects

h. Studies have shown decrease in GI side effects with COX 2 inhibitors.
   i. PGE analog (misoprostol) used for prophylaxis against NSAID-induced GI injury also shown to be protective against indomethacin-induced renal injury

j. H2 blockers, sucralfate, antacids, and proton pump inhibitors may also be protective.

k. Safe when used under appropriate medical supervision
   i. Monitor LFT, hemoglobin, hematocrit, renal function, and testing for occult blood in the stool.

SUGGESTED READINGS

Barash PG, Cullen BF, Stoelting RK. Clinical Anesthesia, 4th ed. Philadelphia, Lippincott Williams & Wilkins, 2001, pp 1435–1462.

Lynch D: Clinical Insights: Region Anesthesia and Pain Management in the Elderly. 20 March 2005 http://www.mdconsult.com.

Miller RD: Anesthesia. Vol. 1, 6th ed. Philadelphia, Elsevier/Churchill Livingstone, 2004.

Morgan GE Jr, Mikhail MS, Murray MJ: Clinical Anesthesiology. New York, McGraw-Hill, 2002, pp 310–312.

1. ABDOMINAL WALL PAIN

a. Early pregnancy: miscarriage
   i. Treatment: OB/GYN consult
b. Hypogastric pain and suprapubic tenderness: ovarian torsion, unruptured ectopic pregnancy
   i. Treatment: OB/GYN consult is advisable.
c. Round ligament stretch or hematoma is a result of the uterus rising in the abdomen. Pain and tenderness are localized over the ligament and radiate to the pubic tubercle.
   i. Treatment: Rest, local warmth, mild analgesic; OB/GYN consult is advisable.
d. Rectus hematoma: overstretching of the abdominal muscles by an expanding uterus.
   i. Severe localized pain usually after a bout of coughing or sneezing
   ii. With patient supine, pain is made worse when the patient lifts her head
      (1) Treatment: Rest, heat mild analgesic; OB/GYN consult may be advisable.

2. LUMBAR BACK PAIN

a. Very common regardless of exercise status: 50% of pregnant women
b. Increased lumbar lordosis
c. Ligament laxity secondary to luteal relaxin may result in pain in the midthoracic, low lumbar, or posterior pelvic locations.
   i. Pain can begin as early as 10 to 12 weeks' gestation.

3. RADICULAR SYMPTOMS

a. Not uncommon.
b. Herniated nucleus pulposus (HNP): 1:10,000
c. Direct pressure of the fetus on the lumbosacral nerves
d. True sciatica: 1%
e. Myofascial in origin

4. POSTERIOR PELVIC PAIN

a. Relaxation of the pelvic girdle, sacroiliac (SI) joint dysfunction
b. Increased mobility of the SI joints and symphysis pubis due to the hormonal changes of pregnancy
c. May occur as early as the 10th to 12th week of pregnancy

d. SI joint pain: radiates down the posterior thigh, sometimes to below the knee, but not as far as the ankle or foot
e. Reassurance, warmth, activity change, Tylenol, physical therapy

5. EVALUATION OF THE BACK PAIN OF PREGNANCY

a. History is the most important tool.
   i. Low-back pain and uterine contractions: preterm labor, ruptured membranes
   ii. Urologic causes of back pain: pyelonephritis, renal calculi, hydronephrosis

6. PHYSICAL EXAMINATION

a. Complete back and neurologic exam
b. Focused exam of the SI joints and pelvis

7. TREATMENT

a. Reassurance
b. Change in activity
c. Physical therapy
d. Massage, heat or ice, muscular conditioning exercises, good posture
e. Aquatic exercises
f. Nonelastic trochanteric belt
g. Wedge-shaped pillow for sleep
h. Epidural steroid injection
   i. Lumbar nerve root impingement consistent with symptoms
   ii. Single injection poses minimal risk to fetus
i. Medications
   i. Tylenol analgesic of choice
   ii. Use of nonsteroidal anti-inflammatory drugs is controversial
   iii. Short courses of opioids are acceptable

SUGGESTED READINGS

Cunningham FG, et al: Prenatal Care. In Williams Obstetrics, 21st ed. New York, McGraw-Hill, 2001, 215, 242, 243.
Wallace M, Staats P: Pain Medicine and Management. New York, McGraw-Hill, 2005, 225–230.

1. TRANSFER OF DRUGS ACROSS THE PLACENTA

a. Maternal cardiac output
b. Placenta binding and metabolism, factors that affect passive placental diffusion
c. Fetal exposure: fetal metabolism, first-pass effect
d. Fetal protein binding
e Fetal cardiac output

2. TERATOGENICITY

a. Gestational age is a major determinant.
b. Structural malformations, functional and behavioral effects secondary to drug effects
c. Interspecies variation: mechanism poorly understood
d. Period of teratogenicity: corresponds with organogenesis: 31 to 71 days after last menstrual period

3. FOOD AND DRUG ADMINISTRATION (FDA) RISK CLASSIFICATION

a. Categories
   i. No increased fetal risk in well-controlled human studies
   ii. Animal studies: no harm or do indicate a teratogenic risk
      (1) Human studies: well-controlled, no risk
   iii. No controlled studies in animals or humans
      (1) Studies have shown embryocidal or teratogenic risk in animals.
   iv. Humans: well-controlled studies or observational, fetal risk
   v. Positive evidence of fetal risk in well controlled human and animal studies
      (1) The drug is contraindicated who are or may be pregnant.
b. Specific drugs
   i. Aspirin: risk of gastroschisis if more than 150 mg/day
      (1) If taken near birth, there is an increased incidence of neonatal intracranial bleed.
   ii. Full dose aspirin and nonsteroidal anti-inflammatory drugs (NSAIDs) are to be avoided in the third trimester.
      (1) Tylenol is the drug of choice.
   iii. Motrin/naproxen in the 1st trimester is acceptable
   iv. Prostaglandin inhibitors
      (1) Reversible narrowing of ductus arteriosus in utero
      (2) May decrease amniotic fluid volume and prolong labor and delivery (aspirin as well)

v. Opioid agonists and agonist-antagonists are not known to be teratogenic. Possible neonatal abstinence syndrome.
vi. Bupivacaine and lidocaine are not teratogenic. Mepivacaine?
vii. Steroids: Oral clefts? Limited trial of epidural steroids has minimal risk.
viii. Selective serotonin reuptake inhibitors, tricyclic antidepressants are not associated with teratogenicity.
ix. Anticonvulsants, such as phenytoin, Tegretol, and valproic acid, can result in fetal dysmorphic syndromes. Risk/benefit must be considered.
x. Beta blockers: possibility of intrauterine growth retardation
xi. Ergotamine: stimulates uterine contractions; possibly teratogenic, therefore contraindicated
c. FDA risk classification of drug examples
i. None
ii. NSAIDs, some opioid (Demerol), steroids, caffeine
iii. Elavil ASA, Ketorolac, codeine, Darvon, Vicodin, gabapentin, lidocaine, Inderal, sumatriptan
iv. Tofranil, Tegretol, cortisone, Valium, phenobarbital, valproic acid, phenytoin
v. Ergotamine

SUGGESTED READING

Wallace M, Staats P: Pain medicine and management. In Benzon H (ed): Essentials of Pain Medicine and Regional Anesthesia, 2nd ed. New York, McGraw-Hill, 2005, pp 565–584.

139 Medication Use During Lactation

1. GENERAL CONSIDERATIONS

a. Neonatal dose of medication is 1% to 2% of the maternal dose.
b. Take medicines after breast-feeding or just before the infant goes to sleep.
c. If possible, avoid long-acting medications.
d. Take the safest drug and only when necessary.
e. If the mother is taking a drug that may potentially harm the infant, it may become necessary to monitor serum levels of the drug from the infant.

2. COMMONLY USED MEDICINES FOR PAIN MANAGEMENT

a. Nonsteroidal anti-inflammatory drugs (NSAIDs)
   i. Generally considered compatible with nursing.
   ii. Aspirin use is controversial.
   iii. Motrin/Ibuprofen is minimally transported into the breast milk, therefore is compatible with breast-feeding.
b. Tylenol
   i. Analgesic of choice for the breast-feeding mother
c. Opioid agonists and agonist-antagonists
   i. Opioids are considered compatible with breast-feeding.
      (1) Methadone: up to 20 mg/day
      (2) Codeine, fentanyl, morphine, and propoxyphene are compatible with breast-feeding.
d. Steroids
   i. Even high doses are unlikely to suppress the infant's adrenal gland.
e. Benzodiazepines
   i. To be avoided, infant may show sedation and poor feeding
f. Anticonvulsants
   i. Phenytoin, Tegretol, and valproic acid are not harmful.
   ii. Gabapentin: no data
g. Tricyclic antidepressants, selective serotonin reuptake inhibitors
   i. Unknown risk during lactation
h. Local anesthetics
   i. Considered safe for use in the nursing mother
i. Ergotamine
   i. Neonatal convulsions, gastrointestinal disturbances; not to be used in the nursing mother
j. Sumatriptan
   i. Not well studied in nursing mothers

k. Caffeine
   i. Two cups a day does not seem to affect the infant.
   ii. Excessive consumption may cause increased irritability or wakefulness.

SUGGESTED READINGS

Benzon H, et al: Pain management during pregnancy and lactation. In: Essentials of Pain Medicine and Regional Anesthesia, 2nd ed. Philadelphia, Elsevier Inc., 2005.

Wallace M, Staats P: Pain Medicine and Management. New York, McGraw-Hill, Inc., 2005, pp 225–230.

140 Diagnostic Imaging During Pregnancy

1. GENERAL

a. No single diagnostic x-ray procedure had been shown to threaten the well-being of the embryo or fetus.
b. X-ray exposure: ionizing radiation
  i. Cell death and teratogenic effects
    (1) High-dose radiation before implantation (much more than is commonly used in diagnostic procedures) is usually lethal to the embryo.
    (2) High-dose radiation in humans can result in growth retardation, microcephaly, and mental retardation.
    (3) The risk of carcinogenesis as a result of in utero exposure is unclear but probably is minimal.
c. Ultrasonography
  i. This involves the use of sound waves and has replaced x-ray as the primary fetal-imaging technique.
  ii. No adverse fetal effects have been documented.
d. Magnetic resonance imaging
  i. Magnets alter the energy state of hydrogen protons.
  ii. May prove valuable in the diagnosis of fetal central nervous system anomalies and placental anomalies.
e. Nuclear medicine studies
  i. Fetal exposure depends on the physical and biochemical properties of the isotope.
  ii. Technetium (Tc-99m) is the most commonly used with less than 0.5m rad exposure.
  iii. Ventilation-perfusion scan to rule out suspected pulmonary embolism utilizes Tc-99m and xenon; minimal exposure of ~50 mrad.
f. Spiral computed tomography scanning
  i. Less fetal radiation exposure than from a ventilation-perfusion scan
  ii. Radioactive iodine may adversely affect the fetal thyroid.
  iii. Radioactive isotopes of iodine are contraindicated during pregnancy.
  iv. Contrast agents: The radiopaque agents studied in animals do not appear to be teratogenic.
  v. Consult an expert in dosimetry if multiple diagnostic x-rays are performed on a pregnant patient.

SUGGESTED READINGS

ACOG Committee Opinion No. 299. Vol.104, No.3, September 2004.
Cunningham FG, Gant NF, Leveno KJ: General considerations and maternal evaluation (Ch 32). In Williams Obstetrics, 21st ed. New York, McGraw-Hill, 2001, pp 143–158.

141 Medicolegal Concerns in Pain Medicine

1. INTRODUCTION

a. Some patients sent to a pain center may be involved in litigation or compensation cases: may impact an outcome of patient care.
b. Malpractice claims: 2% of all anesthesia malpractice claims in the 1970s, 8% in the 1990s: nonoperative management.
c. The greatest risk for major claims is associated with ablative nerve blocks.

2. STANDARD OF CARE

a. Pain physician is a fully responsible provider who must thoroughly evaluate the patient; overlooking an associated or previously undiscovered problem is poor quality medical care and exposes the practitioner to possible litigation.
b. It is inappropriate for a referring physician to order a procedure and irresponsible of the pain physician to perform the procedure if it is not indicated.

3. THE PHYSICIAN-PATIENT RELATIONSHIP

a. Consensual agreement, rarely a contractual agreement.
b. Once this relationship is established, the physician has a duty to the patient.
c. Termination of the relationship:
    i. The physician's services are no longer required.
    ii. The patient terminates the relationship.
    iii. The physician gives the patient a reasonable period of time to find another caregiver.
    iv. The pain physician must remain available for consultation until another caregiver is found.
d. It is not clear what constitutes a relationship.
    i. Making an appointment at the pain center?
    ii. Must be seen by a physician?
e. The physician must send a registered letter to the patient if the intent is to terminate the relationship.
f. The physician is not obliged to see every patient seeking an appointment.

4. PATIENT RECORDS

a. The medical record is the most important factor determining the outcome of a lawsuit.
b. Document facts only; no inflammatory remarks should be entered into the record.

c. All telephone calls with the patient or the patient's pharmacy must be documented.

d. All procedures must be carefully documented as well as the recovery room period and all follow-up visits and phone calls.

e. The medical record must never be altered after it has been initiated.

f. If the record needs to be amended or something in it requires explanation, this may be done in a separate entry that is properly dated and timed.

g. Patient medical information may not be released without the expressed written authorization of the patient.

5. PRESCRIBING CONTROLLED SUBSTANCES

a. Documentation in the medical record of the necessity for prescribing these medications:
  i. Nonopioid medicines have failed.
  ii. The risks, benefits, and alternatives to opioids have been discussed with the patient.
  iii. Goals as a measure of treatment success.
  iv. Periodic assessment as to progress toward these goals.
  v. The patient should receive controlled substances from one physician (or pain center) and one pharmacy.
  vi. Opioid contract: delineates patient's responsibilities for the continued use of controlled substances.
  vii. The condition must warrant the use of a controlled substance.
  viii. Prior use of controlled substances:
    (1) Effects on the patient's ability to function
    (2) History of substance abuse

6. INFORMED CONSENT

a. The following constitutes a complete informed consent:
  i. Why the treatment is being done
  ii. The goals of treatment
  iii. Likely outcome without treatment
  iv. Risks/benefits of treatment
  v. Reasonable alternative therapies
  vi. Likelihood of success of the treatment

Index